Novel Biomarkers of Gastrointestinal Cancer

Novel Biomarkers of Gastrointestinal Cancer

Editor

Takaya Shimura

MDPI • Basel • Beijing • Wuhan • Barcelona • Belgrade • Manchester • Tokyo • Cluj • Tianjin

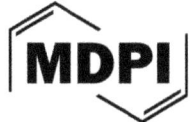

Editor
Takaya Shimura
Nagoya City University Graduate School of Medical Sciences
Japan

Editorial Office
MDPI
St. Alban-Anlage 66
4052 Basel, Switzerland

This is a reprint of articles from the Special Issue published online in the open access journal *Cancers* (ISSN 2072-6694) (available at: https://www.mdpi.com/journal/cancers/special_issues/Gastrointestinal_Biomarkers).

For citation purposes, cite each article independently as indicated on the article page online and as indicated below:

LastName, A.A.; LastName, B.B.; LastName, C.C. Article Title. *Journal Name* **Year**, *Volume Number*, Page Range.

ISBN 978-3-0365-4931-6 (Hbk)
ISBN 978-3-0365-4932-3 (PDF)

© 2022 by the authors. Articles in this book are Open Access and distributed under the Creative Commons Attribution (CC BY) license, which allows users to download, copy and build upon published articles, as long as the author and publisher are properly credited, which ensures maximum dissemination and a wider impact of our publications.

The book as a whole is distributed by MDPI under the terms and conditions of the Creative Commons license CC BY-NC-ND.

Contents

About the Editor vii

Takaya Shimura
Novel Biomarkers of Gastrointestinal Cancer
Reprinted from: *Cancers* **2021**, *13*, 1501, doi:10.3390/cancers13071501 1

Hiroyasu Iwasaki, Takaya Shimura, Mika Kitagawa, Tamaki Yamada, Ruriko Nishigaki, Shigeki Fukusada, Yusuke Okuda, Takahito Katano, Shin-ichi Horike and Hiromi Kataoka
A Novel Urinary miRNA Biomarker for Early Detection of Colorectal Cancer
Reprinted from: *Cancers* **2022**, *14*, 461, doi:10.3390/cancers14020461 5

I-Ting Liu, Chia-Sheng Yen, Wen-Lung Wang, Hung-Wen Tsai, Chang-Yao Chu, Ming-Yu Chang, Ya-Fu Hou and Chia-Jui Yen
Predict Early Recurrence of Resectable Hepatocellular Carcinoma Using Multi-Dimensional Artificial Intelligence Analysis of Liver Fibrosis
Reprinted from: *Cancers* **2021**, *13*, 5323, doi:10.3390/cancers13215323 17

Jae-Yong Park, Chil-Sung Kang, Ho-Chan Seo, Jin-Chul Shin, Sung-Min Kym, Young-Soo Park, Tae-Seop Shin, Jae-Gyu Kim and Yoon-Keun Kim
Bacteria-Derived Extracellular Vesicles in Urine as a Novel Biomarker for Gastric Cancer: Integration of Liquid Biopsy and Metagenome Analysis
Reprinted from: *Cancers* **2021**, *13*, 4687, doi:10.3390/cancers13184687 35

Marina V. Nemtsova, Alexey I. Kalinkin, Ekaterina B. Kuznetsova, Irina V. Bure, Ekaterina A. Alekseeva, Igor I. Bykov, Tatiana V. Khorobrykh, Dmitry S. Mikhaylenko, Alexander S. Tanas and Vladimir V. Strelnikov
Mutations in Epigenetic Regulation Genes in Gastric Cancer
Reprinted from: *Cancers* **2021**, *13*, 4586, doi:10.3390/cancers13184586 49

Ankit Patel, Masanori Oshi, Li Yan, Ryusei Matsuyama, Itaru Endo and Kazuaki Takabe
The Unfolded Protein Response Is Associated with Cancer Proliferation and Worse Survival in Hepatocellular Carcinoma
Reprinted from: *Cancers* **2021**, *13*, 4443, doi:10.3390/cancers13174443 65

Delphine Dayde, Jillian Gunther, Yutaka Hirayama, David C. Weksberg, Adam Boutin, Gargy Parhy, Clemente Aguilar-Bonavides, Hong Wang, Hiroyuki Katayama, Yuichi Abe, Kim-Anh Do, Kazuo Hara, Takashi Kinoshita, Koji Komori, Yasuhiro Shimizu, Masahiro Tajika, Yasumasa Niwa, Alan Y. Wang, Ronald DePinho, Samir Hanash, Sunil Krishnan and Ayumu Taguchi
Identification of Blood-Based Biomarkers for the Prediction of the Response to Neoadjuvant Chemoradiation in Rectal Cancer
Reprinted from: *Cancers* **2021**, *13*, 3642, doi:10.3390/cancers13143642 79

Alessandro Ottaiano, Mariachiara Santorsola, Paola Del Prete, Francesco Perri, Stefania Scala, Michele Caraglia and Guglielmo Nasti
Prognostic Significance of CXCR4 in Colorectal Cancer: An Updated Meta-Analysis and Critical Appraisal
Reprinted from: *Cancers* **2021**, *13*, 3284, doi:cancers13133284 93

Devalingam Mahalingam, Leonidas Chelis, Imran Nizamuddin, Sunyoung S. Lee, Stylianos Kakolyris, Glenn Halff, Ken Washburn, Kristopher Attwood, Ibnshamsah Fahad, Julia Grigorieva, Senait Asmellash, Krista Meyer, Carlos Oliveira, Heinrich Roder, Joanna Roder and Renuka Iyer
Detection of Hepatocellular Carcinoma in a High-Risk Population by a Mass Spectrometry-Based Test
Reprinted from: *Cancers* **2021**, *13*, 3109, doi:10.3390/cancers13133109 105

Elizabeth Herring, Éric Tremblay, Nathalie McFadden, Shigeru Kanaoka and Jean-François Beaulieu
Multitarget Stool mRNA Test for Detecting Colorectal Cancer Lesions Including Advanced Adenomas
Reprinted from: *Cancers* **2021**, *13*, 1228, doi:10.3390/cancers13061228 121

Nadja Niclauss, Ines Gütgemann, Jonas Dohmen, Jörg C. Kalff and Philipp Lingohr
Novel Biomarkers of Gastric Adenocarcinoma: Current Research and Future Perspectives
Reprinted from: *Cancers* **2021**, *13*, 5660, doi:10.3390/cancers13225660 133

Hiroto Tominaga, Juntaro Matsuzaki, Chihiro Oikawa, Kensho Toyoshima, Haruki Manabe, Eriko Ozawa, Atsushi Shimamura, Riko Yokoyama, Yusuke Serizawa, Takahiro Ochiya and Yoshimasa Saito
Challenges for Better Diagnosis and Management of Pancreatic and Biliary Tract Cancers Focusing on Blood Biomarkers: A Systematic Review
Reprinted from: *Cancers* **2021**, *13*, 4220, doi:10.3390/cancers13164220 169

Gary Tincknell, Ann-Katrin Piper, Morteza Aghmesheh, Therese Becker, Kara Lea Vine, Daniel Brungs and Marie Ranson
Experimental and Clinical Evidence Supports the Use of Urokinase Plasminogen Activation System Components as Clinically Relevant Biomarkers in Gastroesophageal Adenocarcinoma
Reprinted from: *Cancers* **2021**, *13*, 4097, doi:10.3390/cancers13164097 181

Sophia Harlid, Marc J. Gunter and Bethany Van Guelpen
Risk-Predictive and Diagnostic Biomarkers for Colorectal Cancer; a Systematic Review of Studies Using Pre-Diagnostic Blood Samples Collected in Prospective Cohorts and Screening Settings
Reprinted from: *Cancers* **2021**, *13*, 4406, doi:10.3390/cancers13174406 201

About the Editor

Takaya Shimura

Takaya Shimura (assistant professor) is an assistant professor in the Department of Gastroenterology and Metabolism at the Nagoya City University Graduate School of Medical Sciences.

He graduated from the Nagoya City University Medical School receiving his MD in 1997. He started his residency in the First Internal Medicine of Nagoya City University Hospital in 1997, and joined as a faculty physician in the Department of Gastroenterology at Iwata Municipal Hospital. He started the Ph.D. program in 2005 and acquired a PhD from the Nagoya City University Graduate School of Medical Sciences in 2009. Additionally, he joined the short residency medical oncology program at the National Cancer Center Hospital East, Japan, in 2008–2009. He was promoted to an assistant professor at the Nagoya City University Graduate School of Medical Sciences in 2009, then becoming a vice director in the Clinical Trial Management Center at the Nagoya City University Hospital in 2011.

Thereafter, he earned an opportunity to work as a post-doctoral research fellow in the Vascular Biology Program and Department of Surgery at Boston Children's Hospital and Harvard Medical School in 2012–2015. He moved back to Japan and restarted his work as an assistant professor in the Department of Gastroenterology and Metabolism at the Nagoya City University Graduate School of Medical Sciences in 2015.

His research interests include the discovery of urinary/serum biomarkers for gastrointestinal cancers, and cover all fields of gastrointestinal cancers, including oncology and endoscopy. He has five patents as a principal investigator in the biomarker field. All his years of study have led to the publication of 112 articles in international peer-reviewed journals, with an H-index of 24.

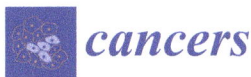

Editorial

Novel Biomarkers of Gastrointestinal Cancer

Takaya Shimura

Department of Gastroenterology and Metabolism, Graduate School of Medical Sciences, Nagoya City University, Nagoya 467-8601, Japan; tshimura@med.nagoya-cu.ac.jp; Tel.: +81-52-853-8211; Fax: +81-52-852-0952

Gastrointestinal (GI) cancer is a major cause of morbidity and mortality worldwide. Among the top seven malignancies with worst mortality, GI cancer consists of five cancers: colorectal cancer (CRC), liver cancer, gastric cancer (GC), esophageal cancer, and pancreatic cancer, which are the second, third, fourth, sixth, and seventh leading causes of cancer death worldwide, respectively [1]. To improve the prognosis of GI cancers, scientific and technical development is required for both diagnostic and therapeutic strategies.

1. Diagnostic Biomarker

As for diagnosis, needless to say, early detection is the first priority to prevent cancer death. The gold standard diagnostic tool is objective examination using an imaging instrument, including endoscopy and computed tomography, and the final diagnosis is established with pathologic diagnosis using biopsy samples obtained through endoscopy, ultrasonography, and endoscopic ultrasonography. Clinical and pathological information is definitely needed before the initiation of treatment because they could clarify the specific type and extent of disease. However, these imaging examinations have not been recommended as screening tests for healthy individuals due to their invasiveness and high cost. Hence, the discovery of novel non-invasive biomarkers is needed in detecting GI cancers. In particular, non-invasive samples, such as blood, urine, feces, and saliva, are promising diagnostic biomarker samples for screening.

Stool-based tests, including guaiac fecal occult blood test (gFOBT) and fecal immunochemical test for hemoglobin (FIT), for CRC have been some of the most successful screening tests for GI cancers. Although the gFOBT is the only non-invasive method that demonstrated a reduction in CRC mortality [2], the FIT recently gained popularity because the FIT has a higher sensitivity for CRC and adenoma than gFOBT [3] due to its specificity for human globin. However, since both gFOBT and FIT aim to detect only blood contamination in feces, which is not cancer-specific, sensitivity for early-stage cancer and advanced adenoma is quite low. Moreover, in handling stool samples, stool-based tests are challenging for both patients and investigators, and the quality of sample collection by patients may affect the results.

Fortunately, recent technical and mechanical developments have enabled the detection of slight differences in factors that are modified in physical condition, which might contribute to novel biomarker discovery for GI cancers. Analytical targets include a wide variety of factors, including DNA mutation, DNA methylation, miRNA, protein, and metabolites [4]. Moreover, many types of body fluids are target samples. Although blood is the most popular biomarker sample, other samples, including urine, saliva, and sweat are also attractive tools because of their non-invasiveness.

Diagnostic biomarkers are mostly developed in the field of CRC, including blood- and stool-based biomarkers. As expected, blood-based test is more preferred than a stool-based test as an alternative noninvasive test, and Epi proColon® 2.0 CE is an FDA-approved blood test for CRC screening, which detects methylated Septin9 DNA [5]. However, this blood-based test has not been recommended as a screening test for CRC due to its low sensitivity and limited data [6]. Presently, many researchers are trying to explore reliable blood-based

Citation: Shimura, T. Novel Biomarkers of Gastrointestinal Cancer. *Cancers* **2021**, *13*, 1501. https://doi.org/10.3390/cancers13071501

Received: 19 March 2021
Accepted: 23 March 2021
Published: 25 March 2021

Publisher's Note: MDPI stays neutral with regard to jurisdictional claims in published maps and institutional affiliations.

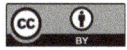

Copyright: © 2021 by the author. Licensee MDPI, Basel, Switzerland. This article is an open access article distributed under the terms and conditions of the Creative Commons Attribution (CC BY) license (https://creativecommons.org/licenses/by/4.0/).

biomarkers for detecting GI cancers. Among these, cell-free DNA, miRNA, and proteomics approaches are the most common targets. However, these novel biomarkers are still under study, and we expect future clinical application with reliable validation.

In contrast, there are far fewer studies on urinary biomarkers than on blood-based biomarkers for GI cancers. We and another group previously reported the usefulness of urinary protein and miRNA biomarkers in detecting GI cancers [4,7–10]. As urine is a completely non-invasive sample, urinary biomarker enables screening tests at home. The advantages of urinary biomarkers with easy access and low cost might improve screening compliance, which may result in a reduction in GI cancer mortalities.

2. Treatment Biomarker

In terms of treatment biomarkers, since patients have already been diagnosed with some types of cancers, invasive sampling from tissue, bile, and pancreatic juice is accepted, which can be generally obtained through close examination. Indeed, some tissue-based biomarkers have already been applied to clinical practices of GC and CRC. Positive expression of human epidermal growth factor receptor 2 (HER2) in GC tissues is a predictive biomarker for anti-HER2 antibody, trastuzumab, in advanced GC [11] as well as HER2-positive breast cancer.

Tumor *RAS* mutation representing mutation in exons 2, 3, and 4 of *KRAS* and *NRAS* is a negative predictive biomarker for anti-EGFR antibody therapy against metastatic CRC [12]. Moreover, BRAF inhibitor has been applied for metastatic CRC with *BRAF* V600E mutation in tumor tissues [13]. Likewise, immune checkpoint inhibitors have been applied for metastatic CRC with high microsatellite instability or mismatch-repair deficiency [14,15]. Precision medicine based on these predictive biomarkers contributes to not only better prognosis and safety but also cost reduction by avoiding unnecessary treatment.

Moreover, liquid biopsy detecting circulating cell-free DNA has been recently applied as an alternative test to the tissue-based *RAS* mutation test, which showed a high concordance rate between plasma and tissue-based results [16]. Liquid biopsy, which comprises body fluid-based biomarkers, has a huge benefit compared to tissue-based biopsy because it easily enables repeated sampling depending on the systemic physical situation. This benefit is especially useful in monitoring during a specific therapy and follow-up observation after tumor resection. Since malignant tumors consist of heterogenous cells, the characteristic of dominant cancer cells might be dynamically changed in a time-dependent manner. Additionally, the microenvironment surrounding tumors also changes dynamically. Since liquid biopsy through circulating body fluid might systemically capture these dynamic changes, it can be applied for monitoring biomarker beyond treatment biomarker. In fact, a Signatera^{TM} test detecting custom-built plasma cell-free DNAs could predict relapse after surgical resection of stage I–III CRC with high sensitivity [17]. Liquid biopsy is presently in the initial phase, and future development is expected in many fields of GI cancers for predicting efficacy, adverse events, and recurrence.

Funding: This research received no external funding.

Conflicts of Interest: The suthors declare no conflict of interest.

References

1. Sung, H.; Ferlay, J.; Siegel, R.L.; Laversanne, M.; Soerjomataram, I.; Jemal, A.; Bray, F. Global cancer statistics 2020: GLOBOCAN estimates of incidence and mortality worldwide for 36 cancers in 185 countries. *CA Cancer J. Clin.* **2021**, *70*. [CrossRef]
2. Hewitson, P.; Glasziou, P.; Watson, E.; Towler, B.; Irwig, L. Cochrane Systematic Review of Colorectal Cancer Screening using the Fecal Occult Blood Test (Hemoccult): An Update. *Am. J. Gastroenterol.* **2008**, *103*, 1541–1549. [CrossRef] [PubMed]
3. Schreuders, E.H.; Ruco, A.; Rabeneck, L.; Schoen, R.E.; Sung, J.J.; Young, G.P.; Kuipers, E.J. Colorectal cancer screening: A global overview of existing programmes. *Gut* **2015**, *64*, 1637–1649. [CrossRef] [PubMed]
4. Iwasaki, H.; Shimura, T.; Yamada, T.; Okuda, Y.; Natsume, M.; Kitagawa, M.; Horike, S.-I.; Kataoka, H. A novel urinary microRNA biomarker panel for detecting gastric cancer. *J. Gastroenterol.* **2019**, *54*, 1061–1069. [CrossRef] [PubMed]
5. Lamb, Y.N.; Dhillon, S. Epi proColon®2.0 CE: A Blood-Based Screening Test for Colorectal Cancer. *Mol. Diagn. Ther.* **2017**, *21*, 225–232. [CrossRef]

6. Shaukat, A.; Kahi, C.J.; Burke, C.A.; Rabeneck, L.; Sauer, B.G.; Rex, D.K. ACG Clinical Guidelines: Colorectal Cancer Screening 2021. *Am. J. Gastroenterol.* **2021**, *116*, 458–479. [CrossRef]
7. Shimura, T.; Dayde, D.; Wang, H.; Okuda, Y.; Iwasaki, H.; Ebi, M.; Kitagawa, M.; Yamada, T.; Yamada, T.; Hanash, S.M.; et al. Novel urinary protein biomarker panel for early diagnosis of gastric cancer. *Br. J. Cancer* **2020**, *123*, 1656–1664. [CrossRef]
8. Shimura, T.; Iwasaki, H.; Kitagawa, M.; Ebi, M.; Yamada, T.; Yamada, T.; Katano, T.; Nisie, H.; Okamoto, Y.; Ozeki, K.; et al. Urinary Cysteine-Rich Protein 61 and Trefoil Factor 3 as Diagnostic Biomarkers for Colorectal Cancer. *Transl. Oncol.* **2019**, *12*, 539–544. [CrossRef]
9. Shimura, T.; Dagher, A.; Sachdev, M. Urinary ADAM12 and MMP-9/NGAL complex detect the presence of gastric cancer. *Cancer Prev. Res.* **2015**, *8*, 240–248. [CrossRef] [PubMed]
10. Roy, R.; Zurakowski, D.; Wischhusen, J.; Frauenhoffer, C.; Hooshmand, S.; Kulke, M.A.; Moses, M. Urinary TIMP-1 and MMP-2 levels detect the presence of pancreatic malignancies. *Br. J. Cancer* **2014**, *111*, 1772–1779. [CrossRef] [PubMed]
11. Bang, Y.-J.; Van Cutsem, E.; Feyereislova, A.; Chung, H.C.; Shen, L.; Sawaki, A.; Lordick, F.; Ohtsu, A.; Omuro, Y.; Satoh, T.; et al. Trastuzumab in combination with chemotherapy versus chemotherapy alone for treatment of HER2-positive advanced gastric or gastro-oesophageal junction cancer (ToGA): A phase 3, open-label, randomised controlled trial. *Lancet* **2010**, *376*, 687–697. [CrossRef]
12. Sorich, M.J.; Wiese, M.D.; Rowland, A.; Kichenadasse, G.; McKinnon, R.A.; Karapetis, C.S. Extended RAS mutations and anti-EGFR monoclonal antibody survival benefit in metastatic colorectal cancer: A meta-analysis of randomized, controlled trials. *Ann. Oncol.* **2015**, *26*, 13–21. [CrossRef] [PubMed]
13. Kopetz, S.; Grothey, A.; Yaeger, R.; Van Cutsem, E.; Desai, J.; Yoshino, T.; Wasan, H.; Ciardiello, F.; Loupakis, F.; Hong, Y.S.; et al. Encorafenib, Binimetinib, and Cetuximab in BRAF V600E–Mutated Colorectal Cancer. *N. Engl. J. Med.* **2019**, *381*, 1632–1643. [CrossRef] [PubMed]
14. André, T.; Shiu, K.-K.; Kim, T.W.; Jensen, B.V.; Jensen, L.H.; Punt, C.; Smith, D.; Garcia-Carbonero, R.; Benavides, M.; Gibbs, P.; et al. Pembrolizumab in Microsatellite-Instability-High Advanced Colorectal Cancer. *N. Engl. J. Med.* **2020**, *383*, 2207–2218. [CrossRef] [PubMed]
15. Overman, M.J.; McDermott, R.; Leach, J.L.; Lonardi, S.; Lenz, H.-J.; Morse, M.A.; Desai, J.; Hill, A.; Axelson, M.A.; Moss, R.; et al. Nivolumab in patients with metastatic DNA mismatch repair-deficient or microsatellite instability-high colorectal cancer (CheckMate 142): An open-label, multicentre, phase 2 study. *Lancet Oncol.* **2017**, *18*, 1182–1191. [CrossRef]
16. Garcia-Foncillas, J.; Tabernero, J.; Elez, E.; Aranda, E.; Benavides, M.; Camps, C.; Vivancos, A. Prospective multicenter real-world RAS mutation comparison between OncoBEAM-based liquid biopsy and tissue analysis in metastatic colorectal cancer. *Br. J. Cancer* **2018**, *119*, 1464–1470. [CrossRef] [PubMed]
17. Reinert, T.; Henriksen, T.V.; Christensen, E.; Sharma, S.; Salari, R.; Sethi, H.; Knudsen, M.; Nordentoft, I.; Wu, H.-T.; Tin, A.S.; et al. Analysis of Plasma Cell-Free DNA by Ultradeep Sequencing in Patients with Stages I to III Colorectal Cancer. *JAMA Oncol.* **2019**, *5*, 1124–1131. [CrossRef] [PubMed]

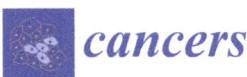

Article

A Novel Urinary miRNA Biomarker for Early Detection of Colorectal Cancer

Hiroyasu Iwasaki [1], Takaya Shimura [1,*], Mika Kitagawa [1], Tamaki Yamada [2], Ruriko Nishigaki [1], Shigeki Fukusada [1], Yusuke Okuda [1], Takahito Katano [1], Shin-ichi Horike [3] and Hiromi Kataoka [1]

[1] Department of Gastroenterology and Metabolism, Nagoya City University Graduate School of Medical Sciences, 1 Kawasumi, Mizuho-cho, Mizuho-ku, Nagoya 467-8601, Japan; hiwasaki@med.nagoya-cu.ac.jp (H.I.); mk313659@med.nagoya-cu.ac.jp (M.K.); nishiga2@med.nagoya-cu.ac.jp (R.N.); a100405@med.nagoya-cu.ac.jp (S.F.); okuda10@med.nagoya-cu.ac.jp (Y.O.); takatano@med.nagoya-cu.ac.jp (T.K.); hkataoka@med.nagoya-cu.ac.jp (H.K.)

[2] Okazaki Public Health Center, 1-3 Harusaki, Harisaki-cho, Okazaki 444-0827, Japan; t-yamada@okazaki-med.or.jp

[3] Advanced Science Research Center, Kanazawa University, 13-1 Takaramachi, Kanazawa 920-8640, Japan; sihorike@staff.kanazawa-u.ac.jp

* Correspondence: tshimura@med.nagoya-cu.ac.jp; Tel.: +81-52-853-8211; Fax: +81-52-852-0952

Simple Summary: Early diagnosis is critically important to achieve life-saving therapy for colorectal cancer (CRC). Since colonoscopy is not suitable as a screening method for CRC due to its invasiveness and high-cost, reliable and non-invasive diagnostic biomarkers are hopeful for CRC. In this case-control study, we established completely non-invasive, novel urinary microRNA (miRNA) biomarker panel combining miR-129-1-3p and miR-566 for the diagnosis of CRC. In the independent age- and sex-matched three cohorts comprising 415 participants, urinary levels of these miRNAs were consistently elevated in the CRC group compared to the healthy controls. Notably, the panel of combining miR-129-1-3p and miR-566 revealed an AUC of 0.845 for stage 0/I CRC that can be treated with endoscopic resection.

Abstract: Since noninvasive biomarkers as an alternative to invasive colonoscopy to detect colorectal cancer (CRC) are desired, we conducted this study to determine the urinary biomarker consisting of microRNAs (miRNAs). In total, 415 age- and sex-matched participants, including 206 patients with CRC and 209 healthy controls (HCs), were randomly divided into three groups: (1) the discovery cohort (CRC, $n = 3$; HC, $n = 6$); (2) the training cohort (140 pairs); and (3) the validation cohort (63 pairs). Among 11 urinary miRNAs with aberrant expressions between the two groups, miR-129-1-3p and miR-566 were significantly independent biomarkers that detect CRC. The panel consisting of two miRNAs could distinguish patients with CRC from HC participants with an area under the curve (AUC) = 0.811 in the training cohort. This panel showed good efficacy with an AUC = 0.868 in the validation cohort. This urinary biomarker combining miR-129-1-3p and miR-566 could detect even stage 0/I CRC effectively with an AUC = 0.845. Moreover, the expression levels of both miR-129-1-3p and miR-566 were significantly higher in primary tumor tissues than in adjacent normal tissue. Our established novel biomarker consisting of urinary miR-129-1-3p and miR-566 enables noninvasive and early detection of CRC.

Keywords: colorectal cancer; biomarker; urinary miRNA; miR-129-1-3p; miR-566

Citation: Iwasaki, H.; Shimura, T.; Kitagawa, M.; Yamada, T.; Nishigaki, R.; Fukusada, S.; Okuda, Y.; Katano, T.; Horike, S.-i.; Kataoka, H. A Novel Urinary miRNA Biomarker for Early Detection of Colorectal Cancer. *Cancers* 2022, 14, 461. https://doi.org/10.3390/cancers14020461

Academic Editors: Mark Molloy and David Kerr

Received: 18 November 2021
Accepted: 14 January 2022
Published: 17 January 2022

Publisher's Note: MDPI stays neutral with regard to jurisdictional claims in published maps and institutional affiliations.

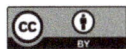

Copyright: © 2022 by the authors. Licensee MDPI, Basel, Switzerland. This article is an open access article distributed under the terms and conditions of the Creative Commons Attribution (CC BY) license (https://creativecommons.org/licenses/by/4.0/).

1. Introduction

Colorectal cancer (CRC) is a frequent cause of cancer deaths worldwide [1]. Because early-stage CRC is curable by minimally invasive therapy in many cases, early detection through mass screening is important for reducing mortality. The gold standard for CRC diagnosis is pathological diagnosis using biopsy samples obtained through a colonoscopy (CS). Although CS screening shows high CRC detection rates and adenomas [2], it has not been widely applied for screening tests due to its invasiveness and high cost. The fecal immunochemical test (FIT) has been established as a widely recommended screening tool to detect CRC [3,4]. However, it has been reported that 20–40% of CRC, especially stage 0/I CRC, is not detectable by FIT [5–7]. In recent years, the multitarget stool DNA screening test that detects CRC-related genetic mutations has been developed to detect CRC [8,9]; however, there is insufficient evidence to warrant its replacement of FIT. In addition, it is challenging to handle stool samples because of bacterial abundance, odor, and contamination of food residues. Although serum tumor markers, such as carcinoembryonic antigen (CEA) and carbohydrate antigen 19-9 (CA19-9), are often used as noninvasive CRC markers during medical checkups, they are inappropriate as screening tools due to their low sensitivity, especially for early disease [10–12]. It is thus important to establish a noninvasive biomarker for the early diagnosis of CRC.

MicroRNAs (miRNAs) are short non-coding RNAs that regulate the expression of target genes through messenger RNA degradation. Their aberrant expression seems to be involved in carcinogenesis [13,14]. Because miRNAs form complexes with Argonaute proteins, some lipids, and microvesicles when transported [15], they are protected from degradation and considered relatively stable under various storage conditions [16–19]. Therefore, they should act as biomarkers. Although many researchers have reported diagnostic biomarkers for CRC using serum or plasma miRNAs [20,21], there are no known biomarkers consisting of urinary miRNAs [22]. Urine is an ideal sample for medical checkups because of its noninvasiveness, easy handling, and low cost. We have made a longstanding effort to discover urinary biomarkers and established urinary protein biomarkers for diagnosing gastric cancer (GC) and CRC [23–26]. Moreover, we have also identified the urinary miRNA biomarker to detect GC [27] and esophageal cancer (EC) [28]. Based on this background, we conducted this study to establish reliable and noninvasive urinary miRNA biomarkers for CRC.

2. Materials and Methods

2.1. Patients and Study Design

We studied 522 urine samples from 223 patients with CRC and 299 healthy controls (HCs). All samples were collected from September 2012 to August 2018 at three Japanese institutions. We included males and females aged 20–90 years. Patients with CRC (CRC group) had an existing cancer diagnosis, established by histological and endoscopic findings, and no prior treatment on entry. HCs were recruited from healthy individuals without any symptoms, and had no neoplasms as confirmed by a medical checkup. Individuals with previous cancer or other malignancies within the past 5 years were excluded from the study. There were no criteria for timing of urine collection and for preparation before urine collection. To ensure the accuracy and comprehensiveness of reporting in this case-control biomarker study, we complied with both the REMARK guidelines [29] and the STROBE statement [30]. This study was registered with the University Hospital Medical Information Network Clinical Trials Registry (UMIN000021350).

2.2. Samples and Definition

Urine samples were collected from each patient with CRC before any treatment and immediately stored at −80 °C until analyzed, as reported previously [23–25,27]. All patients with CRC were classified based on Tumor Node Metastasis staging and the Union for International Cancer Control guidelines, version 7 [31].

2.3. miRNA Extraction

The procedure was described in a previous report [27]. Briefly, 200 µL (600 µL for microarray use) of urine or serum was used for extracting miRNA by miRNeasy Serum/Plasma Kit (Qiagen, Valencia, CA, USA) according to the manufacturer's instructions. Extraction of miRNAs from formalin-fixed paraffin-embedded (FFPE) tissues was conducted using the miRNeasy FFPE Kit (Qiagen).

2.4. miRNA Microarray Assay

The miRNA microarray assay was conducted as described in a previous report [27]. Briefly, Cyanine-3 (Cy3) labeled cRNA were synthesized using the miRNA Complete Labeling and Hyb Kit (Agilent, Santa Clara, CA, USA) according to the manufacturer's protocol. Cy3-labeled miRNA specimens were hybridized to the Agilent Human miRNA Microarrays (G4872A). After overnight for hybridization, microarrays were scanned by the Agilent DNA Microarray Scanner (G2539A). The obtained images were analyzed with Feature Extraction Software 11.0.1.1 (Agilent).

2.5. Quantitative Reverse Transcription-Polymerase Chain Reaction (qRT-PCR)

The protocol was also described previously [27]. Briefly, complementary DNA (cDNA) was prepared from miRNA samples using TaqMan Advanced MicroRNA cDNA Synthesis Kit (Applied Biosystems, Foster, CA, USA), according to the manufacturer's instructions. Quantitative PCRs were conducted in duplicate using the TaqMan Advanced MicroRNA Assay (Applied Biosystems) and TaqMan Fast Advanced Master Mix (Applied Biosystems) by 7500 Fast Real-Time PCR system (Applied Biosystems). We calculated cycle threshold (Ct) values to quantify miRNA expression using the $2^{-\Delta Ct}$ method. Internal controls for normalization in qPCR of urinary miRNA were determined using a global mean normalization method with the microarray results [32]. Therefore, miR-4669 and miR-6756-5p were determined to be the internal normalization controls for qPCR of urinary and serum miRNAs, as shown in the previous study [28]. As the internal normalizer for the qPCR of miRNA in FFPE tissues, we used RNU6B. The reagents used in qRT-PCR were listed in Table S1.

2.6. In Silico Analyses

Kaplan–Meier curves showing the relationship between miRNA expression and survival time of the patients of rectal adenocarcinoma was downloaded from Kaplan–Meier Plotter (https://kmplot.com/analysis/index.php?p=service&cancer=pancancer_mirna (accessed on 17 November 2021)).

2.7. Statistical Analyses

Matching between the CRC and HC groups was conducted using a propensity score (PS) determined by a logistic regression model (age and gender). The two groups were randomly matched one-to-one using the nearest-neighbor method within a caliper width of 25% of the standard deviation of the PS logit.

The Mann–Whitney U test, Student's *t*-test (for serum creatinine values), and chi-squared test were used for detection of the significant differences as appropriate. We evaluated correlation using Spearman's rank method with a coefficient (r). Receiver operating characteristic (ROC) curve analysis was used to calculate the area under the curve (AUC) for each biomarker, and the AUC value with a 95% confidence interval (CI) was shown as the representative value. Logistic regression modeling was used to estimate the odds ratio (OR) with 95% CI and construct a formula for scoring, which, in turn, was used to draw the ROC curve to compute the AUC for the combination biomarker. Instead of the actual measured values, the Z score's adjusted values were used to calculate OR. Statistical analyses were carried out using R software (https://www.R-project.org/, (accessed on 17 November 2021)) or IBM SPSS statistics, version 25 (IBM Corp., Tokyo, Japan), respectively. All *p* values were two-sided, and those <0.05 were considered statistically significant.

3. Results

3.1. Participants

The study flowchart is shown in Figure 1. Among 522 participants comprising 223 patients with CRC and 299 HC subjects, 415 age- and sex-matched participants were enrolled in the study (206 patients from the CRC group and 209 participants from the HC group). Afterward, this cohort was randomly divided into three groups, with nine participants (three patients from CRC group and six participants from HC group) in the discovery cohort, 280 participants (140 pairs) in the training cohort, and 126 participants (63 pairs) in the validation cohort. There were no significant differences for all factors between the two groups. About two-thirds of CRC group had sigmoid or rectal cancer, and 66 patients (32.0%) with CRC had stage 0 or I CRC (Table 1).

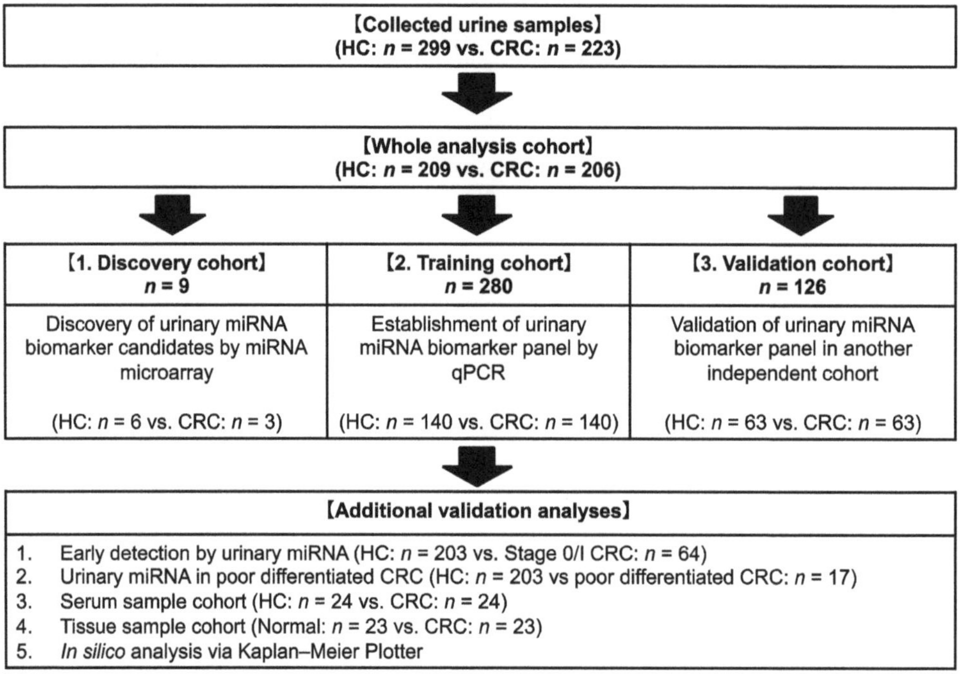

```
           【Collected urine samples】
           (HC: n = 299 vs. CRC: n = 223)
                       ↓
           【Whole analysis cohort】
           (HC: n = 209 vs. CRC: n = 206)
         ↓              ↓              ↓
【1. Discovery    【2. Training    【3. Validation
    cohort】         cohort】          cohort】
    n = 9           n = 280           n = 126

Discovery of     Establishment    Validation of
urinary miRNA    of urinary       urinary miRNA
biomarker        miRNA            biomarker panel
candidates by    biomarker        in another
miRNA            panel by qPCR    independent
microarray                        cohort

(HC: n = 6       (HC: n = 140     (HC: n = 63
vs. CRC: n = 3)  vs. CRC: n = 140) vs. CRC: n = 63)
                       ↓
           【Additional validation analyses】
1. Early detection by urinary miRNA (HC: n = 203 vs. Stage 0/I CRC: n = 64)
2. Urinary miRNA in poor differentiated CRC (HC: n = 203 vs poor differentiated CRC: n = 17)
3. Serum sample cohort (HC: n = 24 vs. CRC: n = 24)
4. Tissue sample cohort (Normal: n = 23 vs. CRC: n = 23)
5. In silico analysis via Kaplan–Meier Plotter
```

Figure 1. Study profile. HC, healthy control; CRC, colorectal cancer; qPCR, quantitative polymerase chain reaction.

Table 1. Patient characteristics.

Item		HC (n = 209)	CRC (n = 206)	p Value
Age (years)	Median (IQR)	69 (63–74)	69.5 (63–75)	0.275
Gender, n	Male	123	117	0.672
	Female	86	89	
Serum Cr (mg/dL)	Mean ± SD	0.78 ± 0.18	0.77 ± 0.26	0.787
Histological grade, n, %	well to mod		189 (91.7)	
	por		17 (8.3)	
Location, n, %	Cecum		20 (9.7)	
	Ascending		29 (14.1)	
	Transverse		22 (10.7)	

Table 1. Cont.

Item		HC (n = 209)	CRC (n = 206)	p Value
	Descending		8 (3.9)	
	Sigmoid		54 (26.2)	
	Rectum		73 (35.4)	
Stage, n, %	0		22 (10.7)	
	I		44 (21.4)	
	II		44 (21.4)	
	III		48 (23.3)	
	IV		48 (23.3)	

HC, healthy control; CRC, colorectal cancer; IQR, interquartile range; Cr, creatinine; SD, standard deviation; well to mod, well to moderately differentiated adenocarcinoma; por, poorly differentiated adenocarcinoma.

3.2. Urinary miRNA Difference between HC and CRC Groups

First, to detect differences in urinary miRNAs between the HC and CRC groups comprehensively, we conducted an miRNA microarray analysis in the discovery cohort (HC = 6 vs. CRC = 3). Eleven urinary miRNAs showed significantly aberrant expressions between the HC and CRC groups (Figure S1).

3.3. Development of Urinary miRNA Biomarker

Among 11 candidate miRNAs identified through microarray analysis, eight miRNAs revealed unstable urine sample expression. Consequently, we quantitated three miRNAs using qRT-PCR in the next training cohort.

Univariate analysis showed that urinary expression levels of miR-129-1-3p, miR-566, and miR-598-5p were significantly higher in the CRC group than in the HC group ($p < 0.001$). Moreover, multivariate analysis revealed that urinary levels of miR-129-1-3p (OR: 5.59 [95% CI, 2.82–11.10]; $p < 0.001$) and miR-566 (OR: 1.64 [95% CI, 1.09–2.45]; $p = 0.017$) were also independent biomarkers for the diagnosis of CRC (Table 2). Based on these results, we established a diagnostic biomarker panel of CRC consisting of urinary miR-129-1-3p and miR-566 using a logistic regression model. This urinary miRNA biomarker panel showed satisfactory power to distinguish patients with CRC from HC participants with an AUC = 0.811 (95% CI, 0.762–0.861), which was higher than that of either miR-129-1-3p or miR-566 alone (Figure 2A). When the cut-off point was determined at the Youden index, this logistic regression model showed good efficacy, with 80.7% sensitivity, 70.7% specificity, and 75.7% accuracy for detecting CRC.

Table 2. Urinary miRNA expression in the training phase.

Variable	$2^{-\Delta Ct}$ (Median, IQR)		Univariate Analysis	Multivariate Analysis	
	HC (n = 140)	CRC (n = 140)	p Value	Odds Ratio (95% CI)	p Value
miR-129-1-3p	0.00054 (0.00019–0.00101)	0.00150 (0.00082–0.00326)	<0.001	5.59 (2.82–11.10)	<0.001
miR-566	0.050 (0.029–0.163)	0.184 (0.071–0.438)	<0.001	1.64 (1.09–2.45)	0.017
miR-598-5p	0.122 (0.070–0.266)	0.273 (0.130–0.402)	<0.001		

IQR, interquartile range; 95% CI, confidence interval.

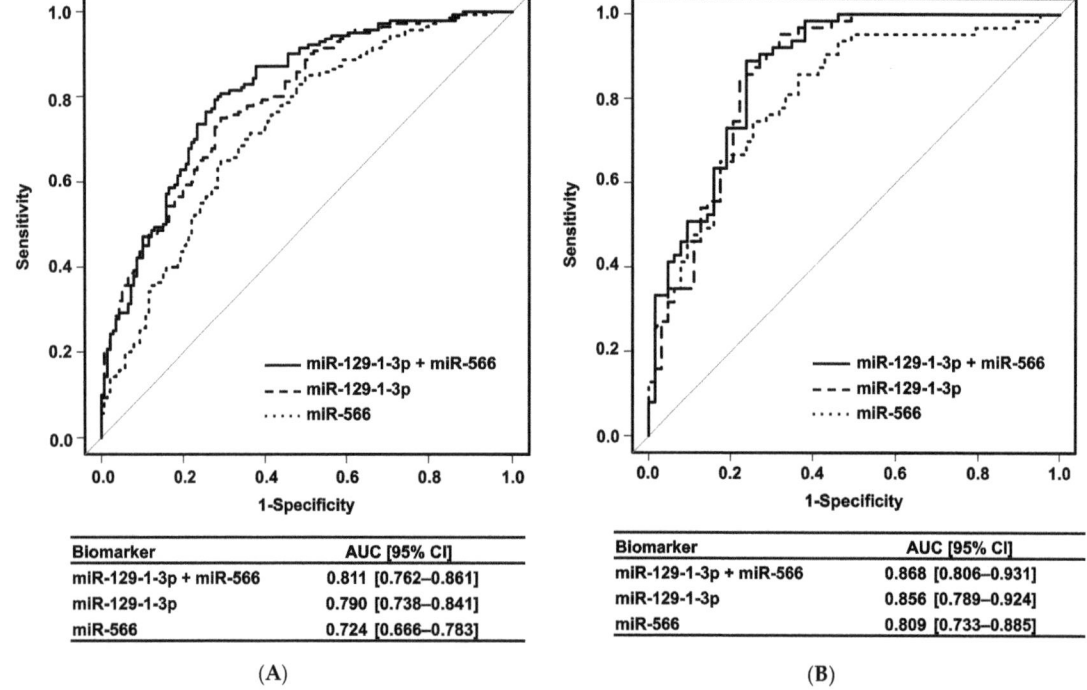

Figure 2. Receiver operating characteristics curves. (**A**) Training cohort. (**B**) Validation cohort. AUC, area under the curve; 95% CI, 95% confidence interval.

3.4. Validation of Urinary miRNA Biomarker

Further validation of this diagnostic biomarker panel was performed in an independent cohort (the validation cohort) to ensure extrapolation. Urinary expression levels of both miR-129-1-3p and miR-566 were significantly higher in the CRC group than in the HC group ($p < 0.001$). These results were consistent with findings in the training cohort (Table 3). The combination biomarker panel also showed a good AUC = 0.868 (95% CI, 0.806–0.931) with 88.9% sensitivity, 76.2% specificity, and 82.5% accuracy in the validation cohort (Figure 2B).

Table 3. Urinary miRNA biomarker in the validation cohort.

Variable	$2^{-\Delta Ct}$ (Median, IQR)		Univariate Analysis	Multivariate Analysis	
	HC	CRC	p Value	Odds Ratio (95% CI)	p Value
	($n = 63$)	($n = 63$)			
miR-129-1-3p	0.00025 (0.00015–0.00079)	0.00141 (0.00095–0.00218)	<0.001	5.03 (1.99–12.70)	<0.001
miR-566	0.040 (0.017–0.105)	0.222 (0.100–0.526)	<0.001	2.99 (1.13–7.89)	0.027

IQR, interquartile range; 95% CI, confidence interval.

Since background factors may affect urinary miRNA expression, we investigated the relationship between urinary levels of these miRNAs and clinical parameters (age, gender, degree of differentiation, and serum creatinine level). Although age, degree of differentiation, and serum creatinine level were not correlated with the expression of urinary miRNAs, both urinary miRNAs were significantly higher in female than in male (Figure S2A). However, gender was not significant upon the multivariate analysis, and our established urinary miRNA biomarker panel showed good efficacy in both the male and female cohorts with an AUC = 0.882 (95% CI, 0.839–0.925) and 0.773 (95% CI, 0.703–0.843), respectively (Figure S2B).

Next, we investigated the diagnostic ability for early-stage CRC. In a comparison between HC participants and patients with early-stage CRC, both urinary miR-129-1-3p and miR-566 showed significantly higher levels in the stage 0/I CRC group than in the HC group ($p < 0.001$) (Figure 3A). This urinary miRNA biomarker panel also showed excellent power to distinguish patients with stage 0/I CRC from HC participants with an AUC = 0.845 (95% CI, 0.798–0.893) (Figure 3B). Conversely, expression levels of both miR-129-1-3p and miR-566 in urine did not correlate to the disease stage (Figure S3). In Kaplan–Meier curves based on the Kaplan–Meier Plotter, both miR-129 (logrank $p = 0.37$) and miR-566 (logrank $p = 0.21$) had no correlation with overall survival of the patients with rectal adenocarcinoma. Regardless of disease stage, this urinary biomarker was superior to currently used tumor markers (serum CEA and CA19-9) (Figure S4). Of note, this urinary combination biomarker panel showed 82.8% sensitivity for stage 0/I CRC, whereas both serum CEA and CA19-9 showed only 11.1% sensitivity for stage 0/I CRC. These results suggest that our established urinary biomarker panel is a useful noninvasive screening tool for the early detection of CRC.

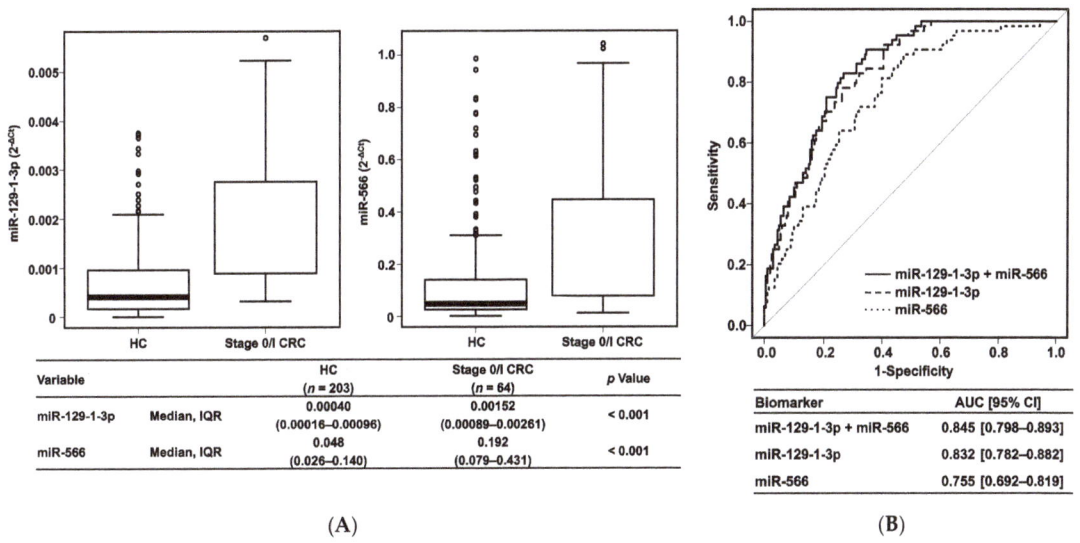

Figure 3. Urinary miRNA biomarker in stage 0/I CRC. (A) Boxplots. (B) Receiver operating characteristics curves. HC, healthy control; CRC, colorectal cancer; IQR, interquartile range; AUC, area under the curve; 95% CI, 95% confidence interval.

In addition, regardless of the degree of differentiation, these urinary miRNA biomarkers showed significantly higher expression levels in the CRC group than in the HC group (Table S2).

3.5. Analysis Using Serum and Tissue Samples

Next, we analyzed serum levels of miR-129-1-3p and miR-566, but no significant correlations were found between urine and serum levels. Nevertheless, serum miR-566 showed a significantly higher expression level in the CRC group than in the HC group, and serum miR-129-1-3p showed the same tendency (Table S3). Because it is unclear whether urinary miR-129-1-3p and miR-566 are derived from CRC tissues, we also measured the expression levels of these miRNAs in tissue samples. Interestingly, expression levels of both miR-129-1-3p and miR-566 were significantly higher in the primary tumor tissues than in the adjacent normal tissues (Figure S5). Table S4 shows the characteristics of patients with CRC for tissue miRNA analysis.

4. Discussion

This large sample study, including three independent cohorts, clearly showed that the urinary biomarker panel combining miR-129-1-3p and miR-566 is a novel diagnostic noninvasive biomarker to detect CRC, even at an early stage. While the sensitivity of FIT for detecting advanced adenoma (i.e., stage 0 CRC) was reportedly 11–56% [5–7], our urinary biomarker showed good sensitivity of 82.8% for detecting stage 0/I CRC patients. Although we cannot simply compare the two methods, our established urinary miRNA biomarker might overcome FIT in point of early detection of CRC.

Urine is an ideal sample for mass screening because of its easy handling and collection. Previous studies have reported the usefulness of urinary methylated or mutated genes for CRC detection [22]; however, additional investigation is needed because of low sensitivity and lack of information for early detection. Moreover, such genetic markers may not be able to pass through the glomerulus because of their high molecular weight [33]. Because miRNAs are small molecules consisting of 20–25 nucleotides, miRNAs have an advantage as urinary biomarker targets. Indeed, miR-129-1-3p and miR-566 expression levels were also elevated in both serum and tissue samples in this study, suggesting that the overexpression of these miRNAs in CRC tissues would be secreted into the serum and finally excreted into the urine. These results were consistent with our previously identified urinary miRNA biomarkers for GC and EC [27,28]. No direct correlations were found for the two urinary miRNAs between urine and serum levels. Similarly, the previous study reported different miRNA profiles between plasma and other fluids [34]. We also showed different signatures between serum and urinary miRNAs in the previous biomarker study of EC [28]. These results have suggested that serum miRNAs might be susceptible to other abundant factors in serum, and the present miRNA urinary biomarkers revealed ideal performance of predictability for the presence of CRC in urine through the selective filtering process.

There are several reports using serum/plasma and fecal miRNAs to detect CRC. One study showed that the expression level of serum miR-1290 is increased in patients with CRC and distinguished patients with CRC efficiently [21]. Another study indicated that the diagnostic panel consisting of fecal miR-421, miR-27a-3p, and hemoglobin showed better efficacy than hemoglobin alone [35]. However, there are no known reports of urinary miRNA biomarkers to detect patients with CRC. Because urine contains only small amounts of miRNA compared with serum/plasma and feces, it would appear to be difficult to detect the small difference in urinary miRNA expression. However, it is also a strong advantage that urine contains very few substances such as bacteria and protein that cause some expression analysis noises. In addition, urinary miRNAs seem stable under various storage conditions [17,36].

miR-129 family members are generally considered tumor suppressors with decreased expression in various cancers, which often refers to miR-129-5p [37–39]. In terms of miR-129-1-3p, its downregulation was associated with tumor progression via the c-Src pathway in CRC cells and tissues [40], in opposition to our results. Another study indicated that miR-129-1-3p promoted cell proliferation via programmed cell death in GC cells [41]. In our study, miR-129-1-3p was overexpressed in CRC tissues, but its inhibition did not affect cell proliferation and migration (data not shown). Although the function of miR-129-1-3p as related to CRC is controversial, overexpressed miR-129-1-3p may be a result accompanied with carcinogenesis and not a key oncogenic driver.

miR-566 stimulates epidermal growth factor receptor pathway via von Hippel–Lindau disease [42]. In addition, another study reported the oncogenic behavior of miR-566 in renal cell carcinoma (RCC) and upregulated expression in RCC tissues and cells [43].

These conclusions support our findings that miR-566 was upregulated in CRC tissues. Conversely, other studies showed that reduced expression of miR-566 was correlated to CRC development [44] and was involved in epithelial–mesenchymal transition (EMT) driven by *Alu* RNA [45]. Our study showed the urinary level of miR-566 was elevated even in the patients with early-stage CRC, which is generally unrelated to EMT, suggesting that miR-566 may be involved in the carcinogenesis of CRC in complicated ways.

This study has two limitations. First, the oncogenic function of miR-129-1-3p and miR-566 in CRC remains unknown. However, the significant results reported here were consistent among the three independent cohorts. Furthermore, our established urinary miRNA biomarker could efficiently detect stage 0/I CRC, which was a major advantage for developing a mass screening tool. Notably, this urinary miRNA biomarker could show a much higher detection rate than the serum tumor markers currently used. Although additional basic studies are also needed to clarify these miRNAs' mechanism as related to CRC, we think that our urinary miRNA biomarker could be the next-generation CRC screening test. Second, we need to set an optimal cut-off value for the future clinical use. A prospective study is essential to validate the efficacy of this urinary biomarker and set a cut-off with well-balanced sensitivity and false positive rate. We are thus planning the prospective cohort study for the future clinical application.

5. Conclusions

In conclusion, a novel urinary biomarker consisting of miR-129-1-3p and miR-566 has made it possible for the early detection of CRC in a completely noninvasive manner.

Supplementary Materials: The following are available online at https://www.mdpi.com/article/10.3390/cancers14020461/s1, Figure S1: Urinary miRNA microarray in the discovery cohort, Figure S2: Receiver operating characteristics curve in the whole cohort, Figure S3: Correlation between urinary miRNA level and disease stage, Figure S4: Comparison between urinary biomarker and serum CEA/CA19-9, Figure S5: Expression of miR-129-1-3p and miR-566 in tissue sample, Table S1: TaqMan Advanced miRNA Assays for qRT-PCR, Table S2: Urinary miRNA biomarker in the patients with well to poorly differentiated CRC, Table S3: Expression of miR-129-1-3p and miR-566 in serum sample, Table S4: Characteristics of the patients with CRC for tissue miRNA analysis.

Author Contributions: Conceptualization, T.S.; methodology, T.S.; software, H.I. and T.S.; validation, H.I. and T.S.; formal analysis, H.I and T.S.; investigation, H.I., Y.O. and S.-i.H.; resources, T.Y. and S.-i.H.; data curation, H.I, R.N., S.F. and T.K.; writing—original draft preparation, H.I.; writing—review and editing, H.I. and T.S.; visualization, H.I.; supervision, H.K.; project administration, H.K.; funding acquisition, T.S. and M.K. All authors have read and agreed to the published version of the manuscript.

Funding: This study was supported, in part, by the Nitto Foundation (to T.S.) and JSPS KAKENHI Grant Number 18K15757 (to M.K.).

Institutional Review Board Statement: The study protocol conforms to the ethical guidelines of the 1975 Declaration of Helsinki (6th revision, 2008) and was approved by the ethics committee at each participating institution (Nagoya City University Hospital Institutional Review Board, Japanese Red Cross Aichi Medical Center Nagoya Daini Hospital Institutional Review Board, and Okazaki Public Health Center Ethical Committee) (approval number, #45-12-0013).

Informed Consent Statement: Informed consent was obtained from all subjects involved in the study.

Data Availability Statement: The data presented in this study are available on request from the corresponding author (T.S.).

Acknowledgments: We thank Masahide Ebi at Aichi Medical University, Tomonori Yamada at Japanese Red Cross Aichi Medical Center Nagoya Daini Hospital, and clinical colleague at Nagoya City University for sample collection. We also thank Yukimi Hashidume-Itoh for handling of urine sample and Yukao Kusaka, Chiaki Tsuzuki, and Kana Saji for data management of enrolled patients in this study (Department of Gastroenterology and Metabolism, Nagoya City University Graduate School of Medical Sciences).

Conflicts of Interest: The authors declare no conflict of interest.

References

1. Fitzmaurice, C.; Akinyemiju, T.F.; al Lami, F.H.; Alam, T.; Alizadeh-Navaei, R.; Allen, C.; Alsharif, U.; Alvis-Guzman, N.; Amini, E.; Anderson, B.O.; et al. Global Burden of Disease Cancer Collaboration. Global, Regional, and National Cancer Incidence, Mortality, Years of Life Lost, Years Lived with Disability, and Disability-Adjusted Life-Years for 29 Cancer Groups, 1990 to 2016: A Systematic Analysis for the Global Burden of Disease Study. *JAMA Oncol.* **2018**, *4*, 1553–1568. [CrossRef] [PubMed]
2. Bretthauer, M.; Kaminski, M.; Løberg, M.; Zauber, A.G.; Regula, J.; Kuipers, E.J.; Hernán, M.; McFadden, E.; Sunde, A.; Kalager, M.; et al. Population-Based Colonoscopy Screening for Colorectal Cancer: A Randomized Clinical Trial. *JAMA Intern. Med.* **2016**, *176*, 894–902. [CrossRef]
3. Halloran, S.; Launoy, G.; Zappa, M. European guidelines for quality assurance in colorectal cancer screening and diagnosis.—First Edition Faecal occult blood testing. *Endoscopy* **2012**, *44* (Suppl. S3), SE65–SE87. [CrossRef]
4. US Preventive Services Task Force; Bibbins-Domingo, K.; Grossman, D.C.; Curry, S.J.; Davidson, K.W.; Epling, J.W., Jr.; García, F.A.R.; Gillman, M.W.; Harper, D.M.; Kemper, A.R.; et al. Screening for Colorectal Cancer: US Preventive Services Task Force Recommendation Statement. *JAMA* **2016**, *315*, 2564–2575. [CrossRef]
5. van Dam, L.; Kuipers, E.J.; van Leerdam, M.E. Performance improvements of stool-based screening tests. *Best Pr. Res. Clin. Gastroenterol.* **2010**, *24*, 479–492. [CrossRef] [PubMed]
6. Gies, A.; Cuk, K.; Schrotz-King, P.; Brenner, H. Direct Comparison of Diagnostic Performance of 9 Quantitative Fecal Immunochemical Tests for Colorectal Cancer Screening. *Gastroenterology* **2018**, *154*, 93–104. [CrossRef]
7. de Klaver, W.; Wisse, P.H.A.; van Wifferen, F.; Bosch, L.J.W.; Jimenez, C.R.; van der Hulst, R.W.M.; Fijneman, R.J.A.; Kuipers, E.J.; Greuter, M.J.E.; Carvalho, B.; et al. Clinical Validation of a Multitarget Fecal Immunochemical Test for Colorectal Cancer Screening: A Diagnostic Test Accuracy Study. *Ann. Intern. Med.* **2021**, *174*, 1224–1231. [CrossRef]
8. Imperiale, T.; Ransohoff, D.F.; Itzkowitz, S.H.; Levin, T.R.; Lavin, P.; Lidgard, G.P.; Ahlquist, D.A.; Berger, B.M. Multitarget Stool DNA Testing for Colorectal-Cancer Screening. *N. Engl. J. Med.* **2014**, *370*, 1287–1297. [CrossRef] [PubMed]
9. Zhai, R.-L.; Xu, F.; Zhang, P.; Zhang, W.-L.; Wang, H.; Wang, J.-L.; Cai, K.-L.; Long, Y.-P.; Lu, X.-M.; Tao, K.-X.; et al. The Diagnostic Performance of Stool DNA Testing for Colorectal Cancer: A Systematic Review and Meta-Analysis. *Medicine* **2016**, *95*, e2129. [CrossRef] [PubMed]
10. Fletcher, R.H. Carcinoembryonic Antigen. *Ann. Intern. Med.* **1986**, *104*, 66–73. [CrossRef]
11. Nicolini, A.; Ferrari, P.; Duffy, M.J.; Antonelli, A.; Rossi, G.; Metelli, M.R.; Fulceri, F.; Anselmi, L.; Conte, M.; Berti, P.; et al. Intensive Risk-Adjusted Follow-up With the CEA, TPA, CA19.9, and CA72.4 Tumor Marker Panel and Abdominal Ultrasonography to Diagnose Operable Colorectal Cancer Recurrences: Effect on survival. *Arch. Surg.* **2010**, *145*, 1177–1183. [CrossRef] [PubMed]
12. Thomas, D.; Fourkala, E.-O.; Apostolidou, S.; Gunu, R.; Ryan, A.; Jacobs, I.; Menon, U.; Alderton, W.; Gentry-Maharaj, A.; Timms, J.F. Evaluation of serum CEA, CYFRA21-1 and CA125 for the early detection of colorectal cancer using longitudinal preclinical samples. *Br. J. Cancer* **2015**, *113*, 268–274. [CrossRef]
13. Calin, G.A.; Croce, C.M. MicroRNA Signatures in Human Cancers. *Nat. Rev. Cancer* **2006**, *6*, 857–866. [CrossRef]
14. Calin, G.; Croce, C.M. Chromosomal Rearrangements and MicroRNAs: A New Cancer Link with Clinical Implications. *J. Clin. Investig.* **2007**, *117*, 2059–2066. [CrossRef] [PubMed]
15. Arroyo, J.D.; Chevillet, J.R.; Kroh, E.M.; Ruf, I.K.; Pritchard, C.C.; Gibson, D.F.; Mitchell, P.S.; Bennett, C.F.; Pogosova-Agadjanyan, E.L.; Stirewalt, D.L.; et al. Argonaute2 complexes carry a population of circulating microRNAs independent of vesicles in human plasma. *Proc. Natl. Acad. Sci. USA* **2011**, *108*, 5003–5008. [CrossRef]
16. Egidi, M.G.; Cochetti, G.; Guelfi, G.; Zampini, D.; Diverio, S.; Poli, G.; Mearini, E. Stability Assessment of Candidate Reference Genes in Urine Sediment of Prostate Cancer Patients for miRNA Applications. *Dis. Markers* **2015**, *2015*, 973597. [CrossRef] [PubMed]
17. Mall, C.; Rocke, D.M.; Durbin-Johnson, B.; Weiss, R.H. Stability of miRNA in human urine supports its biomarker potential. *Biomark. Med.* **2013**, *7*, 623–631. [CrossRef] [PubMed]
18. Andreasen, D.; Fog, J.U.; Biggs, W.; Salomon, J.; Dahslveen, I.K.; Baker, A.; Mouritzen, P. Improved microRNA quantification in total RNA from clinical samples. *Methods* **2010**, *50*, S6–S9. [CrossRef]
19. Mraz, M.; Malinova, K.; Mayer, J.; Pospisilova, S. MicroRNA isolation and stability in stored RNA samples. *Biochem. Biophys. Res. Commun.* **2009**, *390*, 1–4. [CrossRef]
20. Ng, E.K.-O.; Chong, W.W.S.; Jin, H.; Lam, E.K.Y.; Shin, V.Y.; Yu, J.; Poon, T.C.W.; Ng, S.S.M.; Sung, J.J.Y. Differential expression of microRNAs in plasma of patients with colorectal cancer: A potential marker for colorectal cancer screening. *Gut* **2009**, *58*, 1375–1381. [CrossRef]
21. Imaoka, H.; Toiyama, Y.; Fujikawa, H.; Hiro, J.; Saigusa, S.; Tanaka, K.; Inoue, Y.; Mohri, Y.; Mori, T.; Kato, T.; et al. Circulating microRNA-1290 as a novel diagnostic and prognostic biomarker in human colorectal cancer. *Ann. Oncol.* **2016**, *27*, 1879–1886. [CrossRef]
22. Iwasaki, H.; Shimura, T.; Kataoka, H. Current status of urinary diagnostic biomarkers for colorectal cancer. *Clin. Chim. Acta* **2019**, *498*, 76–83. [CrossRef]
23. Shimura, T.; Dagher, A.; Sachdev, M.; Ebi, M.; Yamada, T.; Yamada, T.; Joh, T.; Moses, M.A. Urinary ADAM12 and MMP-9/NGAL Complex Detect the Presence of Gastric Cancer. *Cancer Prev. Res.* **2015**, *8*, 240–248. [CrossRef] [PubMed]

24. Shimura, T.; Ebi, M.; Yamada, T.; Yamada, T.; Katano, T.; Nojiri, Y.; Iwasaki, H.; Nomura, S.; Hayashi, N.; Mori, Y.; et al. Urinary kallikrein 10 predicts the incurability of gastric cancer. *Oncotarget* **2017**, *8*, 29247–29257. [CrossRef]
25. Shimura, T.; Iwasaki, H.; Kitagawa, M.; Ebi, M.; Yamada, T.; Yamada, T.; Katano, T.; Nisie, H.; Okamoto, Y.; Ozeki, K.; et al. Urinary Cysteine-Rich Protein 61 and Trefoil Factor 3 as Diagnostic Biomarkers for Colorectal Cancer. *Transl. Oncol.* **2019**, *12*, 539–544. [CrossRef] [PubMed]
26. Shimura, T.; Dayde, D.; Wang, H.; Okuda, Y.; Iwasaki, H.; Ebi, M.; Kitagawa, M.; Yamada, T.; Yamada, T.; Hanash, S.M.; et al. Novel urinary protein biomarker panel for early diagnosis of gastric cancer. *Br. J. Cancer* **2020**, *123*, 1656–1664. [CrossRef]
27. Iwasaki, H.; Shimura, T.; Yamada, T.; Okuda, Y.; Natsume, M.; Kitagawa, M.; Horike, S.-I.; Kataoka, H. A novel urinary microRNA biomarker panel for detecting gastric cancer. *J. Gastroenterol.* **2019**, *54*, 1061–1069. [CrossRef]
28. Okuda, Y.; Shimura, T.; Iwasaki, H.; Fukusada, S.; Nishigaki, R.; Kitagawa, M.; Katano, T.; Okamoto, Y.; Yamada, T.; Horike, S.-I.; et al. Urinary microRNA biomarkers for detecting the presence of esophageal cancer. *Sci. Rep.* **2021**, *11*, 8508. [CrossRef]
29. McShane, L.M.; Altman, D.G.; Sauerbrei, W.; Taube, S.E.; Gion, M.; Clark, G.M. Reporting Recommendations for Tumor Marker Prognostic Studies. *J. Clin. Oncol.* **2005**, *23*, 9067–9072. [CrossRef] [PubMed]
30. Vandenbroucke, J.P.; von Elm, E.; Altman, D.G.; Gøtzsche, P.C.; Mulrow, C.D.; Pocock, S.J.; Poole, C.; Schlesselman, J.J.; Egger, M. Strengthening the Reporting of Observational Studies in Epidemiology (STROBE). *Epidemiology* **2007**, *18*, 805–835. [CrossRef] [PubMed]
31. Fisseler-Eckhoff, A. New TNM classification of malignant lung tumors 2009 from a pathology perspective. *Der Pathol.* **2009**, *30* (Suppl. S2), 193–199. [CrossRef]
32. Mestdagh, P.; Van Vlierberghe, P.; De Weer, A.; Muth, D.; Westermann, F.; Speleman, F.; Vandesompele, J. A novel and universal method for microRNA RT-qPCR data normalization. *Genome Biol.* **2009**, *10*, 1–10. [CrossRef] [PubMed]
33. Brenner, B.M.; Bohrer, M.P.; Baylis, C.; Deen, W.M. Determinants of glomerular permselectivity: Insights derived from observations in vivo. *Kidney Int.* **1977**, *12*, 229–237. [CrossRef] [PubMed]
34. Weber, J.A.; Baxter, D.H.; Zhang, S.; Huang, D.Y.; How Huang, K.; Jen Lee, M.; Galas, D.J.; Wang, K. The MicroRNA Spectrum in 12 Body Fluids. *Clin. Chem.* **2010**, *56*, 1733–1741. [CrossRef] [PubMed]
35. Sanchon, S.D.; Moreno, L.; Augé, J.M.; Serra-Burriel, M.; Cuatrecasas, M.; Moreira, L.; Martín, A.; Serradesanferm, A.; Pozo, À.; Costa, R.; et al. Identification and Validation of MicroRNA Profiles in Fecal Samples for Detection of Colorectal Cancer. *Gastroenterology* **2020**, *158*, 947–957.e4. [CrossRef]
36. Armstrong, D.A.; Dessaint, J.A.; Ringelberg, C.S.; Hazlett, H.F.; Howard, L.; Abdalla, M.A.; Barnaby, R.L.; Stanton, B.A.; Cervinski, M.; Ashare, A. Pre-Analytical Handling Conditions and Small RNA Recovery from Urine for miRNA Profiling. *J. Mol. Diagn.* **2018**, *20*, 565–571. [CrossRef]
37. Dyrskjøt, L.; Ostenfeld, M.S.; Bramsen, J.B.; Silahtaroglu, A.N.; Lamy, P.; Ramanathan, R.; Fristrup, N.; Jensen, J.L.; Andersen, C.L.; Zieger, K.; et al. Genomic Profiling of MicroRNAs in Bladder Cancer: miR-129 Is Associated with Poor Outcome and Promotes Cell Death In vitro. *Cancer Res.* **2009**, *69*, 4851–4860. [CrossRef] [PubMed]
38. Bandres, E.; Agirre, X.; Bitarte, N.; Ramirez, N.; Zarate, R.; Roman-Gomez, J.; Prosper, F.; Garcia-Foncillas, J. Epigenetic regulation of microRNA expression in colorectal cancer. *Int. J. Cancer* **2009**, *125*, 2737–2743. [CrossRef] [PubMed]
39. Chen, S.; Sun, K.-X.; Liu, B.-L.; Zong, Z.-H.; Zhao, Y. The role of glycogen synthase kinase-3β (GSK-3β) in endometrial carcinoma: A carcinogenesis, progression, prognosis, and target therapy marker. *Oncotarget* **2016**, *7*, 27538–27551. [CrossRef]
40. Okuzaki, D.; Yamauchi, T.; Mitani, F.; Miyata, M.; Ninomiya, Y.; Watanabe, R.; Akamatsu, H.; Oneyama, C. c-Src promotes tumor progression through downregulation of microRNA-129-1-3p. *Cancer Sci.* **2020**, *111*, 418–428. [CrossRef]
41. Du, Y.; Wang, D.; Luo, L.; Guo, J. miR-129-1-3p Promote BGC-823 Cell Proliferation by Targeting PDCD2. *Anat. Rec. Adv. Integr. Anat. Evol. Biol.* **2014**, *297*, 2273–2279. [CrossRef] [PubMed]
42. Zhang, K.-L.; Zhou, X.; Han, L.; Chen, L.-Y.; Chen, L.-C.; Shi, Z.-D.; Yang, M.; Ren, Y.; Yang, J.-X.; Frank, T.S.; et al. MicroRNA-566 activates EGFR signaling and its inhibition sensitizes glioblastoma cells to nimotuzumab. *Mol. Cancer* **2014**, *13*, 63. [CrossRef] [PubMed]
43. Pan, X.; Quan, J.; Li, Z.; Zhao, L.; Zhou, L.; Jinling, X.; Weijie, X.; Guan, X.; Li, H.; Yang, S.; et al. miR-566 functions as an oncogene and a potential biomarker for prognosis in renal cell carcinoma. *Biomed. Pharmacother.* **2018**, *102*, 718–727. [CrossRef] [PubMed]
44. Drusco, A.; Nuovo, G.J.; Zanesi, N.; Di Leva, G.; Pichiorri, F.; Volinia, S.; Fernandez, C.; Antenucci, A.; Costinean, S.; Bottoni, A.; et al. MicroRNA Profiles Discriminate among Colon Cancer Metastasis. *PLoS ONE* **2014**, *9*, e96870. [CrossRef]
45. Di Ruocco, F.; Basso, V.; Rivoire, M.; Mehlen, P.; Ambati, J.; De Falco, S.; Tarallo, V. Alu RNA accumulation induces epithelial-to-mesenchymal transition by modulating miR-566 and is associated with cancer progression. *Oncogene* **2017**, *37*, 627–637. [CrossRef]

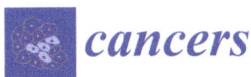

Article

Predict Early Recurrence of Resectable Hepatocellular Carcinoma Using Multi-Dimensional Artificial Intelligence Analysis of Liver Fibrosis

I-Ting Liu [1,2,†], Chia-Sheng Yen [3,†], Wen-Lung Wang [2], Hung-Wen Tsai [4], Chang-Yao Chu [5], Ming-Yu Chang [2], Ya-Fu Hou [2] and Chia-Jui Yen [2,*]

[1] Institute of Clinical Medicine, College of Medicine, National Cheng Kung University, Tainan 70401, Taiwan; tim1226.tw@yahoo.com.tw
[2] Department of Oncology, National Cheng Kung University Hospital, College of Medicine, National Cheng Kung University, Tainan 70403, Taiwan; wwenlung@gmail.com (W.-L.W.); myc1209@gmail.com (M.-Y.C.); yafu0815@gmail.com (Y.-F.H.)
[3] Division of General Surgery, Department of Surgery, Kaohsiung Veterans General Hospital, Kaohsiung 81362, Taiwan; gsvsycs@gmail.com
[4] Department of Pathology, National Cheng Kung University Hospital, College of Medicine, National Cheng Kung University, Tainan 70403, Taiwan; hungwen@mail.ncku.edu.tw
[5] Department of Pathology, Chi-Mei Medical Center, Tainan 71004, Taiwan; b00804@mail.chimei.org.tw
* Correspondence: yencj@mail.ncku.edu.tw
† These authors contributed equally to this work.

Citation: Liu, I.-T.; Yen, C.-S.; Wang, W.-L.; Tsai, H.-W.; Chu, C.-Y.; Chang, M.-Y.; Hou, Y.-F.; Yen, C.-J. Predict Early Recurrence of Resectable Hepatocellular Carcinoma Using Multi-Dimensional Artificial Intelligence Analysis of Liver Fibrosis. *Cancers* 2021, 13, 5323. https://doi.org/10.3390/cancers13215323

Academic Editor: Takaya Shimura

Received: 1 October 2021
Accepted: 21 October 2021
Published: 23 October 2021

Publisher's Note: MDPI stays neutral with regard to jurisdictional claims in published maps and institutional affiliations.

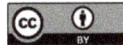

Copyright: © 2021 by the authors. Licensee MDPI, Basel, Switzerland. This article is an open access article distributed under the terms and conditions of the Creative Commons Attribution (CC BY) license (https://creativecommons.org/licenses/by/4.0/).

Simple Summary: Hepatocellular carcinoma (HCC) is the third most commonly diagnosed cancer in the world, and surgical resection is the commonly used curative management of early-stage disease. However, the recurrence rate is high after resection, and liver fibrosis has been thought to increase the risk of recurrence. Conventional histological staging of fibrosis is highly subjective to observer variations. To overcome this limitation, we used a fully quantitative fibrosis assessment tool, qFibrosis (utilizing second harmonic generation and two-photon excitation fluorescence microscopy), with multi-dimensional artificial intelligence analysis to establish a fully-quantitative, accurate fibrotic score called a "combined index", which can predict early recurrence of HCC after curative intent resection. Therefore, we can pay more attention on the patients with high risk of early recurrence.

Abstract: Background: Liver fibrosis is thought to be associated with early recurrence of hepatocellular carcinoma (HCC) after resection. To recognize HCC patients with higher risk of early recurrence, we used a second harmonic generation and two-photon excitation fluorescence (SHG/TPEF) microscopy to create a fully quantitative fibrosis score which is able to predict early recurrence. Methods: The study included 81 HCC patients receiving curative intent hepatectomy. Detailed fibrotic features of resected hepatic tissues were obtained by SHG/TPEF microscopy, and we used multi-dimensional artificial intelligence analysis to create a recurrence prediction model "combined index" according to the morphological collagen features of each patient's non-tumor hepatic tissues. Results: Our results showed that the "combined index" can better predict early recurrence (area under the curve = 0.917, sensitivity = 81.8%, specificity = 90.5%), compared to alpha fetoprotein level (area under the curve = 0.595, sensitivity = 68.2%, specificity = 47.6%). Using a Cox proportional hazards analysis, a higher "combined index" is also a poor prognostic factor of disease-free survival and overall survival. Conclusions: By integrating multi-dimensional artificial intelligence and SHG/TPEF microscopy, we may locate patients with a higher risk of recurrence, follow these patients more carefully, and conduct further management if needed.

Keywords: liver fibrosis; hepatocellular carcinoma; recurrence; SHG/TPEF microscopy; artificial intelligence

1. Introduction

Hepatocellular carcinoma (HCC) is the fourth most common cause of cancer deaths around the world [1]. It is also the fifth most commonly diagnosed cancer and is the second most common cause of cancer deaths in Taiwan [2]. The majority of HCC (75–80%) cases are attributable to persistent viral infections with the hepatitis B virus (HBV) (50–65%) and hepatitis C virus (HCV) (10–15%) in Taiwan [3]. Carcinogenesis of HCC is a very complex multi-factor process, including viral or non-viral causes such as alcoholic hepatitis and nonalcoholic steatohepatitis (NASH) [4]. Chronic hepatitis infection causes liver inflammation and damage, subsequent fibrosis, and liver regeneration that may lead to malignant transformation of the liver [5]. In early-stage HCC, potentially curative treatments are available. They include surgical resection, percutaneous ablation, and liver transplantation. Percutaneous ablation and liver transplantation can only be applied in carefully selected patients depending on the patient's tumor status and general condition as well donor availability. Therefore, surgical resection is the most commonly used curative management of HCC. However, the recurrence rate is high after resection, especially within the first two years [6]. About 50% to 90% of postoperative deaths after curative resection are a result of recurrence of the disease, and intrahepatic recurrence accounts for the majority of cases. Liver fibrosis has been thought to increase the risk of intrahepatic recurrence after hepatectomy in the case of HCC [7].

Conventional histological staging of fibrosis, such as the Ishak fibrotic score, is highly subjective and prone to sampling error and observer variations. Second harmonic generation and two-photon microscopy was first used as a comprehensive, morphology-based, quantified method for scoring liver fibrosis [8–10]. qFibrosis uses a system of second harmonic generation plus two-photon excitation fluorescence (SHG/TPEF) microscopy to image tissue samples and establish an index by (i) identification of different collagen patterns, (ii) extraction of collagen architectural features, and (iii) statistical analysis of features of the respective collagen patterns. qFibrosis scoring has been analyzed employing Metavir and Ishak fibrosis staging as standard references and has been established as a fully-quantitative, innovative method incorporating histological features to facilitate accurate fibrosis scoring in animal models and chronic hepatitis B patients [11]. Besides this, it was also applied to quantitatively identify subtle changes of liver fibrosis in chronic hepatitis B patients following antiviral therapy as well as to accurately assess fibrosis in non-alcoholic fatty liver disease patients in more recent studies [12–14]. Therefore, this study involves the use of this more accurate fibrosis scoring method to evaluate the fibrotic status of the hepatic tissue of patients with HCC after hepatectomy.

The application of qFibrosis is intended enable the prediction of early recurrence after curative intent hepatectomy according to the fibrotic features of hepatic tissue. Thus, patients identified as high-risk for early recurrence can be followed more carefully in shorter intervals following hepatectomy. In this study, we generated a "combined index" using multi-dimensional artificial intelligence analysis of qFibrosis with the features of fibrosis from 81 patients receiving partial hepatectomy. When the combined index is larger than 0.501, early recurrence is more likely.

2. Materials and Methods

2.1. Study Population

Adult patients who were diagnosed and staged by liver tumor biopsy, abdomen triphasic computed tomography (CT), and alpha fetoprotein (AFP) as resectable HCC with known HBV or HCV infection and planning to have curative intent surgical resection were enrolled in this study. Patients with co-infection of HBV and HCV, inadequate tissue samples or history of other malignancy within 2 years prior to screening were excluded (detailed inclusion and exclusion criteria as Table S1). These patients receive regular follow-up with abdomen triphasic CT after surgery. Informed consent regarding use of tissue samples, clinical data, and medical records for this research was obtained from all enrolled patients. The clinical and pathological staging used in this study was The American Joint

Committee on Cancer (AJCC) 7th edition. All experimental protocols and study methods conformed to the ethical guidelines of the Declaration of Helsinki and were approved by the Institutional Review Board of Human Research at National Cheng Kung University Hospital and Chi Mei Medical Center.

2.2. Image Acquisition System

Images were acquired on unstained sections of non-tumor liver samples, using a Genesis (HistoIndex Pte. Ltd, Singapore) system, in which second harmonic generation (SHG) microscopy was used to visualize collagen, and the other cell structures were visualized using two-photon excited fluorescence (TPEF) microscopy.

The samples were laser-excited at 780 nm; SHG signals were recorded at 390 nm, and TPEF signals were recorded at 550 nm. Image acquisition was performed at a 20× magnification for each 200 × 200 µm2 image. Multiple adjacent images were captured to encompass large areas. To cover most of the sample areas, 10 five-by-five multi-tile images were acquired for each human sample, with a final image size of 10 mm² (10 × 1 × 1 mm).

2.3. Image Quantification

Total collagen percentages and other collagen features, including specific collagen strings and collagen connectivity-related measurements, were used to predict early recurrence (disease free (DF) < 1 year) and late recurrence (DF ≥ 1 years) post operation HCC.

A total of 100 morphological features were initially used in this study. Collagen in the overall region was classified into three specific areas: portal collagen (portal expansion), septal collagen (bridging fibrosis), and fibrillar collagen (fine collagen distributed in the pericellular/perisinusoidal space) [11]. Furthermore, in addition to the total measures, collagen was also measured in two different patterns, namely, distributed collagen (fine collagen) and aggregated collagen (large patches). For each pattern in these specific regions (portal, septal, and fibrillar), collagen strings were categorized into short strings, long strings, thin strings, and thick strings according to string length and width (Figure 1a,b). Based on the 100 collagen morphological features, another 76 relativistic features were constructed. Each relativistic feature was the ratio of two morphological features, such as the ratio of the number of short strings to the number of long strings (NoShortStr/NoLongStr) and the ratio of aggregated collagen to distributed collagen (AGG/DIS). Thus, total 176 features were used for model construction (Figure 2a).

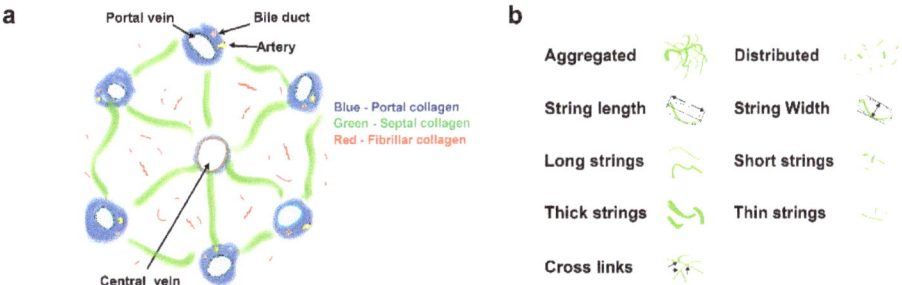

Figure 1. Schematic illustration of the studied collagen features for the prediction of early recurrence. (**a**) Representation of collagen in portal, septal, and fibrillar regions, which are denoted in blue, green, and red, respectively. (**b**) Representation of some features of collagen strings.

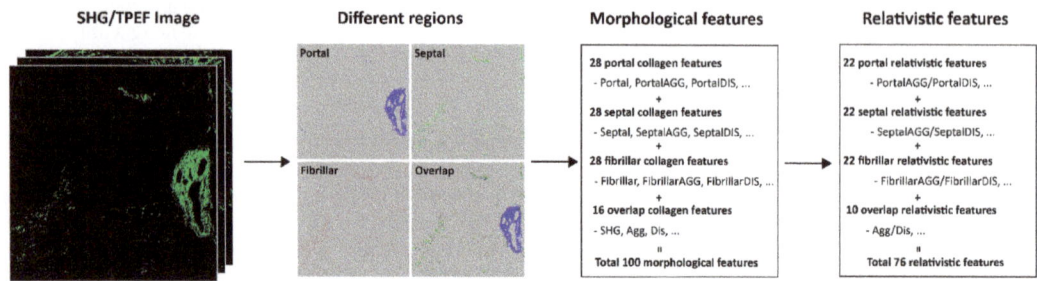

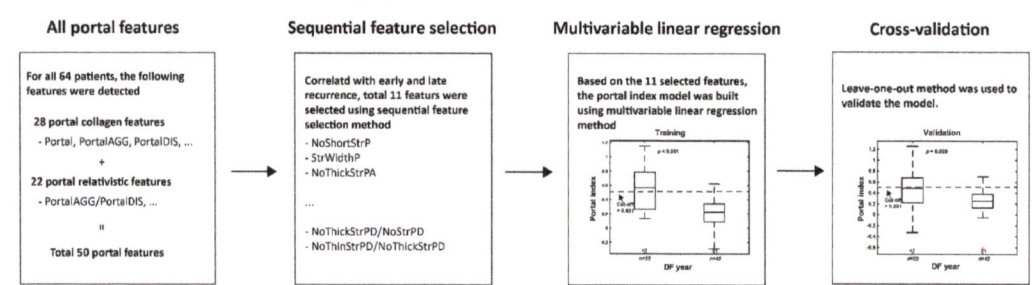

Figure 2. Flowchart of model construction. (**a**) Total 100 morphological features were detected from portal, septal, fibrillar, and overlap regions. Another 76 relativistic features were constructed based on the morphological features. (**b**) The method of portal index is for example. Sequential feature selection method was performed to reduce the dimensionality of data by selecting only a subset of collagen features. A total of 11 features were selected to build the model using multivariable linear regression method. To validate the prediction model, leave-one-out cross-validation method was used. The methods for septa index, fibrillar index, overlap index, and combined index are similar. For combined index, a total of 18 features were selected from 176 features to build the model.

2.4. Model Construction

To predict early recurrence in patients with hepatocellular carcinoma after curative hepatectomy, a prediction model was developed based on the quantified collagen features.

Firstly, each feature was normalized to a value between 0–1 according to its maximum and minimum values. Secondly, feature selection was performed to reduce the dimensionality of data by selecting only a subset of collagen features. A common method of feature selection, named sequential feature selection was used in this study [15]. In the procedure of sequential feature selection, a linear regression model was used whereby the criterion was the residual sum of squares and the search algorithm was sequential forward selection. In total, 64 cases with HBV or HCV but no NASH were used to find the most significant collagen features related with early recurrence.

Next, a model was trained to predict early recurrence in patients with hepatocellular carcinoma after curative hepatectomy using a "combined index", which was constructed from the previously mentioned 64 cases with multivariable linear regression method. To validate the prediction model, leave-one-out cross-validation method was used [16,17]. Briefly, one sample is randomly retained as the validation data while the remaining 63 cases are used as training data to construct the model. The performance of the prediction model is then tested on the single validation case. The cross-validation process is repeated 64 times, with a different case left out each time. The data of combined index for statistical analysis in the study, in the absence of special note was the prediction values by leave-one-out cross-validation method.

Thus, for each HCC patient after hepatectomy, a combined index can be calculated on the SHG/TPEF image using the recurrence prediction model (Figure 2b). This feature indicates that a higher value of the combined index correlates with early recurrence.

2.5. Statistical Analysis

The two-tailed Wilcoxon rank-sum test was performed to estimate the statistical differences of combined index between early and late recurrence. To assess the predictive effect, a receiver operating characteristic curve analysis was used to estimate the area under the curve. Disease-free curves were calculated using the Kaplan–Meier method, and distributions were compared using the log-rank test. Disease-specific overall survival was calculated from the date of diagnosis until disease-caused death or the end of follow-up. A univariate COX regression analysis was used to assess the association between each variable and survival/recurrence. A Cox proportional hazards model was used in the multivariate analyses and was also used to estimate Hazard Ratios (HRs) and their 95% confidence intervals (CIs).

3. Results

3.1. Patient Enrollment and Characteristics

A total of 97 patients who had received curative hepatectomy for HCC from June 2007 to January 2013 at National Cheng Kung University Hospital and Chi Mei Medical Center were screened. Among 97 patients, 81 patients were finally enrolled, and 16 patients were excluded due to co-infection of HBV and HCV, incomplete patient data, inadequate qFibrosis image or inevaluable NASH status. These 81 patients were further separated into 2 groups, 64 patients without NASH and 17 patients with NASH features (Figure A1). The characteristics of the 81 patients studied are summarized in Table A1.

Most of the enrolled patients in this study were treatment naïve. In the non-NASH group, local treatment such as transarterial embolization (TAE), radiofrequency ablation (RFA) or partial hepatectomy were performed previously in 5 patients; TAE and RFA were done in 2 patients in the NASH group. No patients received systemic treatment before enrollment. After recurrence, 16 ptients received RFA, 16 patients received transcatheter arterial chemoembolization (TACE)/TAE, 10 patients had medical treatment, 8 patients received surgical intervention, 8 patients had radiotherapy, 2 patients received hepatic arterial infusion chemotherapy, and 2 patients received percutaneous ethanol injection.

3.2. Features for Constructing the Combined Index

qFibrosis is a powerful automated computer-aided image system intended to assess patterns of collagen and quantify liver fibrosis. We used this new technology to evaluate the fibrotic status of hepatic tissue removed from the enrolled patients. To predict early recurrence of viral infection related to HCC after a hepatectomy, a "combined index" was calculated using qFibrosis with the tissue sample for the 64 non-NASH patients. The acquired SHG/TPEF images of liver sections were processed and the combined index was obtained.

The model construction process selected 18 features to construct the prediction model and compute the combined index. Of the 18 features, 9 were in the 100 features and other 9 features were the relativistic features. The coefficients of features for the linear model were estimated based on the 64 samples (Table 1).

Table 1. The list of estimated coefficients of 18 selected features for constructing the combined index of the HBV or HCV patients without NASH.

No.	Features	Estimated Coefficients	Region
0	Intercept	3.838	-
1	SHG	4.300	Overlap
2	StrOrientation	1.280	Overlap
3	StrAreaPA	−2.413	Portal
4	StrAreaPD	−1.269	Portal
5	NoThickStrS	3.182	Septal
6	NoThinStrSA	−2.486	Septal
7	Fibrillar	−2.591	Fibrillar
8	NoThickStrF	−1.889	Fibrillar
9	NoThickStrFA	1.735	Fibrillar
10	NoShortStr/NoLongStr	−3.733	Overlap/Overlap
11	StrLengthP/StrWidthP	−0.859	Portal/Portal
12	NoThickStrPD/NoStrPD	−0.771	Portal/Portal
13	NoThinStrPD/NoThickStrPD	−0.599	Portal/Portal
14	SeptalAGG/Septal	−1.782	Septal/Septal
15	StrLengthSD/StrWidthSD	−0.761	Fibrillar/Fibrillar
16	NoThinStrFA/NoThickStrFA	0.957	Fibrillar/Fibrillar
17	NoThickStrFD/NoStrFD	−0.443	Fibrillar/Fibrillar
18	StrLengthFD/StrWidthFD	1.067	Fibrillar/Fibrillar

3.3. Using the Combined Index of qFibrosis to Predict Early Recurrence of HCC

We employed qFibrosis to evaluate the fibrotic status of the hepatic tissue from patients with HCC, and the architectural features of the studied collagen were separated into 3 regions: portal, septal, and fibrillar, as illustrated in Figure 1a. In Figure 3, we show the results of hematoxylin and eosin (H&E) staining, Masson staining, and SHG/TPEF images in the HCC liver samples with early and late recurrence. The detailed different collagen regions and part of the modal features used for the combined index were shown in Figure 4. Although the Ishak scale scores were the same (Ishak both = 2 in Figure 4a; both = 6 in Figure 4b), the combined index can be used to tell the difference in the fibrotic status, which may predict early and late recurrence (combined index = 0.564 and 0.121 in Figure 4a; =0.963 and 0.267 in Figure 4b). These results indicate that the combined index was better able to distinguish the fibrotic status compared to the conventional Ishak scale. From the training data, we found that a combined index cut-off value of 0.501 was useful to differentiate early recurrence (<1 year; combined index > 0.501) from late or no recurrence ($\geq$1 year; combined index $\leq$ 0.501) (Figure 5a), where the receiver operator characteristic (ROC) curves for the prediction of early recurrence versus late or no recurrence was 0.986 (AUC = 0.986, Figure 5b). The validation confirmed that the combined index showed high performance (AUC = 0.917, Figure 5c,d).

We also applied the combined index in other 17 patients having HCC with NASH features, and the result suggested that it is a poor predictor for early recurrence in these NASH patients (AUC = 0.336, Table A2 and Figure A2). On the other hand, the current model showed promising performance in the 28 cirrhotic patients (AUC = 0.947, Figure A3).

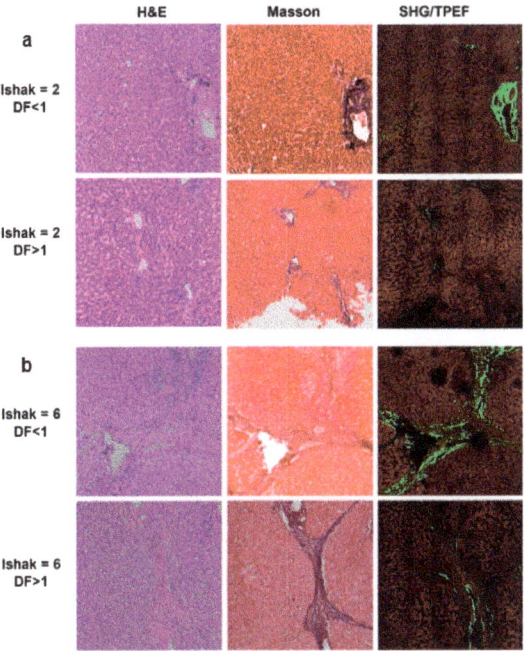

Figure 3. H&E staining, Masson staining, and SHG/TPEF images in the HCC liver samples. (**a**) Ishak score = 2, disease free (DF) < 1 year and > 1 year. (**b**) Ishak score = 6, DF <1 year and >1 year.

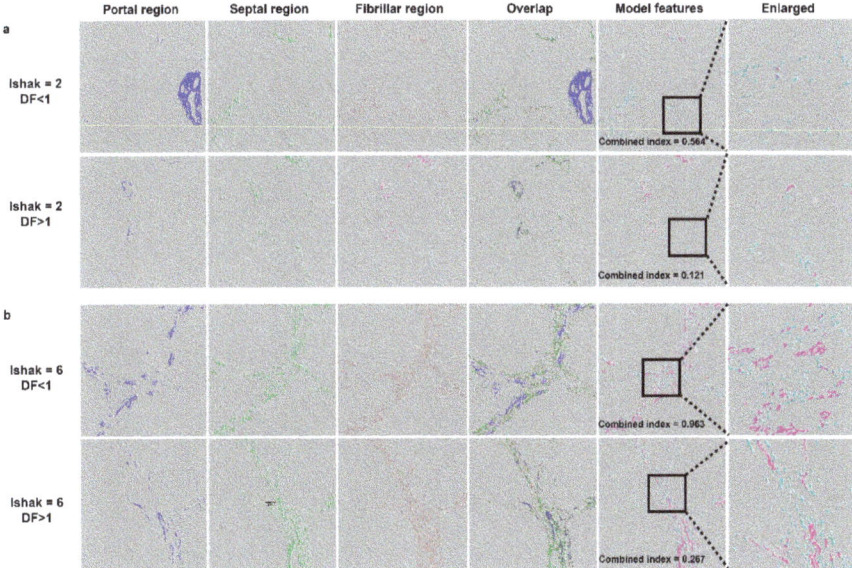

Figure 4. Examples of different collagen regions. (**a**) Ishak score = 2, disease free (DF) < 1 year and > 1 year. (**b**) Ishak score = 6, DF < 1 year and > 1 year. Overlap region includes three collagen patterns (portal/septal/fibrillar). Model features shows two collagen features including aggregated (purple color) and distributed (blue-green color) collagen in septal region used was for the combined index, which is to predict early recurrence in patients with hepatocellular carcinoma after curative hepatectomy.

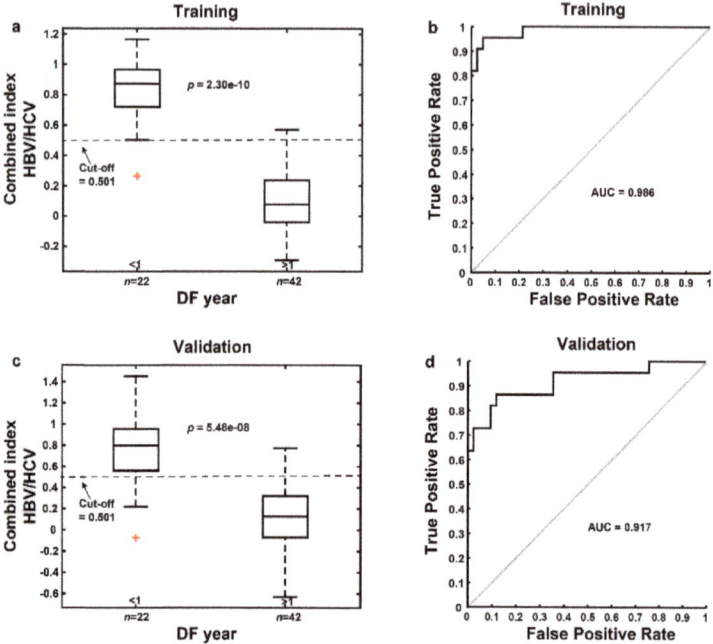

Figure 5. ROC curves for the prediction of early recurrence versus late recurrence for the HBV or HCV patients without NASH. (**a**) A combined index cut-off value of 0.501 is capable of differentiating between early and late recurrence in the training group. (**b**) ROC curve for combined index showed great predictive value of early recurrence (AUC = 0.986) in the training group. (**c**) The predicted combined index values for 64 patients were calculated by leave-one-out cross-validation method. (**d**) ROC curve for the combined index predicted by leave-one-out cross-validation method showed great predictive value of early recurrence (AUC = 0.917). Note: The red plus sign represents outlier.

3.3.1. Combined Index Is a Better Predictor of Early Recurrence than Alpha Fetoprotein

Previous studies reported that HCC patients with high-level serum AFP (>20 ng/mL) had higher postoperative 2-year recurrence rates and lower 24-month survival rates [18,19]. Compared to elevated alpha fetoprotein (AFP >20 ng/mL), the high combined index (>0.501) showed better predictive value for early recurrence, including AUC (0.917 vs. 0.595), sensitivity (81.8% vs. 68.2), specificity (90.5% vs. 47.6%), false positive rate (9.5% vs. 52.4%), and false negative rate (18.2% vs. 31.8%), as shown in Table A3. Disease-free probability was lower in the high-risk group (combined index >0.501, n = 22) than in the low-risk group (combined index $\leq$ 0.501, n = 42), and the p value was 0.035 (Figure 6). In addition, the correlation of the AFP level and combined index was low in patients after hepatectomy using a Pearson's analysis (Figure A4).

In the univariate analysis, vascular invasion (yes vs. no, p = 0.021), tumor size (>5 vs. $\leq$5 cm, p = 0.005), pathological stage (III/IV vs. I/II, p = 0.029), clinical stage (III/IV vs. I/II, p = 0.005), and the combined index (>0.501 vs. $\leq$0.501, p < 0.001) seemed to predict poor survival (Table 2).

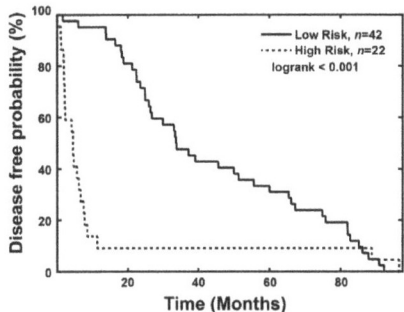

Figure 6. Disease-free probability analysis for HCC patients. A significant difference was noted between the high-risk group (combined-index > 0.501) and low risk group (combined-index ≤0.501) (n = 22 and 42, p < 0.001).

Table 2. Univariate Analysis of Variables Potentially Predictive of Survival in HCC.

Variable	Number of Patients	Death Number	Death Percent	p-Value
Gender				0.126
Male	47	21	44.7	
Female	17	4	23.5	
Groups				0.703
HBV + cirrhosis	20	7	35.0	
HBV	31	13	41.9	
HCV+cirrhosis	8	4	50.0	
HCV	5	1	20.0	
Liver cirrhosis				0.974
No	36	14	38.9	
Yes	28	11	39.3	
Histologic grade				0.431
Well	6	1	16.7	
Moderate	50	20	40.0	
Poor	8	4	50.0	
Vascular invasion				0.021 *
No	37	10	27.0	
Yes	27	15	55.6	
Tumor size (cm)				0.005 *
≤5	37	9	24.3	
>5	27	16	59.3	
AFP (ng/mL)				0.066
≤20	27	7	25.9	
>20	37	18	48.6	
Pathological Stage				0.029 *
Stage I, II	54	18	33.3	
Stage III, IV	10	7	70.0	
Clinical Stage				0.005 *
Stage I, II	50	15	30.0	
Stage III, IV	14	10	71.4	
Combined Index				<0.001 *
≤0.501	42	9	21.4	
>0.501	22	16	72.7	

* p < 0.05.

Using a Cox proportional hazards analysis, we found the combined index (high risk vs. low risk; HR: 3.821, 95% C.I.: 1.596–9.153, p = 0.003) and Model for End-Stage Liver Disease (MELD) score ($\geq$10 vs. $\leq$9; HR: 4.167, 95% C.I.: 1.173–14.803, p = 0.027) to be poor prognostic factors of disease-free survival. We also found the combined index (high risk vs. low risk; HR: 4.509, 95% C.I.: 1.366–12.058, p = 0.012), AFP (>20 vs. $\leq$ 20; HR: 4.639, 95% C.I.: 1.358–15.84, p = 0.014), MELD score ($\geq$10 vs. $\leq$9; HR: 7.628, 95% C.I.: 1.393–41.757, p = 0.019) and Clinical Stage (III/IV vs. I/II; HR: 4.285, 95% C.I.: 1.160–15.825, p = 0.029) to be poor prognostic factors of overall survival (Table 3). According to these data, we conclude that the combined index has better predictive value of early recurrence as compared to the AFP.

Table 3. Cox Proportional Hazards Analysis of Prognostic Parameters in HCC.

Factors	Multivariate			
	HR	95%CI		p-Value
Disease-free survival				
Gender (Female vs. Male)	0.804	0.352	1.838	0.605
Liver cirrhosis (Yes vs. No)	1.344	0.660	2.735	0.415
Histologic grade (Moderate vs. Well)	0.815	0.260	2.554	0.725
Histologic grade (Poor vs. Well)	1.361	0.324	5.709	0.674
Vascular invasion (Yes vs. No)	0.635	0.265	1.518	0.307
Tumor size (>5 vs. $\leq$5)	1.546	0.688	3.476	0.291
AFP (>20 vs. $\leq$20)	1.510	0.651	3.501	0.337
Pathological Stage (III/IV vs. I/II)	1.960	0.692	5.547	0.205
Clinical Stage (III/IV vs. I/II)	2.029	0.816	5.047	0.128
MELD score ($\geq$10 vs. $\leq$9)	4.167	1.173	14.803	0.027 *
BCLC Stage (B/C vs. 0/A)	1.444	0.601	3.466	0.411
Combined Index (High risk vs. Low risk)	3.821	1.596	9.153	0.003 *
Overall survival				
Gender (Female vs. Male)	0.330	0.092	1.176	0.087
Liver cirrhosis (Yes vs. No)	1.517	0.580	3.970	0.395
Histologic grade (Moderate vs. Well)	1.998	0.168	23.790	0.584
Histologic grade (Poor vs. Well)	3.534	0.218	57.208	0.374
Vascular invasion (Yes vs. No)	2.137	0.728	6.277	0.167
Tumor size (>5 vs. $\leq$5)	1.467	0.470	4.584	0.509
AFP (>20 vs. $\leq$20)	4.639	1.358	15.840	0.014 *
Pathological Stage (III/IV vs. I/II)	0.396	0.110	1.425	0.156
Clinical Stage (III/IV vs. I/II)	4.285	1.160	15.825	0.029 *
MELD score ($\geq$10 vs. $\leq$9)	7.628	1.393	41.757	0.019 *
BCLC Stage (B/C vs. 0/A)	1.061	0.367	3.069	0.913
Combined Index (High risk vs. Low risk)	4.059	1.366	12.058	0.012 *

* $p < 0.05$.

3.3.2. The Combined Index Significantly Predicts Early Recurrence as Compared to Other Regions and Features of Fibrosis

To further investigate the correlation with early recurrence, we evaluated fibrotic features in different regions of non-tumor hepatic tissue using qFibrosis. In overlap, portal, septal, and fibrillar regions, 8, 11, 11, and 13 features were selected, respectively (Tables S2–S5). The results of the leave-one-out cross-validation method showed higher correlations in the fibrillar region (AUC = 0.819) than in other (AUC = 0.700 in portal; 0.702 in septal) or overlap regions (AUC = 0.737) (Figure 7a). However, the combined index still exhibited the best correlation (AUC = 0.917). The disease-free probability according to high and low risk by fibrotic features in the overlap, portal, septal, and fibrillar regions of a non-tumor liver are shown in Figure 7b ($p < 0.001$ in four regions). The features of the diagnosis of early recurrence are listed in Table S6. With these data, the combined index is suggested to be most predictive for early recurrence as compared to other regions.

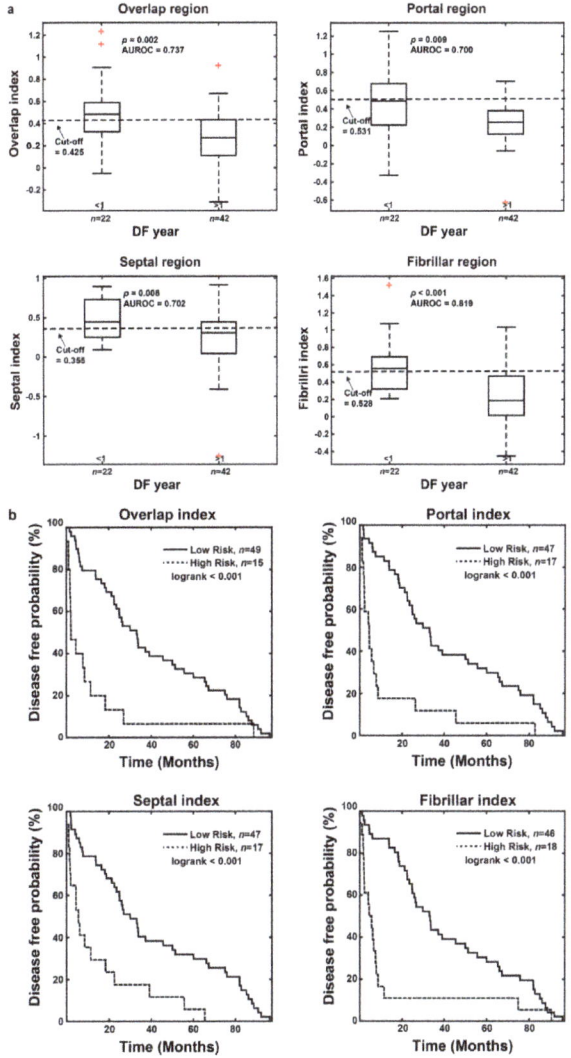

Figure 7. The prediction of early recurrence using features in the overlap, portal, septal, and fibrillar regions by leave-one-out cross-validation method. The features of non-tumor liver in these regions show poorer predictive ability compared with the combined index. (**a**) Box plots. The cut off values were determined by the training data ($n = 64$). (**b**) Disease-free probability analysis. The high-risk group and low risk group were separated by the corresponding cut-off value. Note: The red plus sign represents outlier.

4. Discussion

Currently, HCC is still one of the leading causes of cancer deaths worldwide. Partial hepatectomy remains the most commonly used method to cure patients. However, high recurrence rates have been observed after curative intent hepatectomy. According to previous studies, liver fibrosis increases the risk of intrahepatic recurrence after hepatectomy or radiofrequency ablation for HCC [7,20]. Traditional histological fibrotic staging systems, such as the Ishak fibrotic score, although the current standard, are criticized for their subjective interpretation due to either sampling error or observer variations. qFibrosis provides a fully-quantitative method incorporating histological features to obtain more accurate fibrosis scoring for the liver. Our study results indicated that the combined index calculated using qFibrosis may predict early recurrence of HCC after curative intent hepatectomy.

qFibrosis has shown its ability to perform accurate fibrotic scoring of hepatic tissue in animal models and chronic hepatitis B patients. Besides, it had been established as a better way for screening and enrollment of NASH patients in clinical trials [21,22]. Our results using the recurrence prediction model in 64 HCC patients after hepatectomy indicated that early recurrence can be predicted when the combined index is more than 0.501. Ko et al. reported that histological evidence of fibrosis of the underlying liver tissue is the most significant predictive factor of intrahepatic recurrence. Our novel method can be used to determine differences in fibrotic status when the samples are scored the same by the Ishak system, as shown in Figure 4a,b. Therefore, using this method will make it possible to follow high-risk patients more carefully and also consider other treatment according to the risks of disease recurrence.

It is known that there are also many non-invasive tools for evaluation of fibrotic status [23–27]. Many of them use serum markers, which may be influenced largely by the inflammation status of the patient. In addition, some of these markers may not be specific for the liver. Some image-based non-invasive methods arrive at indeterminate results for fibrotic status in up to 33% of cases, which is not satisfactory by today's medical standards [28]. Artificial intelligence has been widely applied in modern precision medicine for several years, with some applications focusing on digital pathology images [29], others on interpretation of multiple data or radiological images [30–33]. In our study, we simply used qFibrosis to obtain the accurate fibrotic status of the resected liver sample, and processed the specific features with the clinical data using multi-dimensional artificial intelligence analysis. As the result, the "combined index" showed good prediction ability in early recurrence of HCC.

Viral and non-viral related HCC are thought to have different pathologic mechanisms in progression of normal liver tissue to liver cancer. We had applied the combined index, which derived from the viral related non-NASH HCC patients, in other HCC patients with NASH features, and it was unable to predict early recurrence in these NASH patients. Therefore, the fibrotic pattern of liver tissue may be different in the viral and non-viral related HCC patients, and further study is needed.

There were some limitations to this study. First, it was hard for us to collect another group of patients for external validation, so we used a leave-one-out cross-validation method to overcome this problem. Second, although qFibrosis can provide more accurate fibrotic status than conventional histological methods, sampling error may still have some influence on the qFibrosis score. Besides, our study was unable to provide competing risk analysis as Metroticket 2.0 model used in liver transplantation patients owing to the complicated clinical situations and the study design [34,35]. Finally, our method needs liver tissue to obtain its qFibrosis score, so it is not a non-invasive assessment of liver fibrosis.

5. Conclusions

This is the first study using the combined index calculated with qFibrosis to allow accurate quantification of fibrotic status of the peri-tumor liver tissue, and it also provides a good tool for prediction of early hepatocellular carcinoma recurrence after curative intent surgery. Clinically, delayed treatment for recurrent disease may decrease the patient's life expectancy. As a result, patients identified to be at high-risk by the combined index should be monitored in shorter time intervals, and further intervention may be provided earlier if needed.

Supplementary Materials: The following are available online at https://www.mdpi.com/article/10.3390/cancers13215323/s1, Table S1: The inclusion and exclusion criteria, Table S2: The list of estimated coefficients of 8 selected features in the overlap region, Table S3: The list of estimated coefficients of 11 selected features in the portal region, Table S4: The list of estimated coefficients of 11 selected features in the septal region, Table S5: The list of estimated coefficients of 13 selected features in the fibrillar region, Table S6: P values of 100 features for the diagnosis of early recurrence.

Author Contributions: Conceptualization, I.-T.L., C.-S.Y., and C.-J.Y.; methodology, I.-T.L., C.-S.Y., and C.-J.Y.; software, M.-Y.C., Y.-F.H.; validation, I.-T.L., C.-S.Y., H.-W.T., C.-Y.C., and M.-Y.C.; formal analysis, I.-T.L., M.-Y.C., and Y.-F.H.; investigation, I.-T.L., C.-S.Y., and C.-J.Y.; resources, C.-J.Y.; data curation, I.-T.L., C.-S.Y., and C.-J.Y.; writing—original draft preparation, I.-T.L.; writing—review and editing, I.-T.L., C.-S.Y., W.-L.W., H.-W.T., C.-Y.C., M.-Y.C., Y.-F.H., and C.-J.Y.; visualization, I.-T.L., C.-Y.C., and C.-J.Y.; supervision, I.-T.L., C.-S.Y., and C.-J.Y.; project administration, C.-J.Y.; funding acquisition, C.-J.Y. All authors have read and agreed to the published version of the manuscript.

Funding: This research was partly funded by a research grant from the Ministry of Health and Welfare (MOHW106-TDU-B-211-113003).

Institutional Review Board Statement: The study was conducted according to the guidelines of the Declaration of Helsinki, and approved by the Institutional Review Board of Human Research at NCKU Hospital and Chi Mei Medical Center (protocol code B-ER-104-258).

Informed Consent Statement: Informed consent was obtained from all subjects involved in the study. Written informed consent has been obtained from the patients to publish this paper.

Data Availability Statement: The data presented in this study are available in the article and supplementary materials.

Acknowledgments: We would like to thank the non-physician scientist Dean C.S. Tai and Yayun Ren from Hangzhou Choutu Technology Co Ltd for the qFibrosis image acquisition, quantification, and generation of combined index.

Conflicts of Interest: The authors declare no conflict of interest. The funders had no role in the design of the study; in the collection, analyses, or interpretation of data; in the writing of the manuscript, or in the decision to publish the results.

Appendix A

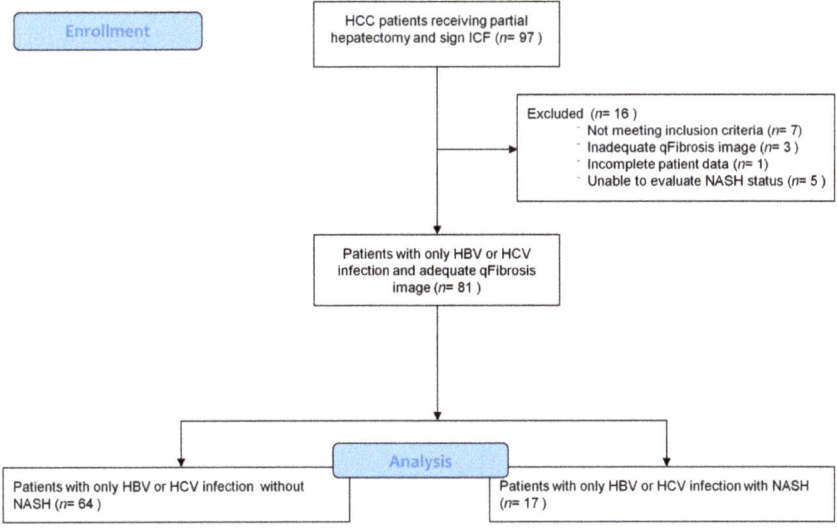

Figure A1. Flowchart for patient enrollment (ICF: Informed Consent Form).

Table A1. Demographic and disease characteristics of the enrolled patients.

Characteristics	NASH Patients (*n* = 64)	Non-NASH Patients (*n* = 17)	Total (*n* = 81)
Age (years) median (range)	55 (27–81)	60 (33–74)	56 (27–81)
Gender			
Male	47 (73%)	10 (59%)	57 (70%)
Female	17 (27%)	7 (41%)	24 (30%)
Viral hepatitis type			
HBV	51 (80%)	13 (76%)	64 (79%)
HCV	13 (20%)	4 (24%)	17 (21%)
Liver cirrhosis			
Yes	28 (44%)	11 (65%)	39 (48%)
No	36 (56%)	6 (35%)	42 (52%)
Histologic grade			
Well	6 (9%)	2 (12%)	8 (10%)
Moderate	50 (78%)	14 (82%)	64 (79%)
Poor	8 (13%)	1 (6%)	9 (11%)
Vascular invasion			
Yes	27 (42%)	2 (12%)	29 (36%)
No	37 (58%)	15 (88%)	52 (64%)
Tumor size (cm)			
≤ 5	37 (58%)	16 (94%)	53 (65%)
>5	27 (42%)	1 (6%)	28 (35%)
AFP (ng/mL)			
≤ 20	27 (42%)	10 (59%)	37 (46%)
>20	37 (58%)	7 (41%)	44 (54%)
Pathological Stage			
I/II	54 (84%)	17 (100%)	71 (88%)
III/IV	10 (16%)	0 (0%)	10 (12%)
Clinical Stage			
I/II	50 (78%)	16 (94%)	66 (81%)
III/IV	14 (22%)	1 (6%)	15 (19%)
MELD score			
≤ 9	59 (92%)	16 (94%)	75 (93%)
≥ 10	5 (8%)	1 (6%)	6 (7%)
BCLC Stage			
0/A	50 (78%)	14 (82%)	64 (79%)
B/C	14 (22%)	3 (18%)	17 (21%)
Child-Pugh class			
A5	62 (97%)	17 (100%)	79 (98%)
A6	2 (3%)	0 (0%)	2 (2%)
ECOG PS			
0	61 (95%)	16 (94%)	77 (95%)
1	3 (5%)	1 (6%)	4 (5%)
Creatinine level (mg/dL)			
Median (IQR)	0.9 (0.79–1.0)	0.8 (0.665–0.94)	0.9 (0.705–0.995)
Liver function enzyme			
AST (mg/dL)			
Median (IQR)	48.5 (33–73)	37 (29–67.5)	47 (33–71)
ALT (mg/dL)			
Median (IQR)	41.5 (31.5–80.25)	33.5 (28.5–37.75)	37.5 (30–64.5)

Table A1. Cont.

Characteristics	NASH Patients (n = 64)	Non-NASH Patients (n = 17)	Total (n = 81)
Comorbidities			
Hypertension	13 (20%)	8 (47%)	21 (26%)
Diabetes mellitus	5 (8%)	3 (18%)	8 (10%)
Chronic kidney disease	4 (6%)	1 (6%)	5 (6%)
Coronary artery disease	1 (2%)	0 (0%)	1 (1%)
Cerebrovascular accident	1 (2%)	0 (0%)	1 (1%)

Abbreviation: AFP: alpha-fetoprotein; MELD score: Model for End-Stage Liver Disease score; BCLC stage: Barcelona Clinic Liver Cancer stage; ECOG PS: Eastern Cooperative Oncology Group performance status; IQR: interquartile range; AST: aspartate aminotransferase; ALT: alanine aminotransferase.

Appendix B

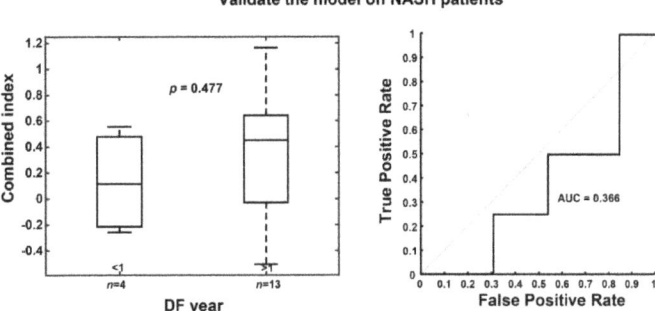

Figure A2. ROC curves for the prediction of early recurrence versus late recurrence for NASH patients.

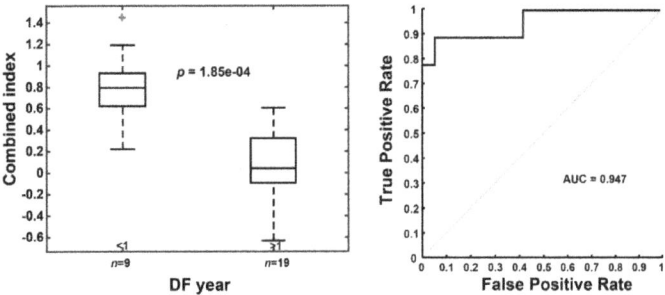

Figure A3. ROC curves for the prediction of early recurrence versus late recurrence for cirrhosis patients. Note: The red plus sign represents outlier.

Table A2. Validation of the model on NASH patients.

Group	p Value between DF Year < 1 and > 1	AUROC
NASH patients (n = 17)	0.477	0.366

Appendix C

Table A3. AUC: sensitivity, specificity, false positive rate (FPR), and false negative rate (FNR) for the combined index and AFP for the prediction of early recurrence.

Characteristics	Combined Index > 0.501	AFP > 20 ng/mL
AUC	0.917	0.595
Sensitivity, %	81.8	68.2
Specificity, %	90.5	47.6
FPR, %	9.5	52.4
FNR, %	18.2	31.8

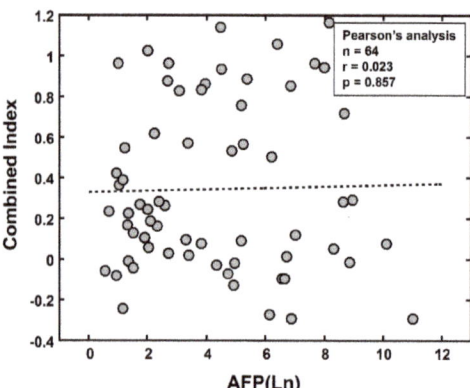

Figure A4. Correlation of AFP level and combined index. In patients after hepatectomy, there is poor correlation shown between the AFP level and combined index as determined with a Pearson's analysis.

References

1. Bray, F.; Ferlay, J.; Soerjomataram, I.; Siegel, R.L.; Torre, L.A.; Jemal, A. Global cancer statistics 2018: GLOBOCAN estimates of incidence and mortality worldwide for 36 cancers in 185 countries. *CA Cancer J. Clin.* **2018**, *68*, 394–424. [CrossRef] [PubMed]
2. Shao, Y.-Y.; Wang, S.-Y.; Lin, S.-M.; Chen, K.-Y.; Tseng, J.-H.; Ho, M.-C.; Lee, R.-C.; Liang, P.-C.; Liao, L.-Y.; Huang, K.-W.; et al. Management consensus guideline for hepatocellular carcinoma: 2020 update on surveillance, diagnosis, and systemic treatment by the Taiwan Liver Cancer Association and the Gastroenterological Society of Taiwan. *J. Formos. Med Assoc.* **2021**, *120*, 1051–1060. [CrossRef]
3. Chen, D.-S. Hepatocellular carcinoma in Taiwan. *Hepatol. Res.* **2007**, *37*, S101–S105. [CrossRef] [PubMed]
4. Anstee, Q.M.; Reeves, H.L.; Kotsiliti, E.; Govaere, O.; Heikenwalder, M. From NASH to HCC: Current concepts and future challenges. *Nat. Rev. Gastroenterol. Hepatol.* **2019**, *16*, 411–428. [CrossRef] [PubMed]
5. Farazi, P.; DePinho, R. Hepatocellular carcinoma pathogenesis: From genes to environment. *Nat. Rev. Cancer* **2006**, *6*, 674–687. [CrossRef] [PubMed]
6. Lau, W.Y.; Lau, S.H.Y. The current role of radiofrequency ablation in the treatment of hepatocellular carcinoma. *Hepatobiliary Pancreat. Dis. Int.* **2017**, *16*, 122–126. [CrossRef]
7. Ko, S.; Kanehiro, H.; Hisanaga, M.; Nagao, M.; Ikeda, N.; Nakajima, Y. Liver fibrosis increases the risk of intrahepatic recur-rence after hepatectomy for hepatocellular carcinoma. *Br. J. Surg.* **2002**, *89*, 57–62. [CrossRef]
8. 8Tai, D.C.; Tan, N.; Xu, S.; Kang, C.H.; Chia, S.M.; Cheng, C.L.; Wee, A.; Wei, C.L.; Raja, A.M.; Xiao, G.; et al. Fibro-C-Index: Comprehensive, morphology-based quantification of liver fibrosis using second harmonic generation and two-photon microscopy. *J. Biomed. Opt.* **2009**, *14*, 044013.
9. He, Y.; Kang, C.H.; Xu, S.; Tuo, X.; Trasti, S.; Tai, D.C.S.; Raja, A.M.; Peng, Q.; So, P.T.C.; Rajapakse, J.C.; et al. Toward surface quantification of liver fibrosis progression. *J. Biomed. Opt.* **2010**, *15*, 056007. [CrossRef] [PubMed]
10. Xu, S.; Tai, D.; Wee, A.; Welsch, R.; So, P.; Yu, H.; Rajapakse, J. Automated scoring of liver fibrosis through combined features from different collagen groups. In Proceedings of the 2011 Annual International Conference of the IEEE Engineering in Medicine and Biology Society, Boston, MA, USA, 30 August–1 September 2011; pp. 4503–4506. [CrossRef]

11. Xu, S.; Wang, Y.; Tai, D.C.; Wang, S.; Cheng, C.L.; Peng, Q.; Yan, J.; Chen, Y.; Sun, J.; Liang, X.; et al. qFibrosis: A fully-quantitative innovative method incorporating histological features to facilitate accurate fibrosis scoring in animal model and chronic hepatitis B patients. *J. Hepatol.* **2014**, *61*, 260–269. [CrossRef] [PubMed]
12. Sun, Y.; Zhou, J.; Wu, X.; Chen, Y.; Piao, H.; Lu, L.; Ding, H.; Nan, Y.; Jiang, W.; Wang, T.; et al. Quantitative assessment of liver fibrosis (qFibrosis) reveals precise outcomes in Ishak "stable" patients on anti-HBV therapy. *Sci. Rep.* **2018**, *8*, 1–11. [CrossRef]
13. Wang, Y.; Wong, G.L.-H.; He, F.-P.; Sun, J.; Chan, A.W.-H.; Yang, J.; Shu, S.S.-T.; Liang, X.; Tse, Y.K.; Fan, X.-T.; et al. Quantifying and monitoring fibrosis in non-alcoholic fatty liver disease using dual-photon microscopy. *Gut* **2019**, *69*, 1116–1126. [CrossRef] [PubMed]
14. Soon, G.; Wee, A. Updates in the quantitative assessment of liver fibrosis for nonalcoholic fatty liver disease: Histological perspective. *Clin. Mol. Hepatol.* **2021**, *27*, 44–57. [CrossRef] [PubMed]
15. Rückstieß, T.; Osendorfer, C.; van der Smagt, P. Sequential feature selection for classification. *Adv. Artif. Intell.* **2011**, *7106*, 132–141.
16. Rushing, C.; Bulusu, A.; Hurwitz, H.I.; Nixon, A.B.; Pang, H. A leave-one-out cross-validation SAS macro for the identification of markers associated with survival. *Comput. Biol. Med.* **2015**, *57*, 123–129. [CrossRef] [PubMed]
17. Wong, T.-T. Performance evaluation of classification algorithms by k-fold and leave-one-out cross validation. *Pattern Recognit.* **2015**, *48*, 2839–2846. [CrossRef]
18. Ma, W.-J.; Wang, H.-Y.; Teng, L.-S. Correlation analysis of preoperative serum alpha-fetoprotein (AFP) level and prognosis of hepatocellular carcinoma (HCC) after hepatectomy. *World J. Surg. Oncol.* **2013**, *11*, 212. [CrossRef] [PubMed]
19. Lai, Q.; Melandro, F.; Pinheiro, R.S.; Donfrancesco, A.; Fadel, B.A.; Sandri, G.B.L.; Rossi, M.; Berloco, P.B.; Frattaroli, F.M. Alpha-Fetoprotein and novel tumor biomarkers as predictors of hepatocellular carcinoma recurrence after surgery: A brilliant star raises again. *Int. J. Hepatol.* **2012**, *2012*, 1–9. [CrossRef]
20. Chung, H.A.; Kim, J.-H.; Hwang, Y.; Choi, H.S.; Ko, S.Y.; Choe, W.H.; Kwon, S.Y. Noninvasive fibrosis marker can predict recurrence of hepatocellular carcinoma after radiofrequency ablation. *Saudi J. Gastroenterol.* **2016**, *22*, 57–63. [CrossRef] [PubMed]
21. Leow, W.-Q.; Bedossa, P.; Liu, F.; Wei, L.; Lim, K.-H.; Wan, W.-K.; Ren, Y.; Chang, J.P.-E.; Tan, C.-K.; Wee, A.; et al. An improved qfibrosis algorithm for precise screening and enrollment into non-alcoholic steatohepatitis (NASH) clinical trials. *Diagnostics* **2020**, *10*, 643. [CrossRef] [PubMed]
22. Liu, F.; Goh, B.B.G.; Tiniakos, D.; Wee, A.; Leow, W.; Zhao, J.; Rao, H.; Wang, X.; Wang, Q.; Wan, W.; et al. qFIBS: An automated technique for quantitative evaluation of fibrosis, inflammation, ballooning, and steatosis in patients with nonalcoholic steatohepatitis. *Hepatology* **2019**, *71*, 1953–1966. [CrossRef] [PubMed]
23. Sebastiani, G.; Castera, L.; Halfon, P.; Pol, S.; Mangia, A.; Di Marco, V.; Pirisi, M.; Voiculescu, M.; Bourliere, M.; Alberti, A. The impact of liver disease aetiology and the stages of hepatic fibrosis on the performance of non-invasive fibrosis biomarkers: An international study of 2411 cases. *Aliment. Pharmacol. Ther.* **2011**, *34*, 1202–1216. [CrossRef]
24. Naveau, S.; Raynard, B.; Ratziu, V.; Abella, A.; Imbert–Bismut, F.; Messous, D.; Beuzen, F.; Capron, F.; Thabut, D.; Munteanu, M.; et al. Biomarkers for the prediction of liver fibrosis in patients with chronic alcoholic liver disease. *Clin. Gastroenterol. Hepatol.* **2005**, *3*, 167–174. [CrossRef]
25. Naveau, S.; Gaudé, G.; Asnacios, A.; Agostini, H.; Abella, A.; Barri-Ova, N.; Dauvois, B.; Prévot, S.; Ngo, Y.; Munteanu, M.; et al. Diagnostic and prognostic values of noninvasive biomarkers of fibrosis in patients with alcoholic liver disease. *Hepatology* **2008**, *49*, 97–105. [CrossRef] [PubMed]
26. Adams, L.; George, J.; Bugianesi, E.; Rossi, E.; De Boer, W.B.; Van Der Poorten, D.; Ching, H.L.; Bulsara, M.; Jeffrey, G.P. Complex non-invasive fibrosis models are more accurate than simple models in non-alcoholic fatty liver disease. *J. Gastroenterol. Hepatol.* **2011**, *26*, 1536–1543. [CrossRef] [PubMed]
27. Guha, I.N.; Parkes, J.; Roderick, P.R.; Harris, S.; Rosenberg, W. Non-invasive markers associated with liver fibrosis in non-alcoholic fatty liver disease. *Gut* **2006**, *55*, 1650–1660. [CrossRef] [PubMed]
28. Almpanis, Z.; Demonakou, M.; Tiniakos, D. Evaluation of liver fibrosis: "Something old, something new . . . ". *Ann. Gastroenterol.* **2016**, *29*, 445–453. [CrossRef] [PubMed]
29. Saito, A.; Toyoda, H.; Kobayashi, M.; Koiwa, Y.; Fujii, H.; Fujita, K.; Maeda, A.; Kaneoka, Y.; Hazama, S.; Nagano, H.; et al. Prediction of early recurrence of hepatocellular carcinoma after resection using digital pathology images assessed by machine learning. *Mod. Pathol.* **2021**, *34*, 417–425. [CrossRef]
30. Schoenberg, M.B.; Bucher, J.N.; Koch, D.; Börner, N.; Hesse, S.; De Toni, E.N.; Seidensticker, M.; Angele, M.K.; Klein, C.; Bazhin, A.V.; et al. A novel machine learning algorithm to predict disease free survival after resection of hepatocellular carcinoma. *Ann. Transl. Med.* **2020**, *8*, 434. [CrossRef]
31. Mai, R.-Y.; Zeng, J.; Meng, W.-D.; Lu, H.-Z.; Liang, R.; Lin, Y.; Wu, G.-B.; Li, L.-Q.; Ma, L.; Ye, J.-Z.; et al. Artificial neural network model to predict post-hepatectomy early recurrence of hepatocellular carcinoma without macroscopic vascular invasion. *BMC Cancer* **2021**, *21*, 1–13. [CrossRef] [PubMed]
32. Huang, Y.; Chen, H.; Zeng, Y.; Liu, Z.; Ma, H.; Liu, J. Development and validation of a machine learning prognostic model for hepatocellular carcinoma recurrence after surgical resection. *Front. Oncol.* **2021**, *10*. [CrossRef] [PubMed]
33. Maruyama, H.; Yamaguchi, T.; Nagamatsu, H.; Shiina, S. AI-based radiological imaging for HCC: Current status and future of ultrasound. *Diagnostics* **2021**, *11*, 292. [CrossRef] [PubMed]

34. Mazzaferro, V.; Sposito, C.; Zhou, J.; Pinna, A.D.; De Carlis, L.; Fan, J.; Cescon, M.; Di Sandro, S.; Yi-Feng, H.; Lauterio, A.; et al. Metroticket 2.0 Model for analysis of competing risks of death after liver transplantation for hepatocellular carcinoma. *Gastroenterology* **2018**, *154*, 128–139. [CrossRef] [PubMed]
35. Centonze, L.; Sandro, S.D.; Lauterio, A.; Carlis, R.D.; Sgrazzutti, C.; Ciulli, C.; Vella, I.; Vicentin, I.; Incarbone, N.; Bagnardi, V.; et al. A retrospective single-centre analysis of the oncological impact of LI-RADS classification applied to Metroticket 2.0 cal-culator in liver transplantation: Every nodule matters. *Transpl. Int.* **2021**, *34*, 1712–1721. [CrossRef] [PubMed]

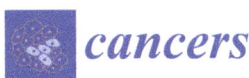

Article

Bacteria-Derived Extracellular Vesicles in Urine as a Novel Biomarker for Gastric Cancer: Integration of Liquid Biopsy and Metagenome Analysis

Jae-Yong Park [1,†], Chil-Sung Kang [2,†], Ho-Chan Seo [2], Jin-Chul Shin [2], Sung-Min Kym [3], Young-Soo Park [4], Tae-Seop Shin [2], Jae-Gyu Kim [1,*] and Yoon-Keun Kim [2,*]

1. Department of Internal Medicine, Chung-Ang University College of Medicine, Seoul 06973, Korea; jay0park@cau.ac.kr
2. Institute of MD Healthcare Inc., Seoul 03923, Korea; cskang@mdhc.kr (C.-S.K.); hcseo@mdhc.kr (H.-C.S.); jcsin@mdhc.kr (J.-C.S.); tsshin@mdhc.kr (T.-S.S.)
3. Division of Infectious Diseases, Department of Internal Medicine, Sejong Chungnam National University Hospital, Sejong 30099, Korea; smkimkor@cnu.ac.kr
4. Department of Internal Medicine, Seoul National University Bundang Hospital, Seongnam 13620, Korea; dkree@snubh.org
* Correspondence: jgkimd@cau.ac.kr (J.-G.K.); ykkim@mdhc.kr (Y.-K.K.); Tel.: +82-2-6299-3147 (J.-G.K.); +82-2-6299-0766 (Y.-K.K.); Fax: +82-2-6299-1137 (J.-G.K.); +82-2-6299-0768 (Y.-K.K.)
† These authors contributed equally to this work.

Simple Summary: Gastric cancer shows an improved prognosis when diagnosed in its early stage. However, non-invasive diagnostic markers for gastric cancer known to date have poor clinical efficacies. Many studies have shown that gastric cancer patients have distinct microbial changes compared to normal subjects. In the present study, we performed metagenome analysis using body fluid samples (gastric juice, blood, and urine) to investigate the distinct microbial composition using bacteria-derived EVs from gastric cancer patients. We could build diagnostic prediction models for gastric cancer with the metagenomic data and analyzed the accuracy of models. Although further validation is required to apply these findings to real clinical practice yet, our study showed the possibility of gastric cancer diagnosis with the integration of liquid biopsy and metagenome analysis.

Abstract: Early detection is crucial for improving the prognosis of gastric cancer, but there are no non-invasive markers for the early diagnosis of gastric cancer in real clinical settings. Recently, bacteria-derived extracellular vesicles (EVs) emerged as new biomarker resources. We aimed to evaluate the microbial composition in gastric cancer using bacteria-derived EVs and to build a diagnostic prediction model for gastric cancer with the metagenome data. Stool, urine, and serum samples were prospectively collected from 453 subjects (gastric cancer, 181; control, 272). EV portions were extracted from the samples for metagenome analysis. Differences in microbial diversity and composition were analyzed with 16S rRNA gene profiling, using the next-generation sequencing method. Biomarkers were selected using logistic regression models based on relative abundances at the genus level. The microbial composition of healthy groups and gastric cancer patient groups was significantly different in all sample types. The compositional differences of various bacteria, based on relative abundances, were identified at the genus level. Among the diagnostic prediction models for gastric cancer, the urine-based model showed the highest performance when compared to that of stool or serum. We suggest that bacteria-derived EVs in urine can be used as novel metagenomic markers for the non-invasive diagnosis of gastric cancer by integrating the liquid biopsy method and metagenome analysis.

Keywords: extracellular vesicles; gastric cancer; liquid biopsy; biomarker; microbiome; 16S rRNA amplicon; metagenomics

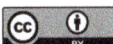

1. Introduction

Although the incidence of gastric cancer has been steadily decreasing worldwide, it still remains one of the most common and fatal causes of cancer death in the world [1]. The 5-year survival rate of gastric cancer is particularly low in the advanced stage [2]. However, the survival rate is much higher in countries where the majority of gastric cancers are newly diagnosed in early stages. This finding is evident in Korea and Japan, where a national screening program for gastric cancer is provided [3,4].

Endoscopic examination with pathologic confirmation is the primary diagnostic modality for gastric cancer. Although relatively safe, endoscopy is an invasive procedure and can cause serious complications occasionally. It can also be a burden in terms of cost. Liquid biopsy is considered the most promising area for cancer diagnosis in that it can be an alternative to traditional tissue biopsy methods, taking advantage of the recent development of next-generation sequencing (NGS) technology [5]. The monitoring system using liquid biopsy was initially studied based on cell-free DNA in blood, but it has recently developed by using body fluids such as stool, urine, or saliva. Several studies have been conducted or are now underway for serological diagnosis of gastric cancer [6]. However, there are no non-invasive markers with significant accuracy in the early diagnosis of gastric cancer yet, which can be used in real clinical settings.

Helicobacter pylori infection is a well-known risk factor for gastric cancer development. Recently, the rapid development of microbiome research has focused much attention on the possibility that microbiome other than *H. pylori* may be involved in the gastric carcinogenesis process [7,8]. The human gastrointestinal tract is the most complex ecosystem well known. The commensal microorganisms in it affect not only the immune system but also numerous physiological and metabolic processes in the human body, suggesting their role in the pathogenesis of various diseases [9,10]. Many studies are underway to establish the relationship between gastric cancer and microbiomes [7,8,11]. Gut microbe-derived extracellular vesicles (EVs) are emerging as novel proof of the relationship between commensal bacteria and host health conditions [12,13]. The EVs can act as intercellular communication mediators carrying various cargoes, including signaling molecules and transcription factors. Many studies have shown that EVs are associated with various immune responses in humans, causing inflammation or inhibiting reactions [14,15]. However, in the context of gastric carcinogenesis, few studies have been reported focusing on microbiome-derived EVs. Studies linking the EVs to early diagnosis of gastric cancer are even more scarce.

In this context, we conducted a metagenome analysis using microbiome-derived EVs in stool, urine, and serum samples from a large number of prospective cohorts of gastric cancer patients and healthy controls. After identifying the potential microbial biomarkers, we developed diagnostic prediction models for gastric cancer with various types of liquid biopsy samples and validated the diagnostic performance of each model.

2. Materials and Methods

2.1. Subjects and Sample Collection

In total, 272 healthy people (159 males and 113 females) and 181 gastric cancer patients (122 males and 59 females) were enrolled from Haewoondae Baek Hospital (Busan, Korea), Chung-Ang University Hospital (Seoul, Korea), and Seoul National University Bundang Hospital (Seongnam, Gyeonggi-do, Korea) between December 2016 and December 2019. Among the patient's medical records, medical history, age, sex, endoscopic diagnosis, and pathologic results were reviewed. The inclusion criteria for the gastric cancer group were patients newly diagnosed with gastric cancer who did not undergo endoscopic or surgical resection or chemotherapy yet. The healthy control group included those without evidence of dysplasia or gastric cancer on the endoscopic examination. Patients were excluded if they had a previous history of gastrointestinal surgery, were pregnant, or were taking antibiotics, probiotics, or acid-suppressing drugs within the previous 3 months, as these conditions can temporarily alter the gut microbial composition. The minimum duration of drug cessation was determined by referring to previous literature [16–19]. This study protocol was approved by the Institutional Review Board of Haewoondae Baek Hospital (IRB No. 129792-2015-064), Chung-Ang University Hospital (IRB No. 1772-001-290), and Seoul National University Bundang Hospital (IRB No. B-1708/412-301). Stool, serum, and urine samples were collected from the subjects for metagenomics analyses. All participants ate a regular Korean diet a day before sampling and did not smoke or drink alcohol. The regular Korean diet is characterized by high levels of whole grains, vegetables, and low levels of animal-derived foods and saturated fat, particularly in contrast to the Western-style diet [20]. The stool sample was collected from the center of the stool, and placed in a sterilized container, and stored at −20 °C. For serum collection, we drew 3 mL of blood from each subject in an SST tube. The tube was then centrifuged (3000× g, 15 min, 4 °C) immediately after collection, and the serum was extracted. The supernatant was stored in Eppendorf tube 1 mL each at −20 °C. For urine, 40 mL of midstream urine was collected at a clean urine container and transferred to a conical tube, which was kept frozen at −20 °C.

2.2. Bacterial and EV Isolation and DNA Extraction from Clinical Samples

Bacteria EVs were isolated from the urine and serum of individuals following the procedure described previously [21,22]. Briefly, each urine sample was centrifuged at 10,000× g for 10 min at 4 °C. The supernatant was taken and passed through a 0.22 μm membrane filter to eliminate foreign particles and then quantified based on protein concentration. For serum, after mixing 100 μL of serum and 900 μL PBS, it was centrifuged at 10,000× g for 10 min at 4 °C to eliminate other components. The supernatant was taken and passed through a 0.22 μm membrane filter to eliminate foreign particles, and it was quantified based on protein concentration. The stool sample was mixed with PBS for dilution in a 1:10 ratio (1 g:10 mL) and maintained at 4 °C for 24 h. After dilution, the sample was centrifuged (10,000× g, 10 min, 4 °C) to separate the bacteria portion and the EV portion. The rest of the procedure was carried out in the same way as urine and serum.

Bacterial DNA extraction from prepared EVs was performed as described previously [23,24]. Briefly, isolated EVs (1 μg by protein, each sample) were boiled at 100 °C for 40 min, centrifuged at 13,000× g for 30 min, and the supernatants were collected. Collected samples were then subjected to bacterial DNA extraction using a DNA extraction kit (PowerSoil DNA Isolation Kit, MO BIO, Carlsbad, CA, USA) following the manufacturer's instructions. Isolated DNA was quantified by using the QIAxpert system (QIAGEN, Hilden, Germany). In the case of stool, DNA was extracted by dividing the pellet (including bacteria portion) and the supernatant (including EV portion) to compare each.

2.3. PCR Amplification, Library Construction, and Sequencing of 16S rRNA Gene Variable Regions

To perform microbiome analysis, 16S rRNA gene amplicon metagenome analysis was conducted. Prepared bacterial DNA was used for PCR amplification of the V3-V4 hypervariable regions of the 16S ribosomal RNA genes using the primer set of 16S_V3_F (5'-TCGTCGGCAGCGTCAGATGTGTATAAGAGACAGCCTACGGGNGGCWGCAG-3') and 16S_V4_R (5'-GTCTCGTGGGCTCGGAGATGTGTATAAGAGACAGGACTACHVGGGTATCT AATCC-3'). The PCR products were used for the construction of 16S rRNA gene libraries following the MiSeq System guidelines (Illumina Inc., San Diego, CA, USA). The 16S rRNA gene libraries for each sample were quantified using QIAxpert (QIAGEN, Germany), pooled at the equimolar ratio, and used for pyrosequencing with the MiSeq System (Illumina Inc., San Diego, CA, USA) according to the manufacturer's recommendations.

2.4. Analysis of Bacterial Composition in the Microbiome

Paired-end reads were trimmed by cutadapt (ver. 1.1.6). The resulting FASTQ files containing paired-end reads were merged using CASPER and then quality filtered by Phred (Q) score. After merging, any reads under 350 bp or over 550 bp were also discarded. Next, a reference-based chimera detection step was performed using VSEARCH against the SILVA gold database. The sequence reads were clustered into operational taxonomic units (OTUs) using the de novo clustering algorithm, and the threshold was 97% sequence similarity. Finally, OTUs were classified using UCLUST under default parameters with SILVA 132 database.

2.5. Diagnostic Prediction Models for Gastric Cancer

The selection of biomarkers for the diagnostic model was based on relative abundances at the genus level. Candidates for bacterial biomarkers were chosen based on two criteria: the statistically significant difference ($p < 0.05$) between control and cancer subjects, the average relative abundance of 0.1% or more for each group. The whole data sets were randomly divided into training sets and test set in a ratio of 8:2. The prediction model was constructed using logistic regression models for each sample type, using the training set. The biomarkers to be used in the model were selected through a stepwise method by eliminating unnecessary variables, and Akaike's information criterion (AIC) was used as a criterion for selection variables in the prediction model. After the diagnostic prediction models were built, the performance was evaluated on the test set for validation.

2.6. Statistical Analysis

To clarify the species abundancy between healthy control and gastric cancer group, alpha diversity of the variance within each clinical sample was assessed using the alpha diversity test in the phyloseq package in R for the total observed OTUs, richness estimates Chao1, and the Shannon and Simpson diversity indices. In order to avoid the alpha diversity bias, we rarified with the minimum read value for each sample. Dimension reduction was conducted to assess the beta diversity between clinical samples based on the Bray–Curtis dissimilarity using principal coordinate analysis (PCoA) and multiple dimension scale (MDS) in the stats package in R. Permutational multivariate analysis of variance (PERMANOVA) was used to validate either the centroid or the spread of each sample are different between the groups. The significant difference between the control group and the gastric cancer group was determined using a t-test, and p-values were adjusted using the Benjamini–Hochberg method to reduce the false discovery rates. Receiver operating characteristic (ROC) curves of gastric cancer diagnostic prediction models were developed through stepwise selection of significantly altered genera. The performance of the models was evaluated by assessing the area under the ROC curve (AUC), sensitivity, specificity, and accuracy. p value < 0.05 was considered statistically significant.

3. Results

3.1. Clinical Characteristics of Subjects

A total of 453 subjects were registered, including 181 gastric cancer patients and 272 healthy controls. Age and sex were matched between each sample group. A total of 813 samples from enrolled subjects were used for analysis. There was no statistical difference in sex and age between the gastric cancer group and control group in all four sample types: ST-Bac (bacteria portion extracted by using centrifuged pellet in stool), ST-EV (EV portion extracted by using centrifuged supernatant in stool), urine, and serum (Table 1).

Table 1. Basal clinical characteristics of each sample group.

Sample Type	Age & Sex	Control	Gastric Cancer	*p*-Value
ST-Bac	Age (mean ± SD)	63.6 ± 8.3	63.6 ± 9.5	0.9815
	Sex (M:F)	127 (93:34)	140 (95:45)	0.4088
ST-EV	Age (mean ± SD)	63.6 ± 8.3	63.6 ± 9.5	0.9853
	Sex (M:F)	127 (93:34)	141 (96:45)	0.4307
Urine	Age (mean ± SD)	63.5 ± 9.8	63.8 ± 9.8	0.8207
	Sex (M:F)	164 (114:50)	168 (114:54)	0.8362
Serum	Age (mean ± SD)	62.3 ± 9.4	63.7 ± 10.3	0.2891
	Sex (M:F)	105 (74:31)	108 (73:35)	0.7590

SD, standard deviation; M, male; F, female.

3.2. Comparison of Alpha and Beta Diversity between Healthy Controls and Gastric Cancer Patients

Read numbers of 16S rRNA amplicons and OTU counts derived from the NGS results are shown in Table 2. In stool samples, alpha diversity did not show significant differences between the two groups for all the diversity indices (Figure S1A,B). In urine and serum samples, Simpson index and Chao1 index showed significant differences between the two groups, respectively (Figure S1C,D). However, the differences in alpha diversity were generally not obvious. To evaluate the alpha diversity that includes all samples, a rarefaction curve analysis was performed with the Chao1 index to calculate species abundance per sequence. The slope of the rarefaction curve was steeper in the healthy control group than in the gastric cancer group in all sample types, indicating higher alpha diversity in the control group than in the gastric cancer group (Figure 1A–D).

Table 2. Read numbers of 16S rRNA amplicons and OTU counts from the NGS results.

Sample Type	Group	Read Count			OTU		
		Mean	Median	SE	Mean	Median	SE
ST-Bac	Control	18,352.6	16,243.0	±1062.7	939.4	810.0	±64.5
	Gastric cancer	19,987.9	16,138.5	±1420.5	890.4	763.5	±46.6
ST-EV	Control	19,262.0	18,378.0	±961.6	550.7	453.0	±32.7
	Gastric cancer	22,555.8	19,753.0	±1227.5	556.9	510.0	±22.7
Urine	Control	12,766.7	12,412.5	±598.8	176.6	140.5	±11.6
	Gastric cancer	12,968.7	9282.0	±787.5	167.4	141.5	±8.6
Serum	Control	11,340.4	10,642.0	±841.3	189.6	144.0	±17.3
	Gastric cancer	14,259.4	10,763.0	±977.6	226.8	181.0	±16.8

OTU, operational taxonomic unit; SE, standard error.

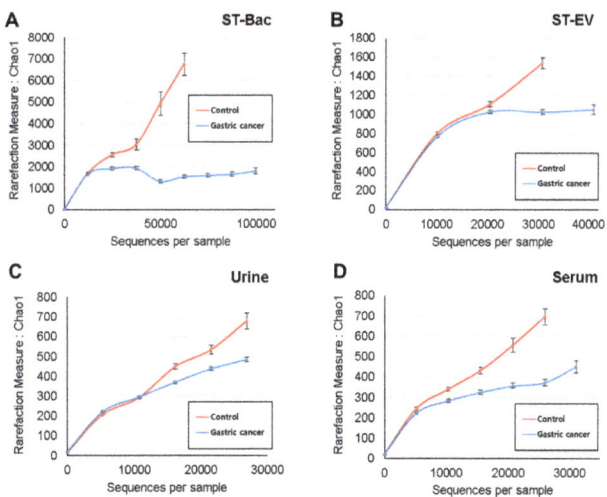

Figure 1. Comparison of alpha diversity between healthy controls and gastric cancer patients in 4 sample types. Estimated species richness (Chao1 measure) is demonstrated for the two groups (**A**) in stool bacteria (ST-Bac) isolated from stool pellet, (**B**) in stool-derived extracellular vesicle (ST-EV) isolated from stool supernatant, (**C**) in urine, and (**D**) in serum.

At the phylum level, the beta diversity showed significant differences between the control group and the gastric cancer group in all sample types (Figure 2A). At the genus level, these differences were repeatedly confirmed, with even higher statistical significances (Figure 2B). Although we could not detect a significant reduction in microbial diversity in gastric cancer, the microbial composition in the gastric cancer group was significantly different from that in healthy controls.

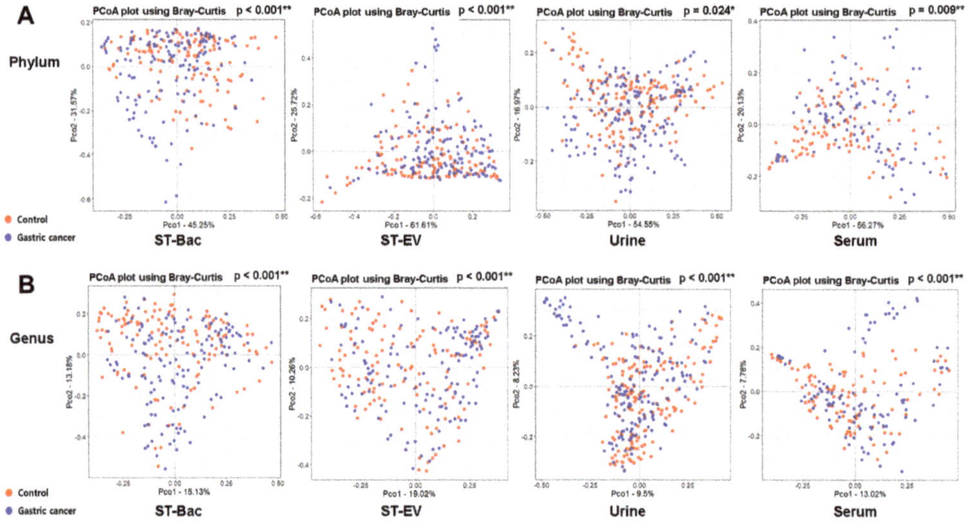

Figure 2. Comparison of beta diversity in phylum and genus levels between healthy controls and gastric cancer patients in 4 sample types. PCoA results based on Bray–Curtis similarity for beta diversity of bacteria are shown (**A**) in phylum level and (**B**) in genus level.

3.3. Relative Abundance Differences between Healthy Controls and Gastric Cancer Patients

We compared the relative abundances of microbiome between the control group and the gastric cancer group to identify the taxa that were differentially represented in the two groups of subjects. In the comparison of phylum levels, heatmaps using ST-Bac samples showed that *Bacteroidetes* were reduced, while *Firmicutes* were increased in gastric cancer (Figures 3A and S2A). In ST-EV samples, *Bacteroidetes* were reduced, while *Actinobacteria* were increased in gastric cancer (Figures 3B and S2B). In urine samples, *Bacteroidetes* and *Fusobacteria* were both increased in gastric cancer, differently from ST-Bac and ST-EV samples (Figures 3C and S2C). In serum samples, *Verrucomicrobia* were reduced, while *Actinobacteria* were increased in gastric cancer (Figures 3D and S2D).

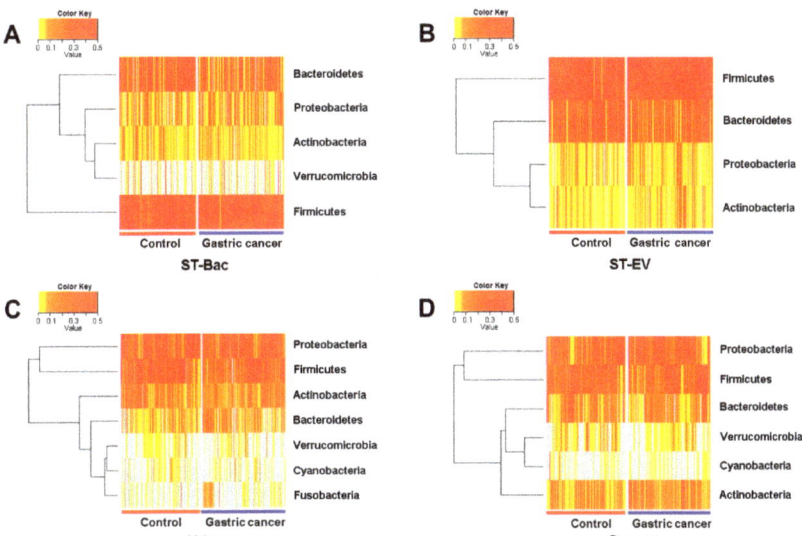

Figure 3. Relative abundance differences in phylum level between healthy controls and gastric cancer patients in 4 sample types. Heatmaps representing the relative abundances of microbiome between the two groups (**A**) in stool bacteria (ST-Bac) isolated from stool pellet, (**B**) in stool-derived extracellular vesicle (ST-EV) isolated from stool supernatant, (**C**) in urine, and (**D**) in serum.

When we compared the relative abundances in genus level, more bacteria became candidates showing the differences between the control group and gastric cancer group. In ST-Bac samples, *Prevotella 9* was decreased, while *Streptococcus, Subdoligranulum, Enterobacter, Lactobacillus, Klebsiella, Ruminiclostridium 9* were increased in gastric cancer (Figures 4A and 5A). In ST-EV samples, *Acinetobacter* was increased in gastric cancer (Figures 4B and 5B). In urine samples, the largest number of bacterial candidates were detected, revealing that *Acinetobacter, Stayphylococcus, Bifidobacterium,* and *Sphingomonas* were decreased, while *Corynebacterium 1, Neisseria, Fusobacterium, Diaphorobacter, Actinomyces, Porphyromonas, Cloacibacterium,* and *Peptoniphilus* were increased in gastric cancer (Figures 4C and 5C). In serum samples, *Bacteroides, Akkermansia, Muribaculaceae(f),* and *Lachnospiraceae NK4A136* were decreased, while *Corynebacterium 1, Rhodococcus, Diaphorobacter, Haemophilus,* and *Cloacibacterium* were increased in gastric cancer (Figures 4D and 5D).

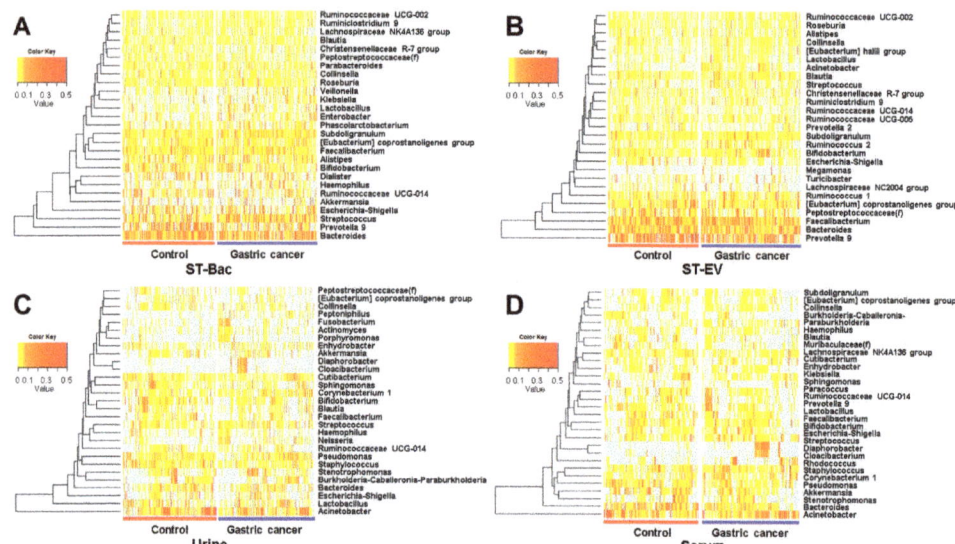

Figure 4. Relative abundance differences in genus level between healthy controls and gastric cancer patients in 4 sample types. Heatmaps representing the relative abundances of microbiome between the two groups (**A**) in stool bacteria (ST-Bac) isolated from stool pellet, (**B**) in stool-derived extracellular vesicle (ST-EV) isolated from stool supernatant, (**C**) in urine, and (**D**) in serum.

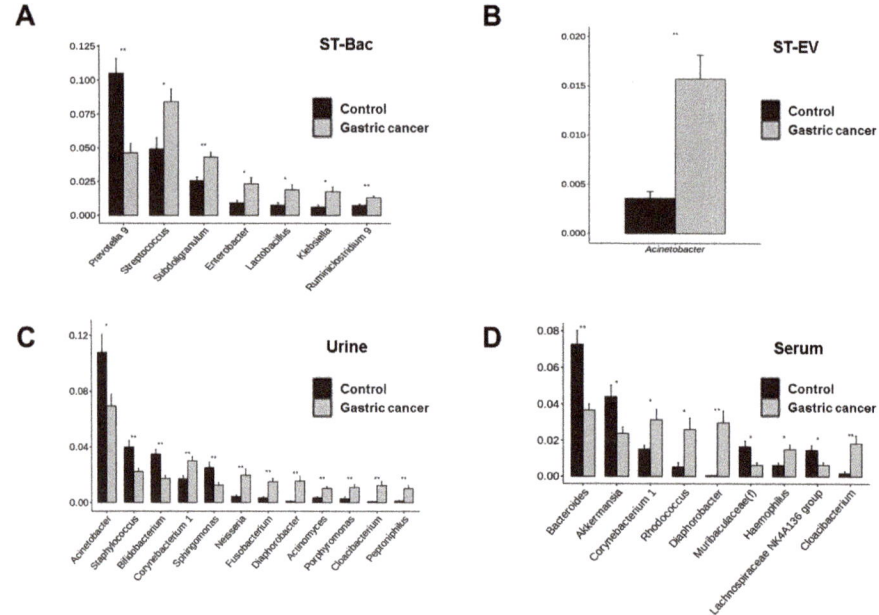

Figure 5. Compositional differences in genus level between healthy controls and gastric cancer patients in 4 sample types. The bar plots highlight the average relative abundance of individual key taxa between the two groups (**A**) in stool bacteria (ST-Bac) isolated from stool pellet, (**B**) in stool-derived extracellular vesicle (ST-EV) isolated from stool supernatant, (**C**) in urine, and (**D**) in serum. *, $p < 0.05$; **, $p < 0.01$.

3.4. Comparison of Diagnostic Prediction Models for Gastric Cancer between Healthy Controls and Gastric Cancer Patients

To further define useful biomarkers from metagenomic biomarkers, optimal models were built using biomarkers to distinguish between gastric cancer group and control group using logistic regression analysis (Figure 6A–D). Selected variables included in the prediction models according to each sample type were as follows: ST-Bac-based model, *Klebsiella, Subdoligranulum, Prevotella 9, Streptococcus, Ruminiclostridium 9*; stool EV-based model, *Acinetobacter*; urine-based model, *Peptoniphilus, Diaphorobacter, Neisseria, Staphylococcus, Bifidobacterium, Corynebacterium 1, Actinomyces, Acinetobacter, Sphingomonas*; serum-based model, *Diaphorobacter, Bacteroides, Corynebacterium 1, Rhodococcus, Cloacibacterium, Haemophilus, Muribaculaceae(f), Akkermansia*.

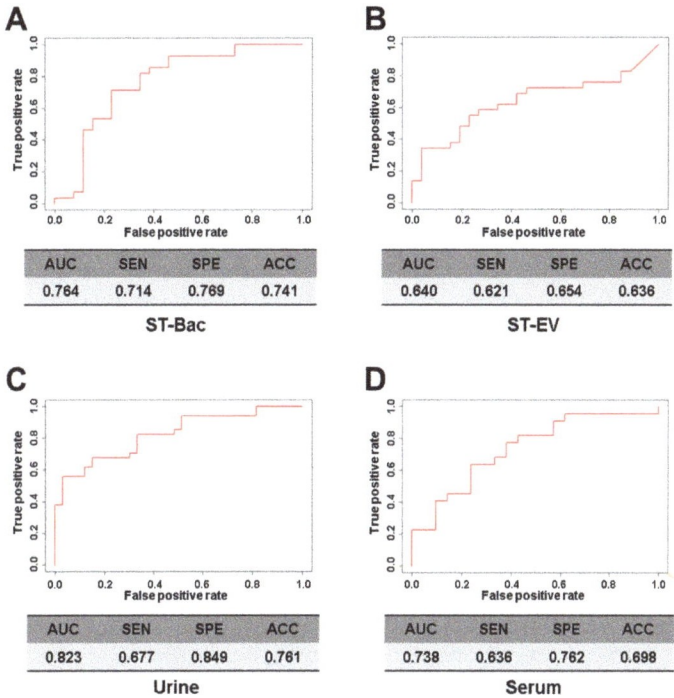

Figure 6. Comparison of gastric cancer diagnostic prediction models between healthy controls and gastric cancer patients in 4 sample types. ROC curves of gastric cancer diagnostic prediction models were developed through stepwise selection of significantly altered genera. Models were validated by performance evaluation in the test set by assessing the area under the curve (AUC), sensitivity, specificity, and accuracy. Performance indices of each model are demonstrated: (**A**) stool bacteria (ST-Bac) isolated from stool pellet, (**B**) stool-derived extracellular vesicle (ST-EV) isolated from stool supernatant, (**C**) urine, and (**D**) serum. SEN, sensitivity; SPE, specificity; ACC, accuracy.

As a result, the model using the urine samples showed the highest AUC value of 0.823 (Figure 6C). Although the sensitivity was rather low (67.7%) in this model, the specificity (84.9%) and accuracy (76.1%) were high when compared to other models. The ST-Bac-based model showed an AUC score of 0.764, lower than the urine-based model, but their sensitivity (71.4%), specificity (76.9%), and accuracy (74.1%) were generally high (Figure 6A). The ST-EV-based model and serum-based model revealed lower AUC values and accuracies than the two models mentioned above (Figure 6B,D).

To further analyze the performance of prediction models according to disease stages, we divided the gastric cancer group into early gastric cancer (EGC) and advanced gastric cancer (AGC) groups. The performance of the prediction model was higher in the AGC group than in the EGC group in all sample types except for ST-Bac Figure S3A–H). For EGC, the ST-Bac prediction model showed the highest AUC value of 0.830.

4. Discussion

We performed microbiome profiling of gastric cancer using various types of samples through analyzing the bacteria-derived EVs to find out diagnostic biomarkers for gastric cancer in correlation with gut microbes. There were significant differences in microbial composition between the gastric cancer group and the control group in all of the sample types. Diagnostic prediction models for gastric cancer were generated based on this information on metagenomic biomarkers, and the model using the urine samples showed the highest performance for the diagnosis of gastric cancer.

In this study, although there seemed to be a trend for reduced alpha diversity in gastric cancer, further analysis with various indices showed that the differences in microbial diversity between the two groups were not consistent among various sample types. This could also be indirectly inferred from the finding that the OTU values of the gastric cancer group and control group showed high standard deviations, which means that the number of microbial taxa in the two groups overlapped each other to some extent. This finding is different from previous reports, which suggest that reduced microbial diversity is often a characteristic feature of diseased status [25,26]. Several studies showed dysbiotic cancer-associated microbiome in gastric cancer, implying the role of microbial dysbiosis in gastric carcinogenesis [8,25]. This discrepancy may be due to several reasons. We used samples from extragastric area that reflect systemic circulation in this study, whereas samples obtained from the stomach (gastric juice, gastric mucosa, etc.) were mainly used in previous studies. Indirect analysis of microbiome using bacteria-derived EVs rather than direct identification of microbiome might also be a possible explanation. However, a comparison of beta diversity between the gastric cancer group and the control group revealed that microbial composition in the gastric cancer group was significantly different from that in healthy controls, which was evident with all four types of samples.

The composition of microbiota was further investigated with a relative abundance of taxa. The five most dominant bacterial phyla in stool were *Bacteroidetes*, *Proteobacteria*, *Actinobacteria*, *Verrucomicrobia*, and *Firmicutes*, which are consistent with previous literature [27,28]. EVs from these phyla were also highly abundant in urine and serum samples. This finding implies that bacteria-derived EVs in systemic circulation can roughly reflect the microbial composition of gastrointestinal microbes. Interestingly, *Proteobacteria* were dominant in urine and serum EVs, while *Firmicutes* and *Bacteroidetes* were the most abundant in stool samples at the phylum level. *Firmicutes* and *Bacteriodetes* generally comprise more than 90% of the human gut microbiome, according to previous studies [28], similar to the results from our study. In addition, *Firmicutes* were increased in stool, while EVs from *Firmicutes* did not show a significant change in serum in gastric cancer. The relative abundances of *Bacteroidetes* in stool and urine EVs also showed conflicting results. The difference in microbial composition was even more evident at the genus level. *Acinetobacter* (phylum *Proteobacteria*) were the most dominant in urine and serum EVs identically, whereas *Prevotella* and *Bacteroides* (phylum *Bacteriodetes*) were the most dominant in stool samples. Representative strains showing changes in gastric cancer were largely different between stool and urine/serum samples. Moreover, the gross pattern of the microbiome from urine and serum samples was similar, which can easily be inferred from the fact that urine is basically filtrated from blood during systemic circulation. This result shows that the microbial composition directly identified from the bacteria present in the gut lumen differs from the composition of bacteria indirectly inferred from the EVs, which are absorbed through the gut mucosa into the systemic circulation. It is recently recognized that bacteria secrete EVs, which are intercellular communicasomes between the host and commensal microbes, that can act as biologically active metabolites or as mediators of host-microbiome interaction [15,29,30]. Considering this, it can be inferred that there is a significant difference between the microbiome simply existing in the gastrointestinal tract and the core microbiome that are deeply involved in host-microbiome interaction, actually affecting the health of the host. In fact, gastric juice and feces contain lots of dead strains and strains with little clinical significance [31,32]. This might partly explain why the microbial diversity between the gastric cancer group and the control group was not consistent among various sample types. Although reduced microbial diversity in the gastrointestinal tract is often a characteristic feature of diseased status, this does not necessarily mean that the bacteria related to systemic circulation should also be less diverse in exactly the same manner. We do not yet fully understand which bacteria play major roles by host-microbiome interaction in certain diseases and how they systemically influence the disease pathogenesis. In fact, blood was known as a sterile specimen except for sepsis, but recent studies have shown that 16S rRNA gene-targeted NGS is possible with normal human blood, suggesting the presence of bacteria-derived EVs in blood. It is known that there is a difference in the EV composition in serum and plasma, and each of them has its inherent advantage according to the type of EVs and purpose of EV analysis [33–35]. Especially in terms of platelet richness in the plasma, there are reports that platelet-rich plasma (PRP) has some antibacterial effect [36,37]. Since 16s rRNA NGS analysis is based on bacteria, the platelet-poor plasma would be preferred over PRP in metagenome analysis using bacteria-derived EVs if plasma is used instead of serum. In brief, when performing microbiome analysis from the perspective of systemic effect on the host, it should be noted that circulating EVs found in blood or urine can have a greater meaning than analyzing samples directly obtained from the gastrointestinal tract.

We tried to explore the possibility of a prediction model that can be used for the early diagnosis of gastric cancer by using the microbiome data derived through EV analysis. Currently, some Asian countries, such as Korea and Japan, where the incidence of gastric cancer is very high, have been operating national cancer screening programs aiming to detect gastric cancer early. These programs increased the early detection of gastric cancer and lowered the mortality rate [3]. However, considering the socioeconomic costs of mass screening for a large number of people and the discomfort or complications from invasive procedures such as endoscopy, other new non-invasive diagnostic methods need to be developed. With the results of microbiome analysis, we investigate the possibility of liquid biopsy using diluted stool, urine, and serum.

In this study, prediction models were established for each sample type to distinguish gastric cancer patients from normal controls, and they were validated to evaluate the performance. The AUC value was higher than 0.7 in urine- and ST-Bac-based models, which is good performance according to the evaluation criteria (0.9–1.0 = excellent, 0.8–0.9 = very good, 0.7–0.8 = good, 0.6–0.7= sufficient, 0.5–0.6 = bad, <0.5). = not useful) [38], and the prediction model with urine showed the highest AUC value. However, although the specificity (84.9%) of the urine-based model was high, the sensitivity (67.7%) of this model was lower compared to that of the ST-Bac-based model (71.4%). When EGC and AGC groups were separately analyzed, although the ST-Bac-based prediction model showed the highest AUC value of 0.830 for EGC, the performances of prediction models were generally higher in the AGC group than in the EGC group except for ST-Bac. This indicates that the performances of prediction models differ by cancer stage and sample type. Accurate prediction of EGC seemed more difficult than AGC as one might easily expect, considering that the microbial changes would be more prominent in a more advanced state of the disease. In order to evaluate the suitability as a diagnostic test, it is necessary to consider various factors such as sensitivity, disease prevalence, cost-effectiveness, and convenience of sample collection. Especially, an ideal screening method should show adequate sensitivity and specificity, and there is typically a trade-off between these two performance metrics. High sensitivity is especially important in this situation, as a low value can lead to increased false-negative results, which means missing more cases with the disease of interest. Although the specificity of the urine-based model in our study was about 85%, the low sensitivity of the model prevents it from being a suitable screening method as it stands. However, despite the relatively low sensitivity of the urine-based model, it should also be considered that urine is much easier to collect than stool samples. Recent studies have also shown that the bacteria-derived EVs in urine samples contain characteristic features in allergic airway disease with a significant correlation with total IgE and eosinophil count, which further supports the possible role of microbial EVs in the implication of microbiota in the diseased state [39,40]. To further investigate the effect of *H. pylori* on the performance of the prognostic models, we tried to use stool samples to detect *H. pylori* first. However, *H. pylori* was detected in ST-Bac samples in only 13.6% of the cases. Furthermore, among the *H. pylori*-positive gastric cancer samples, the relative abundance of *H. pylori* was lower than 0.1% in all but one case. These findings made us assume that the validity of the analysis according to *H. pylori* status might be quite limited, especially when the detection rate and relative abundance of *H. pylori* are low. It is reasonable to investigate the gastric microbiome as a whole, the members of which influence each other and change the adjacent environment. Therefore, we decided to assess the diagnostic ability of prediction models using the whole integrated metagenome data, including *H. pylori*, as a comprehensive biomarker.

This study has some limitations. First, we did not perform the microbiome analysis according to *H. pylori* status. As *H. pylori* is the single most important pathogen for the gastric carcinogenesis process, this might have influenced the interpretation of study results. As the control subjects were recruited from health check-up programs, detailed histological information on the degree of mucosal atrophy was not available. Hypoacidity due to atrophic gastritis could alter the gut microbial composition, which is important in regions with high *H. pylori* prevalence, such as Korea. Therefore, the findings of the present study do not necessarily separate gastric cancer from atrophic pangastritis without cancer. Nevertheless, we showed a possibility of discriminating between gastric cancer patients and the general population without gastric cancer, using metagenomic data from a relatively large number of subjects. Further biomarker studies are needed for the detection of gastric cancer, and mucosal atrophy and *H. pylori* infection should be considered. Second, the performances of diagnostic prediction models were suboptimal. The urine-based model, which had the highest AUC value, showed rather low sensitivity. The results of our study further need to be verified through external validation.

5. Conclusions

In this study, we have shown that bacteria-derived EVs in systemic circulation can be used for demonstrating the changes in microbial composition in gastric cancer. Bacteria-derived EVs in urine harbors a potential as a new diagnostic biomarker for gastric cancer, suggesting that EVs might be a new standard substance for cancer diagnosis. Although it would be difficult to directly apply the results from this study to real clinical practice yet due to the suboptimal sensitivity and specificity of the diagnostic prediction models, these findings still have great significance in that they showed the possibility of integrating a liquid biopsy method with metagenome analysis for gastric cancer diagnosis.

Supplementary Materials: The following are available online at https://www.mdpi.com/article/10.3390/cancers13184687/s1, Figure S1: Alpha diversity of microbiome defined by various indices in 4 sample types, Figure S2: Changes in the relative abundances of individual phyla in gastric cancer in 4 sample types, Figure S3: Comparison of gastric cancer diagnostic prediction models between healthy controls and EGC or AGC in 4 sample types.

Author Contributions: Conceptualization, J.-G.K. and Y.-K.K.; methodology, C.-S.K. and T.-S.S.; software, Y.-K.K.; validation, H.-C.S. and J.-C.S.; formal analysis, H.-C.S. and J.-C.S.; investigation, S.-M.K., Y.-S.P. and J.-G.K.; data curation, J.-Y.P. and C.-S.K.; writing—original draft preparation, J.-Y.P. and C.-S.K.; writing—review and editing, T.-S.S., Y.-K.K. and J.-G.K.; visualization, H.-C.S.; funding acquisition, Y.-S.P. All authors have read and agreed to the published version of the manuscript.

Funding: This research was supported by the Bio & Medical Technology Development Program of the National Research Foundation (NRF), funded by the Ministry of Science & ICT under grant number NRF-2017M3A9F3047495.

Institutional Review Board Statement: The study was conducted according to the guidelines of the Declaration of Helsinki and approved by the Institutional Review Board of Haewoondae Baek Hospital (IRB No. 129792-2015-064) on 22 June 2015, Chung-Ang University Hospital (IRB No. 1772-001-290) on 28 August 2017, and Seoul National University Bundang Hospital (IRB No. B-1708/412-301) on 16 July 2017.

Informed Consent Statement: Informed consent was obtained from all subjects involved in the study.

Data Availability Statement: The data presented in this study are available on request from the corresponding author.

Acknowledgments: Special thanks to MD Healthcare Inc. for providing the sequencing and analysis services for this study.

Conflicts of Interest: The authors declare no conflict of interest. The funders had no role in the design of the study, in the collection, analyses, or interpretation of data, in the writing of the manuscript, or in the decision to publish the results.

References

1. Bray, F.; Ferlay, J.; Soerjomataram, I.; Siegel, R.L.; Torre, L.A.; Jemal, A. Global cancer statistics 2018: GLOBOCAN estimates of incidence and mortality worldwide for 36 cancers in 185 countries. *CA Cancer J. Clin.* **2018**, *68*, 394–424. [CrossRef] [PubMed]
2. Jung, K.W.; Won, Y.J.; Kong, H.J.; Oh, C.M.; Shin, A.; Lee, J.S. Survival of korean adult cancer patients by stage at diagnosis, 2006–2010: National cancer registry study. *Cancer Res. Treat.* **2013**, *45*, 162–171. [CrossRef]
3. Jun, J.K.; Choi, K.S.; Lee, H.Y.; Suh, M.; Park, B.; Song, S.H.; Jung, K.W.; Lee, C.W.; Choi, I.J.; Park, E.C.; et al. Effectiveness of the Korean National Cancer Screening Program in Reducing Gastric Cancer Mortality. *Gastroenterology* **2017**, *152*, 1319–1328.e1317. [CrossRef]
4. Jung, K.W.; Won, Y.J.; Kong, H.J.; Lee, E.S. Cancer Statistics in Korea: Incidence, Mortality, Survival, and Prevalence in 2016. *Cancer Res. Treat.* **2019**, *51*, 417–430. [CrossRef]
5. Domínguez-Vigil, I.G.; Moreno-Martínez, A.K.; Wang, J.Y.; Roehrl, M.H.A.; Barrera-Saldaña, H.A. The dawn of the liquid biopsy in the fight against cancer. *Oncotarget* **2018**, *9*, 2912–2922. [CrossRef]
6. Werner, S.; Chen, H.; Tao, S.; Brenner, H. Systematic review: Serum autoantibodies in the early detection of gastric cancer. *Int. J. Cancer* **2015**, *136*, 2243–2252. [CrossRef]
7. Coker, O.O.; Dai, Z.; Nie, Y.; Zhao, G.; Cao, L.; Nakatsu, G.; Wu, W.K.; Wong, S.H.; Chen, Z.; Sung, J.J.Y.; et al. Mucosal microbiome dysbiosis in gastric carcinogenesis. *Gut* **2018**, *67*, 1024–1032. [CrossRef]
8. Park, C.H.; Lee, A.R.; Lee, Y.R.; Eun, C.S.; Lee, S.K.; Han, D.S. Evaluation of gastric microbiome and metagenomic function in patients with intestinal metaplasia using 16S rRNA gene sequencing. *Helicobacter* **2019**, *24*, e12547. [CrossRef]
9. Brestoff, J.R.; Artis, D. Commensal bacteria at the interface of host metabolism and the immune system. *Nat. Immunol.* **2013**, *14*, 676–684. [CrossRef]
10. Nicholson, J.K.; Holmes, E.; Kinross, J.; Burcelin, R.; Gibson, G.; Jia, W.; Pettersson, S. Host-gut microbiota metabolic interactions. *Science* **2012**, *336*, 1262–1267. [CrossRef] [PubMed]
11. Noto, J.M.; Peek, R.M., Jr. The gastric microbiome, its interaction with *Helicobacter pylori*, and its potential role in the progression to stomach cancer. *PLoS Pathog.* **2017**, *13*, e1006573. [CrossRef]
12. Macia, L.; Nanan, R.; Hosseini-Beheshti, E.; Grau, G.E. Host- and Microbiota-Derived Extracellular Vesicles, Immune Function, and Disease Development. *Int. J. Mol. Sci* **2019**, *21*, 107. [CrossRef]
13. Yang, J.; Moon, H.E.; Park, H.W.; McDowell, A.; Shin, T.S.; Jee, Y.K.; Kym, S.; Paek, S.H.; Kim, Y.K. Brain tumor diagnostic model and dietary effect based on extracellular vesicle microbiome data in serum. *Exp. Mol. Med.* **2020**, *52*, 1602–1613. [CrossRef]
14. Jing, H.; Tang, S.; Lin, S.; Liao, M.; Chen, H.; Zhou, J. The role of extracellular vesicles in renal fibrosis. *Cell Death Dis.* **2019**, *10*, 367. [CrossRef]
15. Choi, J.P.; Jeon, S.G.; Kim, Y.K.; Cho, Y.S. Role of house dust mite-derived extracellular vesicles in a murine model of airway inflammation. *Clin. Exp. Allergy* **2019**, *49*, 227–238. [CrossRef]
16. Raymond, F.; Ouameur, A.A.; Déraspe, M.; Iqbal, N.; Gingras, H.; Dridi, B.; Leprohon, P.; Plante, P.L.; Giroux, R.; Bérubé, È.; et al. The initial state of the human gut microbiome determines its reshaping by antibiotics. *ISME J.* **2016**, *10*, 707–720. [CrossRef] [PubMed]
17. Palleja, A.; Mikkelsen, K.H.; Forslund, S.K.; Kashani, A.; Allin, K.H.; Nielsen, T.; Hansen, T.H.; Liang, S.; Feng, Q.; Zhang, C.; et al. Recovery of gut microbiota of healthy adults following antibiotic exposure. *Nat. Microbiol.* **2018**, *3*, 1255–1265. [CrossRef] [PubMed]

18. Elvers, K.T.; Wilson, V.J.; Hammond, A.; Duncan, L.; Huntley, A.L.; Hay, A.D.; van der Werf, E.T. Antibiotic-induced changes in the human gut microbiota for the most commonly prescribed antibiotics in primary care in the UK: A systematic review. *BMJ Open* **2020**, *10*, e035677. [CrossRef]
19. Morales-Marroquin, E.; Hanson, B.; Greathouse, L.; de la Cruz-Munoz, N.; Messiah, S.E. Comparison of methodological approaches to human gut microbiota changes in response to metabolic and bariatric surgery: A systematic review. *Obes. Rev.* **2020**, *21*, e13025. [CrossRef]
20. Song, Y.; Joung, H. A traditional Korean dietary pattern and metabolic syndrome abnormalities. *Nutr. Metab. Cardiovasc. Dis.* **2012**, *22*, 456–462. [CrossRef] [PubMed]
21. Yoo, J.Y.; Rho, M.; You, Y.A.; Kwon, E.J.; Kim, M.H.; Kym, S.; Jee, Y.K.; Kim, Y.K.; Kim, Y.J. 16S rRNA gene-based metagenomic analysis reveals differences in bacteria-derived extracellular vesicles in the urine of pregnant and non-pregnant women. *Exp. Mol. Med.* **2016**, *48*, e208. [CrossRef] [PubMed]
22. Yang, J.; McDowell, A.; Seo, H.; Kim, S.; Min, T.K.; Jee, Y.K.; Choi, Y.; Park, H.S.; Pyun, B.Y.; Kim, Y.K. Diagnostic Models for Atopic Dermatitis Based on Serum Microbial Extracellular Vesicle Metagenomic Analysis: A Pilot Study. *Allergy Asthma Immunol. Res.* **2020**, *12*, 792–805. [CrossRef]
23. Yang, J.; McDowell, A.; Kim, E.K.; Seo, H.; Yum, K.; Lee, W.H.; Jee, Y.K.; Kim, Y.K. Consumption of a Leuconostoc holzapfelii-enriched synbiotic beverage alters the composition of the microbiota and microbial extracellular vesicles. *Exp. Mol. Med.* **2019**, *51*, 1–11. [CrossRef]
24. Kim, D.J.; Yang, J.; Seo, H.; Lee, W.H.; Ho Lee, D.; Kym, S.; Park, Y.S.; Kim, J.G.; Jang, I.J.; Kim, Y.K.; et al. Colorectal cancer diagnostic model utilizing metagenomic and metabolomic data of stool microbial extracellular vesicles. *Sci Rep.* **2020**, *10*, 2860. [CrossRef]
25. Ferreira, R.M.; Pereira-Marques, J.; Pinto-Ribeiro, I.; Costa, J.L.; Carneiro, F.; Machado, J.C.; Figueiredo, C. Gastric microbial community profiling reveals a dysbiotic cancer-associated microbiota. *Gut* **2018**, *67*, 226–236. [CrossRef]
26. Ahn, J.; Sinha, R.; Pei, Z.; Dominianni, C.; Wu, J.; Shi, J.; Goedert, J.J.; Hayes, R.B.; Yang, L. Human gut microbiome and risk for colorectal cancer. *J. Natl. Cancer Inst.* **2013**, *105*, 1907–1911. [CrossRef]
27. Huse, S.M.; Dethlefsen, L.; Huber, J.A.; Mark Welch, D.; Relman, D.A.; Sogin, M.L. Exploring microbial diversity and taxonomy using SSU rRNA hypervariable tag sequencing. *PLoS Genet.* **2008**, *4*, e1000255. [CrossRef]
28. Eckburg, P.B.; Bik, E.M.; Bernstein, C.N.; Purdom, E.; Dethlefsen, L.; Sargent, M.; Gill, S.R.; Nelson, K.E.; Relman, D.A. Diversity of the human intestinal microbial flora. *Science* **2005**, *308*, 1635–1638. [CrossRef]
29. Tang, W.H.; Kitai, T.; Hazen, S.L. Gut Microbiota in Cardiovascular Health and Disease. *Circ. Res.* **2017**, *120*, 1183–1196. [CrossRef]
30. Iraci, N.; Gaude, E.; Leonardi, T.; Costa, A.S.H.; Cossetti, C.; Peruzzotti-Jametti, L.; Bernstock, J.D.; Saini, H.K.; Gelati, M.; Vescovi, A.L.; et al. Extracellular vesicles are independent metabolic units with asparaginase activity. *Nat. Chem. Biol.* **2017**, *13*, 951–955. [CrossRef] [PubMed]
31. Fu, X.; Zeng, B.; Wang, P.; Wang, L.; Wen, B.; Li, Y.; Liu, H.; Bai, S.; Jia, G. Microbiome of Total Versus Live Bacteria in the Gut of Rex Rabbits. *Front. Microbiol.* **2018**, *9*, 733. [CrossRef]
32. Emerson, J.B.; Adams, R.I.; Román, C.M.B.; Brooks, B.; Coil, D.A.; Dahlhausen, K.; Ganz, H.H.; Hartmann, E.M.; Hsu, T.; Justice, N.B.; et al. Schrödinger's microbes: Tools for distinguishing the living from the dead in microbial ecosystems. *Microbiome* **2017**, *5*, 86. [CrossRef]
33. Palviainen, M.; Saraswat, M.; Varga, Z.; Kitka, D.; Neuvonen, M.; Puhka, M.; Joenväärä, S.; Renkonen, R.; Nieuwland, R.; Takatalo, M.; et al. Extracellular vesicles from human plasma and serum are carriers of extravesicular cargo-Implications for biomarker discovery. *PLoS ONE* **2020**, *15*, e0236439. [CrossRef]
34. Coumans, F.A.W.; Brisson, A.R.; Buzas, E.I.; Dignat-George, F.; Drees, E.E.E.; El-Andaloussi, S.; Emanueli, C.; Gasecka, A.; Hendrix, A.; Hill, A.F.; et al. Methodological Guidelines to Study Extracellular Vesicles. *Circ. Res.* **2017**, *120*, 1632–1648. [CrossRef]
35. Chiam, K.; Mayne, G.C.; Wang, T.; Watson, D.I.; Irvine, T.S.; Bright, T.; Smith, L.T.; Ball, I.A.; Bowen, J.M.; Keefe, D.M.; et al. Serum outperforms plasma in small extracellular vesicle microRNA biomarker studies of adenocarcinoma of the esophagus. *World J. Gastroenterol.* **2020**, *26*, 2570–2583. [CrossRef]
36. Yeaman, M.R. The role of platelets in antimicrobial host defense. *Clin. Infect. Dis.* **1997**, *25*, 951–968. [CrossRef]
37. Drago, L.; Bortolin, M.; Vassena, C.; Romanò, C.L.; Taschieri, S.; Del Fabbro, M. Plasma components and platelet activation are essential for the antimicrobial properties of autologous platelet-rich plasma: An in vitro study. *PLoS ONE* **2014**, *9*, e107813. [CrossRef]
38. Šimundić, A.M. Measures of Diagnostic Accuracy: Basic Definitions. *EJIFCC* **2009**, *19*, 203–211. [PubMed]
39. Samra, M.S.; Lim, D.H.; Han, M.Y.; Jee, H.M.; Kim, Y.K.; Kim, J.H. Bacterial Microbiota-derived Extracellular Vesicles in Children with Allergic Airway Diseases: Compositional and Functional Features. *Allergy Asthma Immunol. Res.* **2021**, *13*, 56–74. [CrossRef]
40. Samra, M.; Nam, S.K.; Lim, D.H.; Kim, D.H.; Yang, J.; Kim, Y.K.; Kim, J.H. Urine Bacteria-Derived Extracellular Vesicles and Allergic Airway Diseases in Children. *Int. Arch. Allergy Immunol.* **2019**, *178*, 150–158. [CrossRef] [PubMed]

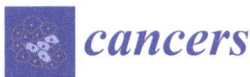

Article

Mutations in Epigenetic Regulation Genes in Gastric Cancer

Marina V. Nemtsova [1,2], Alexey I. Kalinkin [2], Ekaterina B. Kuznetsova [1,2], Irina V. Bure [1], Ekaterina A. Alekseeva [1,2], Igor I. Bykov [3], Tatiana V. Khorobrykh [3], Dmitry S. Mikhaylenko [1,2], Alexander S. Tanas [2] and Vladimir V. Strelnikov [2,*]

[1] Laboratory of Medical Genetics, I.M. Sechenov First Moscow State Medical University, 119991 Moscow, Russia; nemtsova_m_v@mail.ru (M.V.N.); kuznetsova.k@bk.ru (E.B.K.); bureira@mail.ru (I.V.B.); ekater.alekseeva@gmail.com (E.A.A.); dimserg@mail.ru (D.S.M.)

[2] Laboratory of Epigenetics, Research Centre for Medical Genetics, 115522 Moscow, Russia; akalinkin@epigenetic.ru (A.I.K.); atanas@med-gen.ru (A.S.T.)

[3] Department No. 1, Medical Faculty, Faculty Surgery, I.M. Sechenov First Moscow State Medical University, 119991 Moscow, Russia; igor-vr@mail.ru (I.I.B.); horobryh68@list.ru (T.V.K.)

* Correspondence: vstrel@list.ru

Simple Summary: Epigenetic mechanisms, such as DNA methylation/demethylation, covalent modifications of histone proteins, and chromatin remodeling, create specific patterns of gene expression. Epigenetic deregulations are associated with oncogenesis, relapse of the disease and metastases, and can serve as a useful clinical marker. We assessed the clinical relevance of integrity of the genes coding for epigenetic regulator proteins by mutational profiling of 25 genes in 135 gastric cancer (GC) samples. Overall, mutations in the epigenetic regulation genes were found to be significantly associated with reduced overall survival of patients in the group with metastases and in the group with tumors with signet ring cells. We have also discovered mutual exclusivity of somatic mutations in the *KMT2D*, *KMT2C*, *ARID1A*, and *CHD7* genes in our cohort. Our results suggest that mutations in epigenetic regulation genes may be valuable clinical markers and deserve further exploration in independent cohorts.

Abstract: We have performed mutational profiling of 25 genes involved in epigenetic processes on 135 gastric cancer (GC) samples. In total, we identified 79 somatic mutations in 49/135 (36%) samples. The minority ($n = 8$) of mutations was identified in DNA methylation/demethylation genes, while the majority ($n = 41$), in histone modifier genes, among which mutations were most commonly found in *KMT2D* and *KMT2C*. Somatic mutations in *KMT2D*, *KMT2C*, *ARID1A* and *CHD7* were mutually exclusive ($p = 0.038$). Mutations in *ARID1A* were associated with distant metastases ($p = 0.03$). The overall survival of patients in the group with metastases and in the group with tumors with signet ring cells was significantly reduced in the presence of mutations in epigenetic regulation genes ($p = 0.036$ and $p = 0.041$, respectively). Separately, somatic mutations in chromatin remodeling genes correlate with low survival rate of patients without distant metastasis ($p = 0.045$) and in the presence of signet ring cells ($p = 0.0014$). Our results suggest that mutations in epigenetic regulation genes may be valuable clinical markers and deserve further exploration in independent cohorts.

Keywords: gastric cancer; epigenetic regulation genes; somatic mutations; molecular genetic markers

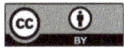

1. Introduction

Gastric cancer (GC) is the 5th most common tumor in the world, and is the 3rd leading cause of cancer-related deaths worldwide. In 2018, more than 1,000,000 new GC patients were identified [1].

Recently, knowledge about the molecular mechanisms of gastric carcinogenesis has been intensively expanded. By using genome-wide approaches, The Cancer Genome Atlas (TCGA) Research Network divided GC into four molecular subtypes: Epstein-Barr associated (EBV), microsatellite instability (MSI), genomically stable (GS), and chromosomal instable (CIN) [2]. Next-generation sequencing (NGS) technologies have allowed identification of genes with an increased frequency of somatic mutations in different types of tumors. Those are the driver genes of carcinogenesis. Being used as targets for a therapy, such genes allow effective treatment of patients. However, GC is not enriched with mutations in known driver genes. Therefore, the targeted drugs that are useful in the treatment of other types of tumors are not effective in GC. Despite the intensive search for new drugs for cancer therapy, only trastuzumab and ramucirumab targeting HER2 and VEGFR2, respectively, are currently approved for GC treatment. Therefore, the search for novel genes with an increased somatic mutation frequency in GC is urgent to identify new clinical and prognostic markers, as well as new targets for treatment.

Epigenetic mechanisms, including DNA methylation/demethylation, covalent modifications of histone proteins (methylation, adenylation, phosphorylation, etc.), chromatin remodeling, and the action of non-coding RNAs create stable and clear patterns of gene expression during cell life. Epigenetic mechanism deregulations are associated with carcinogenesis, relapse of the disease, and metastasis, and can also serve as a useful clinical marker and a marker of response to therapy [3]. Application of NGS allowed identification of tumors without mutations in the known cancer driver genes that are, however, characterized by mutations in genes encoding epigenetic factors and chromatin-modifying enzymes. Today, deregulation of epigenetic mechanisms in different types of tumors has been confirmed, but its causes are insufficiently studied [4,5].

Somatic mutation profiling of epigenetic regulation genes will help to identify causes of epigenetic deregulation in GC and to suggest potential targets for successful therapy.

Using an NGS panel of 25 genes (*DNMT1, MBD1, TET1, DNMT3A, DNMT3B, EZH2, KDM6A, EP300, JARID1B, CREBBP, HDAC2, SIRT1, SMARCB1, SMARCA2, SMARCA4, ARID1A, ARID2, BRD7, PBRM1, CHD5, CHD7, CHD4, KMT2A, KMT2D and KMT2C*), we performed somatic mutation profiling in 135 tumor samples obtained from patients with GC.

2. Materials and Methods

2.1. Patients and Tumor Samples

The study included 135 patients with locally advanced GC who were treated in N.N. Burdenko Faculty Surgery Clinic, I.M. Sechenov First Moscow State Medical University from 2007 to 2015. The study was conducted in accordance with the Declaration of Helsinki and was approved by the Institutional Ethics Committee of I.M. Sechenov First Moscow State Medical University. Written informed consent was obtained from each participant in this study. All patients underwent surgical treatment, and resected tumor samples, as well as non-malignant gastric mucosa samples, were used in the study. GC was confirmed in all patients by morphological examination of the surgical material. For TNM staging, ESMO Clinical Practice Guidelines for diagnosis, treatment, and follow-up for gastric cancer [6] were used. The distribution of patients in clinical groups is presented in Table 2.

2.2. Mutation Screening by NGS

A total of 5 to 7, 10 μm paraffin sections were manually dissected to ensure that each sample contained at least 70% of neoplastic cells. Genomic DNA was isolated from archived samples using a QIAamp DNA FFPE Tissue Kit (Qiagen, Hilden, Germany), as recommended by the manufacturer.

Deep sequencing was performed using the Ion Torrent platform (ThermoFisher, Waltham, MA, USA) following established protocol [7]. The protocol includes the preparation of libraries of genomic DNA fragments, clonal emulsion PCR, sequencing, and bioinformatic analysis of obtained results. DNA fragment libraries were prepared using Ion Ampliseq ultra-multiplex PCR technology.

An epigenetic regulation genes panel with 1376 primer pairs was designed to amplify all coding regions, noncoding regions of the terminal exons, and putative splice site gene regions for 25 human genes: *DNMT1, MBD1, TET1, DNMT3A, DNMT3B, EZH2, KDM6A,*

EP300, JARID1B, CREBBP, HDAC2, SIRT1, SMARCB1, SMARCA2, SMARCA4, ARID1A, ARID2, BRD7, PBRM1, CHD5, CHD7, CHD4, KMT2A, KMT2D and *KMT2C*. The panel was designed by using the Ion Ampliseq Designer v. 7.03 (ThermoFisher, Waltham, MA, USA). The total length of human genome sequences covered by the panel was 250,900 bp. The panel reached 98.09% coverage by design; this applies to exons and 25 bp flanking intron sequences. The information of the panel is shown in Tables S3 and S4. The selection of epigenetic regulation genes for the panel was based on the estimation of the frequency of their somatic mutations in GC, obtained from the COSMIC database and from the literature. Genes reported to be mutated in >3.5% of GC samples were included in the panel.

Multiplex PCR and subsequent stages of the fragment library preparation were performed using an Ion AmpliSeq Library Kit 2.0 (ThermoFisher, Waltham, MA, USA), according to the manufacturer's protocol. Aliquots from the prepared libraries were subjected to clonal amplification on microspheres in the emulsion on the Ion Chef Instrument (ThermoFisher, Waltham, MA, USA). Sequencing was performed on the Ion S5 genomic sequencer according to the manufacturer's protocol (ThermoFisher, Waltham, MA, USA) with the targeted sequencing depth of 1000×. The results were analyzed with Torrent Suite software consisting of Base Caller (the primary analysis of the sequencing results); Torrent Mapping Alignment Program—TMAP (alignment of the sequences to the reference genome GRCh37/hg19); and Torrent Variant Caller (analysis of variations in nucleotide sequences) with the cut-off for variant allele frequency set at 0.1, and minimum read depth of the variant allele set at 5. Genetic variants were annotated with ANNOVAR software [8]. Visual data analysis, manual filtering of sequencing artifacts, and sequence alignment were performed using the Integrative Genomics Viewer (IGV) [9].

2.3. Sanger Sequencing

Sanger sequencing was performed in order to (1) validate mutations detected by NGS screening and (2) distinguish somatic vs. germline mutations. For the second purpose, DNA samples extracted from archived non-malignant gastric mucosa of the same patients were used. The direct sequencing of individual PCR products from primers that flank areas of specific mutations were performed on the automatic genetic analyzer ABI PRISM 3500 (ThermoFisher, Waltham, MA, USA) according to the manufacturer's protocols.

2.4. Statistical Analysis

Samples were compared using Fisher's exact test. For more than 3 groups comparison Chi-squared test was used. Overall survival probability (OS) was calculated by the Kaplan–Meier product-limit method from the date of surgery till death by any cause and compared statistically using Mantel–Haenszel (log-rank) test. A groupwise mutual exclusivity test was carried out using the DISCOVER (Discrete Independence Statistic Controlling for Observations with Varying Rates) method, which is based on overall tumor-specific alteration rates to decide if alterations co-occur more or less than expected by chance and preventing spurious associations in co-occurrence detection with increasing statistical power to detect mutual exclusivities [10]. All calculations were conducted using R version 3.6.3 [R Core Team (2020). R: A language and environment for statistical computing. R Foundation for Statistical Computing, Vienna, Austria. URL https://www.R-project.org/ accessed on 7 August 2021].

2.5. Pathogenicity Prediction for Novel Mutations

To predict the pathogenicity of identified novel missense variants, a combination of PolyPhen2, PROVEAN, SIFT, and MutPred2 tools was used. I-Mutant 3.0 software was used to calculate the stability of the mutant protein. Loss of protein function effects were assessed with MutPred-LOF software. The effect of nonsynonymous substitutions on the structure was illustrated using the Project HOPE3D portal.

3. Results

3.1. The Spectrum of Detected Somatic Mutations

Using a targeted NGS panel for 25 epigenetic regulation genes, we performed mutational profiling in 135 tumor samples obtained from patients with GC. Our panel included the *DNMT1, MBD1, TET1, DNMT3A, DNMT3B* genes that control DNA methylation/demethylation; the *EZH2, UTX, EP300, JARID1B, CREBBP, HDAC2, SIRT1, KMT2A, KMT2D,* and *KMT2C* genes encoding histone modifiers; and the *SMARCB1, SMARCA2, SMARCA4, ARID1A, ARID2, BRD7, PBRM1, CHD5, CHD7, CHD4* genes responsible for chromatin remodeling. Mapped data depth and coverage for each sample are presented in Table S5. For the analysis, we selected missense substitutions that were not annotated in the ClinVar, COSMIC, dbSNP databases and/or substitutions with a population frequency of MAF < 0.0005, as well as nonsense mutations and frameshift mutations. A total of 79 different mutations found in our cohort fulfilled the selection criteria. The variant allele frequency, total read depth, reference, and variant allele read depths, etc., for each of these mutations, are presented in Table S1. No appropriate mutations were found in the *DNMT1, DNMT3A, EZH2, UTX, SMARCB1* and *SIRT1* genes. The identified mutations and their characteristics are presented in Table 1.

Table 1. Somatic mutations detected in epigenetic regulation genes in 135 gastric tumors.

№	Gene/Mutation	Position According to hg19	rsID	MAF (gnomAD Exomes)	ClinVar	# of Cases
1	ARID1A:exon1:c.G544A:p.A182T	chr1:27023438	-	-	-	1
2	ARID1A:exon16:c.G3902A:p.S1301N	chr1:27100106	rs989613588	A = 4×10^{-6}	Not Reported	1
3	ARID1A:exon18:c.G4245C:p.Q1415H	chr1:27100963	-	-	Not Reported	1
4	ARID1A:exon20:c.C6706T:p.R2236C	chr1:27107095	rs763691986	T = 2×10^{-5}	Not Reported	1
5	ARID1A:exon20:c.C5483G:p.S1828X	chr1:27105872	-	-	Not Reported	1
6	ARID1A:exon20:c.C5129T:p.P1710L	chr1:27105518	-	-	Not Reported	1
7	ARID1A:exon2:c.G1330A:p.G444S	chr1:27056334	rs541301347	A = 2.4×10^{-5}	Not Reported	1
8	ARID1A:exon20:c.5881_5887del:p.S1961fs	chr1:27106270	-	-	Not Reported	1
9	ARID1A:exon18:c.4713_4714del:p.N1571fs	chr1:27101431	-	-	Not Reported	1
10	ARID2:exon1:c.53_57del:p.A18fs	chr12:46123672	-	-	Not Reported	1
11	ARID2:exon8:c.C820T:p.R274X	chr12:46230571	-	-	Likely pathogenic	1
12	ARID2:exon8:c.C985T:p.Q329X	chr12:46230736	-	-	Not Reported	1
13	SMARCA2:exon7:c.C734T:p.T245M	chr9:2192726	rs753433101	A = 3×10^{-5}	Not Reported	1
14	SMARCA2:exon7:c.A1256G:p.K419R	chr9:2056754	-	-	Not Reported	1
15	SMARCA2:exon7:c.G1202A:p.R401H	chr9:2056700	rs745500947	T = 8×10^{-6}	Not Reported	1
16	SMARCA4:exon18:c.C2738T:p.P913L	chr19:11132522	rs778175819	T = 4×10^{-6}	Not Reported	1
17	SMARCA4:exon3:c.C430T:p.Q144X	chr19:11096939	-	-	Not Reported	1
18	SMARCA4:exon3:c.583delC:p.P195fs	chr19:11097092	-	-	Not Reported	1
19	KDM5B:exon17:c.C2392T:p.R798W	chr1:202711581	rs1189771603	A = 2.8×10^{-5}	Not Reported	1
20	CHD4:exon28:c.C4216T:p.R1406C	chr12:6692034	-	-	Not Reported	1
21	CHD4:exon4:c.417_419del:p.139_140del	chr12:6711145	rs71584865	del(TCC)3 = 8×10^{-6}	Not Reported	2
22	CHD4:exon4:c.C421G:p.P141A	chr12:6710929	-	-	Not Reported	1
23	CHD5:exon2:c.119delT:p.F40fs	chr1:6228298	-	-	Not Reported	1
24	CHD5:exon15:c.C2257A:p.L753M	chr1:6202367	-	-	Not Reported	1
25	CHD5:exon7:c.G910A:p.A304T	chr1:6211176	rs768430028	T = 1.3×10^{-4}	Not Reported	2
26	CHD5:exon2:c.A156T:p.K52N	chr1:6228261	rs964095593	A = 3×10^{-5}	Not Reported	1

Table 1. *Cont.*

№	Gene/Mutation	Position According to hg19	rsID	MAF (gnomAD Exomes)	ClinVar	# of Cases
27	CHD7:exon31:c.G6112A:p.D2038N	chr8:61765396	rs747846723	A = 6×10^{-5}	Uncertain Significance	1
28	CHD7:exon35:c.A7819G:p.S2607G	chr8:61773673	rs1424434796	G = 5×10^{-6}	Not Reported	2
29	CHD7:exon22:c.G4859A:p.R1620Q	chr8:61757431	rs768497646	A = 2.9×10^{-5}	Not Reported	1
30	CHD7:exon1:c.G749A:p.R250H	chr8:61654740	rs767475667	A = 6×10^{-5}	Not Reported	1
31	CHD7:exon22:c.G5017A:p.D1673N	chr8:61757589	rs769563309	A = 2.4×10^{-5}	Not Reported	1
32	CHD7:exon29:c.G5828A:p.R1943Q	chr8:61764740	rs753723769	A = 2.8×10^{-5}	Uncertain Significance	1
33	EP300:exon3:c.A752G:p.N251S	chr22:41521890	rs142009367	G = 2.2×10^{-4}	Benign	2
34	HDAC2:exon13:c.C1430A:p.T477N	chr6:114262878	rs1341257540	-	Not Reported	1
35	HDAC2:exon6:c.G511A:p.V171I	chr6:114274569	-	-	Not Reported	1
36	CREBBP:exon30:c.C6335T:p.P2112L	chr16:3778599	rs587783512	A = 1.6×10^{-5}	Uncertain Significance	1
37	CREBBP:exon2:c.C458T:p.P153L	chr16:3900638	rs146538907	A = 3.35×10^{-4}	Likely Benign	1
38	CREBBP:exon3:c.C922T:p.P308S	chr16:3860657	-	-	Not Reported	1
39	CREBBP:exon18:c.A3421C:p.K1141Q	chr16:3807998	-	-	Not Reported	1
40	BRD7:exon7:c.A871G:p.S291G	chr16:50368638	rs200218240	C = 1.6×10^{-4}	Not Reported	1
41	BRD7:exon5:c.C571T:p.Q191X	chr16:50383954	-	-	Not Reported	1
42	PBRM1:exon17:c.C2032T:p.R678C	chr3:52643864	rs1422119249	-	Not Reported	1
43	KMT2A:exon27:c.T9737C:p.I3246T	chr11:118376344	rs1259638674	C = 3×10^{-5}	Not Reported	1
44	KMT2A:exon27:c.C9947T:p.A3316V	chr11:118376554	rs201447376	T = 1.3×10^{-4}	Not Reported	1
45	KMT2A:exon27:c.G10181A:p.G3394E	chr11:118376788	rs782460936	A = 3×10^{-5}	Not Reported	1
46	KMT2A:exon21:c.G5726A:p.W1909X	chr11:118368712	-	-	Not Reported	1
47	KMT2A:exon27:c.G9247A:p.V3083I	chr11:118375854	-	-	Not Reported	1
48	KMT2A:exon30:c.A10984G:p.S3662G	chr11:118380746	rs201724738	G = 5.6×10^{-5}	Not Reported	1
49	KMT2A:exon36:c.G11903A:p.R3968Q	chr11:118392871	rs369182428	A = 3×10^{-5}	Not Reported	1
50	KMT2A:exon30:c.A10975G:p.S3659G	chr11:118380746	rs201724738	G = 1×10^{-4}	Not Reported	1
51	KMT2C:exon43:c.G9987A:p.M3329I	chr7:151860675	rs200804156	T = 6×10^{-5}	Not Reported	1
52	KMT2D:exon10:c.T2284C:p.S762P	chr12:49445182	-	-	Not Reported	1
53	KMT2C:exon10:c.C1384T:p.Q462X	chr7:151949716	-	-	Not Reported	1
54	KMT2C:exon36:c.C6836T:p.P2279L	chr7:151878109	rs150844259	A = 6×10^{-5}	Not Reported	1
55	KMT2C:exon36:c.A6919G:p.R2307G	chr7:151878026	rs772283102	C = 2.4×10^{-5}	Not Reported	1
56	KMT2C:exon36:c.G5858A:p.C1953Y	chr7:151879087	-	-	Not Reported	1
57	KMT2C:exon18:c.A2917G:p.R973G	chr7:151927067	rs60244562	-	Not Reported	2
58	KMT2C:exon18:c.G2877A:p.M959I	chr7:151927107	rs4024402	-	Not Reported	1
59	KMT2D:exon31:c.A7954C:p.M2652L	chr12:49433599	rs147706410	G = 4.5×10^{-4}	Likely Benign	1
60	KMT2D:exon41:c.G13780C:p.A4594P	chr12:49424443	rs545972414	G = 2.5×10^{-4}	Not Reported	2
61	KMT2D:exon28:c.C5921T:p.T1974M	chr12:49436060	rs777415982	A = 6×10^{-5}	Not Reported	1
62	KMT2D:exon48:c.G14893A:p.A4965T	chr12:49420856	rs200747934	T = 1.53×10^{-4}	Uncertain Significance	2
63	KMT2D:exon39:c.G12686A:p.R4229Q	chr12:49445262	rs753607446	T = 3.2×10^{-5}	Not Reported	1
64	KMT2D:exon31:c.T7829C:p.L2610P	chr12:49433724	rs200998047	G = 1.85×10^{-4}	Uncertain Significance	1
65	KMT2D:exon31:c.6673delG:p.E2225fs	chr12:49434880	-	-	Not Reported	1
66	KMT2D:exon31:c.C7516T:p.L2506F	chr12:49434037	rs749670394	A = 4×10^{-6}	Not Reported	1

Table 1. Cont.

№	Gene/Mutation	Position According to hg19	rsID	MAF (gnomAD Exomes)	ClinVar	# of Cases
67	KMT2D:exon39:c.C11179T:p.R3727C	chr12:49427309	rs566069597	A = 3.6 × 10^{-5}	Not Reported	1
68	KMT2D:exon10:c.C1628T:p.S543L	chr12:49445838	rs776242478	A = 8 × 10^{-6}	Not Reported	1
69	KMT2D:exon31:c.G8026T:p.E2676X	chr12:49433527	-	-	Not Reported	1
70	KMT2D:exon31:c.C7136T:p.A2379V	chr12:49434417	rs200842315	A = 6 × 10^{-5}	Likely benign	1
71	KMT2D:exon39:c.C11495G:p.S3832C	chr12:49426993	-	-	Not Reported	1
72	MBD1:exon9:c.G796A:p.E266K	chr18:47801382	rs142015383	T = 5 × 10^{-4}	Not Reported	1
73	MBD1:exon8:c.734delC:p.P245fs	chr18:47801527	rs1173827934	-	Not Reported	1
74	TET1:exon4:c.G2407A:p.A803T	chr10:70404893	rs765094207	A = 2.4 × 10^{-5}	Not Reported	1
75	TET1:exon2:c.G320A:p.R107Q	chr10:70332415	rs1419371452	A = 8 × 10^{-6}	Not Reported	1
76	TET1:exon4:c.G3476A:p.R1159Q	chr10:70405962	rs140289196	A = 2.2 × 10^{-4}	Not Reported	1
77	DNMT3B:exon19:c.G2138A:p.R713Q	chr20:31390243	rs747182299	A = 3 × 10^{-5}	Likely Pathogenic	1
78	DNMT3B:exon6:c.A680G:p.Y227C	chr20:31379501	-	-	Not Reported	1
79	DNMT3B:exon17:c.G1855A:p.E619K	chr20:31388054	rs576798456	A = 8 × 10^{-6}	Not Reported	1

In total, we revealed 79 somatic mutations that fulfilled the selection criteria in 49/135 (36%) samples, and no mutations were found in the remaining samples. Among the identified variants, 29/79 were not annotated in dbSNP, 32/79 were not mentioned in gnomAD Exomes, and 68/79 were not mentioned in ClinVar.

The largest number of mutations was determined in histone modifier genes (41), and in chromatin remodeling genes (37). The smallest number was in DNA methylation/demethylation genes (8). Taking into consideration variation in the gene size, we normalized the mutation numbers in these three groups. Of the genes under study, histone modifier genes contained collectively 24,207 codons; chromatin remodeling genes, 16,891 codons, and DNA methylation/demethylation genes, 6188 codons. Thus, frequencies of mutations in these three groups were 0.0017, 0.0022, and 0.0013 per codon, respectively. These figures support a somewhat lower somatic mutation burden on the DNA methylation/demethylation genes, although the differences were not statistically significant. The distribution of variants in the epigenetic regulation genes in our patient samples was as follows: *KMT2D*-16, *ARID1A*-9, *KMT2A*-8, *KMT2C*-8, *CHD7*-7, *CHD5*-5, *CHD4*, *CREBBP*-4 each, *ARID2*, *SMARCA2*, *SMARCA4*, *DNMT3B* and *TET1*-3 each, *HDAC2*, *EP300*, *BRD7* and *MBD1*-2 each, and *PBRM1*, *JARID1B*-1. In 23/49 samples, a combination of more than one mutation in different genes was demonstrated, but mutations in *KMT2D*, *KMT2C*, *ARID1A*, and *CHD7* were significantly rarely found in one and the same sample ($p = 0.038$).

3.2. Pathogenicity Analysis of the Detected Mutations by Prediction Programs

For all novel mutations that fulfilled the selection criteria, pathogenicity analysis was performed by using prediction programs. By in silico analysis of pathogenicity for somatic alterations, we determined that 15/63 alterations were pathogenic according to more than two prediction tools. PolyPhen2-HumDiv predicted 26 of those as 'Probably damaging', and the other 15 were 'Possibly Damaging', whereas PolyPhen2-HumVar predicted 17 alterations as 'Probably damaging', 11 alterations as 'Possibly damaging', while other 35 alterations were 'Benign'. However, it should be noticed that PolyPhen2-HumVar is more effective in mutations pathogenicity prediction for Mendelian disorders. 26/63 somatic alterations were predicted as 'Deleterious' by PROVEAN prediction tool; 42/63 variants were indicated as 'Damaging' by SIFT.

MutPred2 and MutPred-LOF are machine learning approaches, which incorporate genetic and molecular information to predict whether the alteration is pathogenic or not. We assigned a threshold value of 0.68 for pathogenic, as recommended by developers, because it yields a false positive rate of 10%. With this assumption, 11/63 somatic missense variants were predicted as pathogenic, as well as and 10/16 nonsense and frameshift variants, by MutPred-LOF with a cut-off value of 0.50 (as recommended for MutPred-LOF).

I-Mutant 3.0 predicts protein stability changes based on a protein sequence or protein structure by using a support vector machine training algorithm. The I-Mutant 3.0 predicted a decrease in protein structure stability for 44 somatic alterations and an increase for the other 19 (Table S2).

3.3. Analysis of Clinical Significance of Mutations in Epigenetic Regulation Genes

The distribution of mutations in our patient cohort aligned to clinical features is shown in Figure 1.

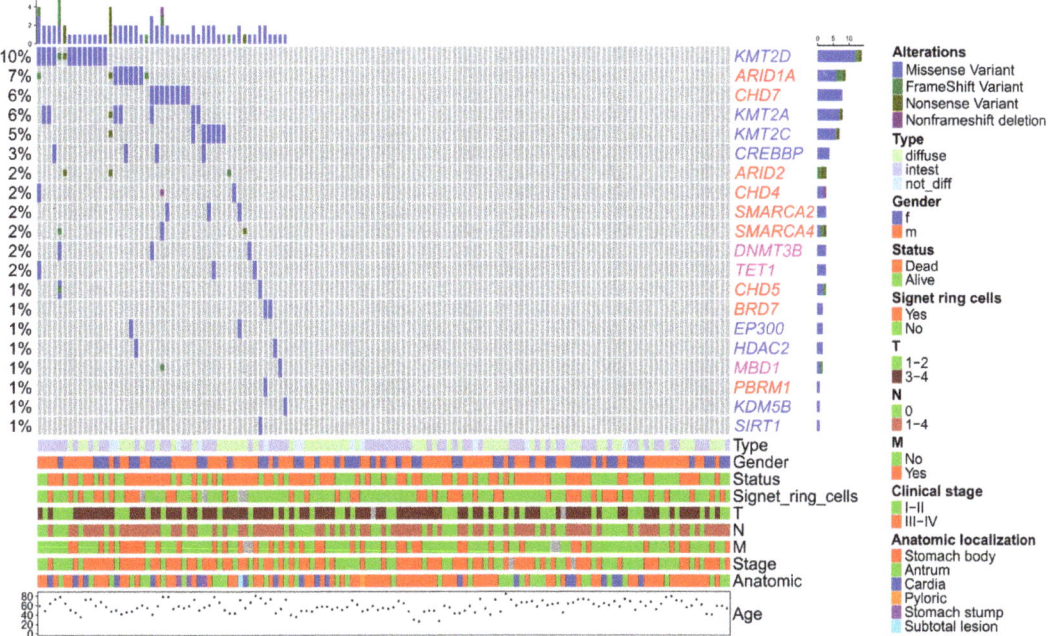

Figure 1. Spectrum of epigenetic regulation genes somatic mutations in gastric cancer. Gene names are marked according to functions of the encoded proteins: histone modifiers, blue; chromatin remodeling, red; DNA methylation/demethylation, magenta.

We found no associations of overall somatic mutation status (absence of mutations vs. presence of at least one mutation) of epigenetic regulation genes with gender, age, tumor size, lymph node metastases, stage, anatomical localization, Lauren type, distant metastases, and presence of signet ring cells (Table 2). As for individual genes, we have only discovered that mutations in *ARID1A* were associated with distant metastases ($p = 0.03$).

Table 2. Clinical characteristics of patients and their distribution by groups with mutations (mut+) and without mutations (mut−) in epigenetic regulation genes.

Parameters		Total Cases	Mut−	Mut+	p-Value *
		135	86	49	
Age	<50	35	22	13	1
	>50	100	64	36	
Sex	m	83	51	32	0.58
	f	52	35	17	
Survival status	Alive	59	42	17	0.14
	Dead	76	44	32	
5-year survival status	Alive	60	42	18	0.19
	Dead	69	40	29	
	<5 years follow-up	6	4	2	
T	T1-2	49	33	16	0.46
	T3-4	84	51	33	
	is	2	2	-	
N	N0	56	37	19	0.71
	N1-3	79	49	30	
M	M0	89	59	30	0.55
	M1	42	25	17	
	Unknown	4	-	-	
Lauren classification	Diffuse	59	41	18	0.26
	Intestinal	64	38	26	
	Not Differentiate	12	7	5	
Stage	I-II	57	39	18	0.36
	III-IV	76	45	31	
	Unknown	2	-	-	
Anatomical localization	Stomach body	75	52	23	0.10
	Antrum	36	22	14	
	Cardia	20	11	8	
	Stomach stump	3	0	3	
	Subtotal lesion	1	0	1	
	Pyloric	1	1	0	
Signet ring cells	yes	42	29	13	0.69
	no	89	57	32	
	Unknown	4	0	4	

* patients group with mutations in epigenetic regulation genes (mut+) vs. without mutations (mut−).

In the analysis of survival using the Kaplan–Meier method, we found that the overall survival of patients in the group with metastases and the group of tumors with signet ring cells was significantly reduced in the presence of mutations in the epigenetic regulation genes ($p = 0.036$ and $p = 0.042$, respectively) comparing with patients without mutations (Figure 2).

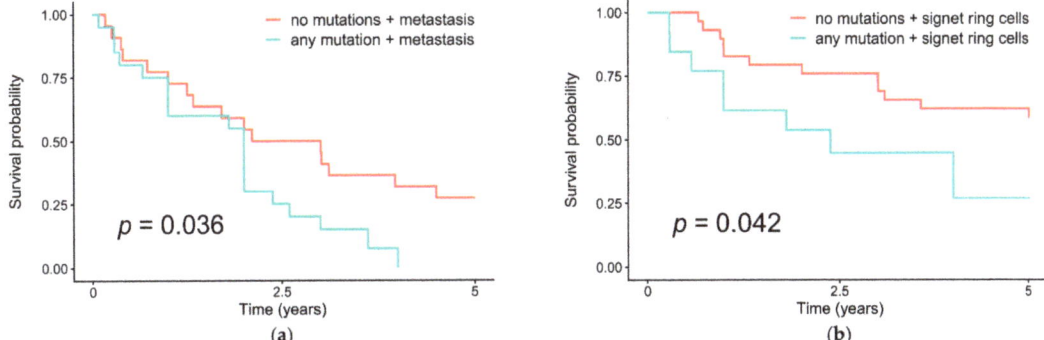

Figure 2. Overall survival in patients with and without somatic mutations of the epigenetic regulation genes in their gastric tumors, and (**a**) with distant metastases; (**b**) with the presence of signet ring cells in tumors.

Somatic mutations in the chromatin remodeling genes correlate with a low survival rate of patients in the absence of distant metastases (p = 0.045) and with the presence of signet ring cells in tumors (p = 0.0014) (Figure 3).

For the group of histone-modifying genes, no significant clinical correlations were found. The group with mutations in the DNA methylation/demethylation genes included only 8 patients and was too small to perform statistical analysis.

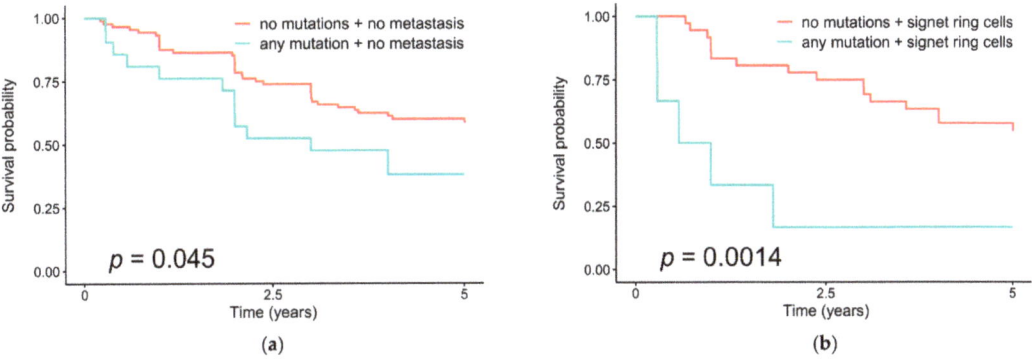

Figure 3. Overall survival in patients with and without somatic mutations of the chromatin remodeling genes in their gastric tumors, and (**a**) with distant metastases; (**b**) with the presence of signet ring cells in tumors.

4. Discussion

Somatic mutations in epigenetic regulation genes are not very common in GC and were determined only in 36% samples (49/135) in our study. Mutations were most rarely detected in genes regulating DNA methylation/demethylation. We have not found any somatic mutations in *DNMT1* and *DNMT3A*. Besides, the group of patients with mutations in the DNA methylation-related genes (*MBD1*, *TET1*, *DNMT3B*) was the smallest one with only 8 out of 135 patients. Such a low frequency may be a result of the cancer type being investigated. Chai-Jin Lee et al. demonstrated that frequencies of somatic mutations in genes associated with DNA methylation and demethylation (*DNMT1*, *DNMT3A*, *MBD1*, *MBD4*, *TET1*, *TET2* and *TET3*) significantly varied in different types of cancers. Thus, in myeloid leukemia samples, the frequency of *DNMT1* and *DNMT3A* mutations was high, whereas, in glioblastoma, renal cell carcinoma, and colon carcinoma, the total mutation rate was less than 9% [11]. The low frequency of mutations in the DNA methylation drivers in solid tumors is consistent with our results. Many studies have been published demonstrating DNA methylation as a clinical marker of carcinogenesis; however, the role of somatic mutations in genes regulating methylation/demethylation in solid tumors has not yet been sufficiently investigated. Moreover, although we did not find any *DNMT3A* mutations in our samples, they were identified in other solid tumors. In 1.2% of papillary thyroid carcinoma cases, mutations and/or loss of *DNMT3A* expression were associated with aggressive clinical course and poor outcome [12].

In our work, the largest number of mutations was detected in histone modification genes (52%, 41/79), with 16 mutations in *KMT2D*, 8 in *KMT2C*, and 8 in *KMT2A*. The proteins encoded by these KMT2 (histone-lysine N-methyltransferases subclass 2) genes were components of a COMPASS-like complex that performs mono-, di-, and trimethylation of lysine 4 (H3K4) in histone 3 and is associated with transcription activation, facilitating access of transcription factors to the promoter and enhancer regions of genes [13]. The functions of COMPASS complexes are vitally important for the normal development of an organism, and mutations in genes encoding their protein components are associated with carcinogenesis [14]. KMT2C and KMT2D proteins restrain cell proliferation and could be considered tumor suppressors [15]. In addition to lysine methylation associated with transcription activation, methyltransferases KMT2C and KMT2D play an important role in the maintenance of genomic stability and DNA repair [16]. Besides, these proteins, together with PTIP (PAX transactivation-domain interacting protein), a subunit of the KMT2C/KMT2D complexes, were found to increase the instability and induce the degradation of the MRE11-dependent replication fork in BRCA-deficient cells [17].

The *KMT2D* and *KMT2C* genes are among the most frequently mutated in cancers, which is also confirmed by our study. Mutations were detected in various types of solid tumors, such as melanoma, urothelial carcinoma, lung cancer, as well as in esophageal and stomach cancers [18].

In our study, *KMT2D* mutations had the highest frequency of 12% and were distributed throughout the gene (Figure 4). Mutations of the *KMT2D* gene are mainly localized in the central part of the gene coding sequence, which corresponds to the protein region between the PHD-finger domain and the SET domain. This is also in concordance with the data obtained by other authors [19].

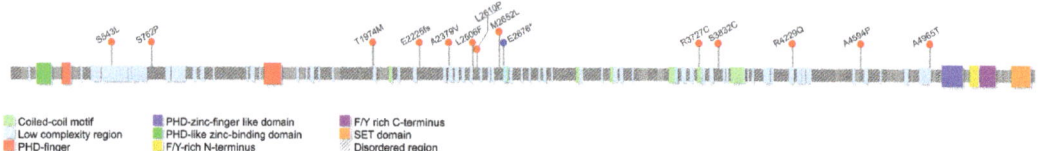

Figure 4. Distribution of the *KMT2D* mutations detected in this study, along the gene.

According to the analysis by pathogenicity prediction programs, one of the novel somatic missense mutations that we identified in the *KMT2D* gene, p.R3727C, was determined as pathogenic by almost all prediction tools. This substitution results in disruption of the leucine zipper motif, which was necessary for the protein–protein interactions or dimerization [20]. Disruption of the leucine zipper motif seriously alters the function of proteins, which leads to a deregulation of protein interactions and blocking transcription. Directed alterations of the leucine zipper motif are currently created in synthetic proteins that are used as antitumor drugs [21].

The analysis of pathogenicity of unannotated mutations identified by us in *KMT2C* revealed three mutations (p.R973G, p.M959I, p.C1953Y) that were pathogenic according to three or more prediction tools. The first two of them were located in the PHD-finger domain of the gene, and p.C1953Y was located in the disorder domain. Disorder domains are characterized by high instability, and substitutions in this region can change the protein conformation. Recent studies have demonstrated that around 20% of mutations in cancers are located in these regions, causing abnormalities of protein conformations and functions [22]. Mutations in *KMT2C* in diffuse GC are associated with epithelial–mesenchymal transition (EMT) and acquisition of the mesenchymal phenotype by cells and are also markers of a poor prognosis [23]. Mutation distribution along the *KMT2C* gene is shown in Figure 5.

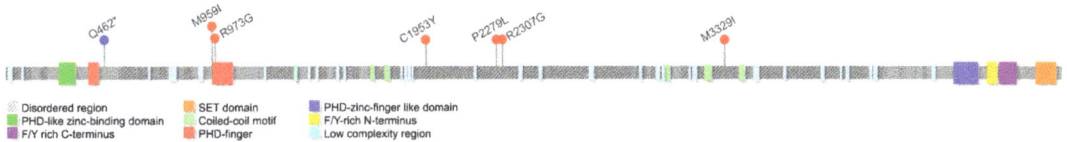

Figure 5. Distribution of the *KMT2C* mutations detected in this study, along the gene.

In our study, mutations in the *KMT2D* and *KMT2C* were significantly rarely combined in one sample (p = 0.038). There is a hypothesis that mutually exclusive genomic events are functionally related by common biological pathways, and mutually exclusive genes act on the same downstream effectors, thereby demonstrating functional redundancy. Therefore, the aberration of one of these genes is enough to completely disrupt their common pathways [24]. The *KMT2D* and *KMT2C* are components of similar COMPASS complexes that perform the same function. Deregulation of either *KMT2C* or *KMT2D* separately can serve as a driver mutation at the early stages of carcinogenesis, leading to changes in the epigenomic landscape. As was demonstrated for bladder cancer, tumor cells with low KMT2C activity experienced a deficiency of DNA repair mediated by homologous recombination and suffer from endogenous DNA damage and genomic instability, and their treatment with the PARP1/2 inhibitor olaparib leads to synthetic lethality [16]. The high frequency of *KMT2D* and *KMT2C* mutations in GC and its associations with repair processes allows considering them as targets for tumor treatment using PARP inhibitors, causing the lethality of tumor cells.

We compared our result on mutual exclusivity of *KMT2D* and *KMT2C* mutations with other GC mutation databases. Three datasets were acquired using cBioPortal (http://cbioportal.org accessed on 7 August 2021): Gastric Cancer (OncoSG, 2018), Stomach Adenocarcinoma (Pfizer and UHK), and TCGA PanCancer Stomach Adenocarcinoma (STAD). Visual analysis suggested that *KMT2D* and *KMT2C* mutations in these datasets were not mutually exclusive (Figure 6). For statistical analysis, we retained only sequenced samples with mutation data (without Copy-Number Alterations) in all three studies. For the groupwise mutual exclusive test, p-values were as follows: 0.088 for Onco SG, 0.016 for TCGA STAD, and 0.5 for the Pfizer study. Using the wFisher p-value combination method [25] with sample size for each experiment, we obtained the p-value of the mutual exclusive test under the nominal significance level of 0.05 (Figure 6a). Another interesting observation was that considering missense mutations only, mutations in *KMT2D* and *KMT2C* visually were almost mutually exclusive in these three datasets, as they were in our study (Figure 6b), although calculated differences did not approach a significance level of 0.05, which we attributed to the sample sizes. In this respect, we paid attention to the studies of bigger sample size, though of another cancer localization, namely, Breast Cancer METABRIC, Nature 2012, and Nat Commun 2016 (2509 samples) and Breast Cancer MSK, Cancer Cell 2018 (1918 samples), and in these datasets, we witnessed obvious mutual exclusivity of somatic mutations in *KMT2D*, *KMT2C*, and *ARID1A*. Although this may be a cancer type-specific observation, we altogether cannot rule out sample size effect and/or peculiarities of mutation detection/interpretation in different studies.

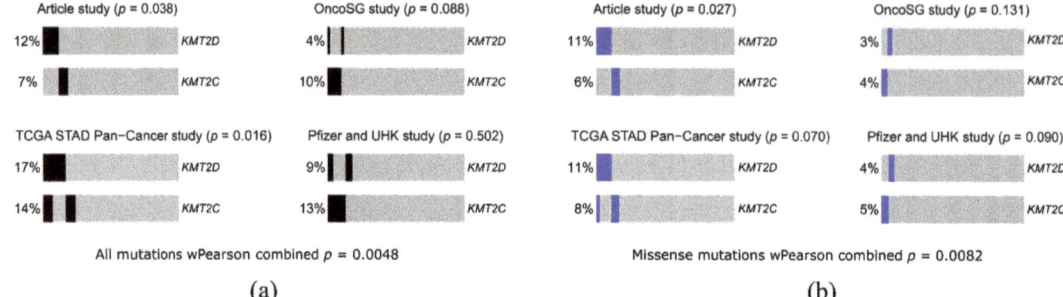

Figure 6. Analysis of mutual exclusivity of *KMT2D* and *KMT2C* mutations on the data presented in this article and in other gastric cancer mutation databases. Portions of samples without mutations in *KMT2D* or *KMT2C* are shown in grey; (a) analysis of all types of mutations, excluding amplification and deep deletions, portions of samples with mutations in *KMT2D* or *KMT2C* are colored black; (b) analysis of missense mutations only, portions of samples with missense mutations in *KMT2D* or *KMT2C* are colored blue.

The *ARID1A* and *CHD7* genes that are related to chromatin remodeling were often mutated in our patient samples. The *ARID1A* is often mutated in esophageal and gastric cancers and is the canonical cancer gene according to the Cosmic Cancer Gene Census [26]. The proteins encoded by the *ARID1A*, *SMARCA1*, *SMARCA2*, and *SMARCA4* are subunits of the conservative multisubunit SWI/SNF complex, which uses the energy of ATP hydrolysis to mobilize nucleosomes and remodel chromatin. The expression of these genes is often deregulated in the esophagus and gastric cancers [27].

ARID1A substitutions that we identified in gastric tumors, not annotated in human mutation databases, namely p.R2236C, p.Q1415H, and p.P1710L, are of interest since they can lead to deregulation of molecular mechanisms important for cancer progression. According to the results of in silico analysis, the p.R2236C substitution results in aberration of ADP-ribosylation, which is important for the DNA damage repair, as well as for the formation of an allosteric site at p.R2233 that can be used to bind therapeutic agents. Today, the search and targeting of allosteric sites are one of the strategies in the development of antitumor drugs [28].

ARID1A:p.Q1415H and ARID1A:p.P1710L amino acid substitutions demonstrate an overall predicted loss of O- and C-linked glycosylation. Post-translational modifications, such as glycosylation, affect the transport, stability, and folding of the protein, changing its biochemical and biophysical properties. Numerous studies confirmed that changes in protein glycosylation have a great impact on carcinogenesis and contribute to the appearance of more aggressive cell phenotypes [29].

Recent studies demonstrated that mutations in genes and abnormal expression of the ISO/SNF complex proteins that participate in chromatin remodeling were associated with a more aggressive course of the disease, as well as with EBV and MSI subtypes of GC [30]. In our study, somatic mutations in the chromatin remodeling genes were also found to be associated with worse overall survival in patients (without distant metastases, $p = 0.045$; and in the presence of signet ring cells, an indicator of the aggressive course in GC, $p = 0.00011$). H. Takeshima et al. investigated the role of chromatin remodelers in GC and suggested that deregulations of chromatin remodeling occur at an early stage of gastric carcinogenesis and are involved in the formation of the field cancerization [31].

Investigation of GC using NGS previously revealed that 47% of gastric adenocarcinomas were characterized by mutations of chromatin remodeling genes, and somatic mutations of *ARID1A* had a high frequency, as it was in our study. It was shown that gastrointestinal tumors with *ARID1A* mutations demonstrated high immune activity [32]. Gastric carcinomas with somatic *ARID1A* mutations were characterized by a more intense PD-L1 expression than tumors without mutations. PD-L1 overexpression contributes to a more active response to immunotherapy and a better prognosis of survival for patients with mutations in *ARID1A* compared to tumors with wild-type *ARID1A*. *ARID1A* mutations can serve as a biomarker for the identification of patients with gastrointestinal cancer who are sensitive to immunotherapy [33]. Clinically, the loss of *ARID1A* expression was correlated with larger tumor size, deeper invasion, lymph node metastasis, and a poor prognosis [34]. In line with these observations, in our study, mutations in *ARID1A* were associated with distant metastases ($p = 0.03$).

5. Conclusions

As a result of somatic mutation profiling of epigenetic regulation genes in GC, we have revealed associations of the presence of such mutations in tumors with a decrease in patient survival and the risk of developing distant metastasis, making the presence of mutations a marker of a poor prognosis. Studying mutations in epigenetic regulation genes can also contribute to the development of new approaches to drug therapy for GC treatment, adding to them PARP inhibitors for the treatment of tumors with mutations in genes of the *KMT2* family and immunotherapy for the treatment of tumors with *ARID1A* mutations. According to our results, this may be a significant group of patients, as the total frequency of mutations in the chromatin remodeling genes and histone modifiers in our sample were approximately 25% of all patients with mutations in epigenetic regulation genes.

Supplementary Materials: The following are available online at https://www.mdpi.com/article/10.3390/cancers13184586/s1, Table S1: variant allele frequency, total read depth, reference, and variant allele read depths for each mutation, Table S2: in silico analysis of somatic mutations found in gastric cancer samples, Tables S3 and S4: designed coverage of the NGS panel, Table S5: mapped data depth and coverage for each sample.

Author Contributions: Conceptualization, M.V.N.; data curation, M.V.N. and I.V.B.; funding acquisition, M.V.N.; investigation, M.V.N., A.I.K., I.I.B. and T.V.K.; methodology, E.B.K. and E.A.A.; software, A.I.K. and A.S.T.; supervision, M.V.N.; validation, E.B.K. and D.S.M.; visualization, A.I.K. and V.V.S.; writing—review and editing, I.V.B. and V.V.S. All authors have read and agreed to the published version of the manuscript.

Funding: This work was supported by the Russian Foundation for Basic Research (project 18-29-09020) and the Ministry of Science and Higher Education of the Russian Federation.

Institutional Review Board Statement: The study was conducted according to the guidelines of the Declaration of Helsinki, and approved by the Ethics Committee of Sechenov First Moscow State Medical University (Sechenov University), 13 July 2016 (protocol 04-19).

Informed Consent Statement: Informed consent was obtained from all subjects involved in the study.

Data Availability Statement: The data presented in this study are available in the article and supplementary files.

Conflicts of Interest: The authors declare no conflict of interest. The funders had no role in the design of the study; in the collection, analyses, or interpretation of data; in the writing of the manuscript, or in the decision to publish the results.

References

1. Bray, F.; Ferlay, J.; Soerjomataram, I.; Siegel, R.L.; Torre, L.A.; Jemal, A. Global Cancer Statistics 2018: GLOBOCAN Estimates of Incidence and Mortality Worldwide for 36 Cancers in 185 Countries. *CA Cancer J. Clin.* **2018**, *68*, 394–424. [CrossRef]
2. Cancer Genome Atlas Research Network. Comprehensive Molecular Characterization of Gastric Adenocarcinoma. *Nature* **2014**, *513*, 202–209. [CrossRef] [PubMed]
3. Thomas, M.; Marcato, P. Epigenetic Modifications as Biomarkers of Tumor Development, Therapy Response, and Recurrence across the Cancer Care Continuum. *Cancers* **2018**, *10*, 101. [CrossRef] [PubMed]
4. You, J.S.; Jones, P.A. Cancer Genetics and Epigenetics: Two Sides of the Same Coin? *Cancer Cell* **2012**, *22*, 9–20. [CrossRef] [PubMed]
5. Nemtsova, M.V.; Mikhaylenko, D.S.; Kuznetsova, E.B.; Bykov, I.I.; Zamyatnin, A.A. Inactivation of Epigenetic Regulators Due to Mutations in Solid Tumors. *Biochemistry* **2020**, *85*, 735–748. [CrossRef] [PubMed]

6. Smyth, E.C.; Verheij, M.; Allum, W.; Cunningham, D.; Cervantes, A.; Arnold, D. Gastric Cancer: ESMO Clinical Practice Guidelines for Diagnosis, Treatment and Follow-Up. *Ann. Oncol.* **2016**, *27*, v38–v49. [CrossRef] [PubMed]
7. Scarpa, A.; Sikora, K.; Fassan, M.; Rachiglio, A.M.; Cappellesso, R.; Antonello, D.; Amato, E.; Mafficini, A.; Lambiase, M.; Esposito, C.; et al. Molecular Typing of Lung Adenocarcinoma on Cytological Samples Using a Multigene Next Generation Sequencing Panel. *PLoS ONE* **2013**, *8*, e80478. [CrossRef]
8. Wang, K.; Li, M.; Hakonarson, H. ANNOVAR: Functional Annotation of Genetic Variants from High-Throughput Sequencing Data. *Nucleic Acids Res.* **2010**, *38*, e164. [CrossRef]
9. Robinson, J.T.; Thorvaldsdóttir, H.; Winckler, W.; Guttman, M.; Lander, E.S.; Getz, G.; Mesirov, J.P. Integrative Genomics Viewer. *Nat. Biotechnol.* **2011**, *29*, 24–26. [CrossRef]
10. Cerami, E.; Gao, J.; Dogrusoz, U.; Gross, B.E.; Sumer, S.O.; Aksoy, B.A.; Jacobsen, A.; Byrne, C.J.; Heuer, M.L.; Larsson, E.; et al. The CBio Cancer Genomics Portal: An Open Platform for Exploring Multidimensional Cancer Genomics Data. *Cancer Discov.* **2012**, *2*, 401–404. [CrossRef]
11. Lee, C.-J.; Ahn, H.; Jeong, D.; Pak, M.; Moon, J.H.; Kim, S. Impact of Mutations in DNA Methylation Modification Genes on Genome-Wide Methylation Landscapes and Downstream Gene Activations in Pan-Cancer. *BMC Med. Genom.* **2020**, *13*, 27. [CrossRef] [PubMed]
12. Siraj, A.K.; Pratheeshkumar, P.; Parvathareddy, S.K.; Bu, R.; Masoodi, T.; Iqbal, K.; Al-Rasheed, M.; Al-Dayel, F.; Al-Sobhi, S.S.; Alzahrani, A.S.; et al. Prognostic Significance of DNMT3A Alterations in Middle Eastern Papillary Thyroid Carcinoma. *Eur. J. Cancer* **2019**, *117*, 133–144. [CrossRef]
13. Fagan, R.J.; Dingwall, A.K. COMPASS Ascending: Emerging Clues Regarding the Roles of MLL3/KMT2C and MLL2/KMT2D Proteins in Cancer. *Cancer Lett.* **2019**, *458*, 56–65. [CrossRef] [PubMed]
14. Herz, H.-M.; Hu, D.; Shilatifard, A. Enhancer Malfunction in Cancer. *Mol. Cell* **2014**, *53*, 859–866. [CrossRef] [PubMed]
15. Chen, C.; Liu, Y.; Rappaport, A.R.; Kitzing, T.; Schultz, N.; Zhao, Z.; Shroff, A.S.; Dickins, R.A.; Vakoc, C.R.; Bradner, J.E.; et al. MLL3 Is a Haploinsufficient 7q Tumor Suppressor in Acute Myeloid Leukemia. *Cancer Cell* **2014**, *25*, 652–665. [CrossRef] [PubMed]
16. Rampias, T.; Karagiannis, D.; Avgeris, M.; Polyzos, A.; Kokkalis, A.; Kanaki, Z.; Kousidou, E.; Tzetis, M.; Kanavakis, E.; Stravodimos, K.; et al. The Lysine-specific Methyltransferase KMT 2C/MLL 3 Regulates DNA Repair Components in Cancer. *EMBO Rep.* **2019**, *20*, 6821. [CrossRef] [PubMed]
17. Poreba, E.; Lesniewicz, K.; Durzynska, J. Aberrant Activity of Histone–Lysine N-Methyltransferase 2 (KMT2) Complexes in Oncogenesis. *Int. J. Mol. Sci.* **2020**, *21*, 9340. [CrossRef]
18. Gao, J.; Aksoy, B.A.; Dogrusoz, U.; Dresdner, G.; Gross, B.; Sumer, S.O.; Sun, Y.; Jacobsen, A.; Sinha, R.; Larsson, E.; et al. Integrative Analysis of Complex Cancer Genomics and Clinical Profiles Using the CBioPortal. *Sci. Signal.* **2013**, *6*, pl1. [CrossRef]
19. Ding, B.; Yan, L.; Zhang, Y.; Wang, Z.; Zhang, Y.; Xia, D.; Ye, Z.; Xu, H. Analysis of the Role of Mutations in the KMT 2D Histone Lysine Methyltransferase in Bladder Cancer. *FEBS Open Bio* **2019**, *9*, 693–706. [CrossRef]
20. Manna, P.R.; Dyson, M.T.; Stocco, D.M. Role of Basic Leucine Zipper Proteins in Transcriptional Regulation of the Steroidogenic Acute Regulatory Protein Gene. *Mol. Cell Endocrinol.* **2009**, *302*, 1–11. [CrossRef]
21. Inamoto, I.; Shin, J.A. Peptide Therapeutics That Directly Target Transcription Factors. *Pept. Sci.* **2019**, *111*, e24048. [CrossRef]
22. Mészáros, B.; Hajdu-Soltész, B.; Zeke, A.; Dosztányi, Z. Mutations of Intrinsically Disordered Protein Regions Can Drive Cancer but Lack Therapeutic Strategies. *Biomolecules* **2021**, *11*, 381. [CrossRef]
23. Cho, S.-J.; Yoon, C.; Lee, J.H.; Chang, K.K.; Lin, J.-X.; Kim, Y.-H.; Kook, M.-C.; Aksoy, B.A.; Park, D.J.; Ashktorab, H.; et al. KMT2C Mutations in Diffuse-Type Gastric Adenocarcinoma Promote Epithelial-to-Mesenchymal Transition. *Clin. Cancer Res.* **2018**, *24*, 6556–6569. [CrossRef]
24. Deng, Y.; Luo, S.; Deng, C.; Luo, T.; Yin, W.; Zhang, H.; Zhang, Y.; Zhang, X.; Lan, Y.; Ping, Y.; et al. Identifying Mutual Exclusivity across Cancer Genomes: Computational Approaches to Discover Genetic Interaction and Reveal Tumor Vulnerability. *Brief. Bioinform.* **2019**, *20*, 254–266. [CrossRef] [PubMed]
25. Yoon, S.; Baik, B.; Park, T.; Nam, D. Powerful P-Value Combination Methods to Detect Incomplete Association. *Sci. Rep.* **2021**, *11*, 6980. [CrossRef] [PubMed]
26. Dietlein, F.; Weghorn, D.; Taylor-Weiner, A.; Richters, A.; Reardon, B.; Liu, D.; Lander, E.S.; Van Allen, E.M.; Sunyaev, S.R. Identification of Cancer Driver Genes Based on Nucleotide Context. *Nat. Genet.* **2020**, *52*, 208–218. [CrossRef]
27. Schallenberg, S.; Bork, J.; Essakly, A.; Alakus, H.; Buettner, R.; Hillmer, A.M.; Bruns, C.; Schroeder, W.; Zander, T.; Loeser, H.; et al. Loss of the SWI/SNF-ATPase Subunit Members SMARCF1 (ARID1A), SMARCA2 (BRM), SMARCA4 (BRG1) and SMARCB1 (INI1) in Oesophageal Adenocarcinoma. *BMC Cancer* **2020**, *20*, 12. [CrossRef]
28. Ye, F.; Huang, J.; Wang, H.; Luo, C.; Zhao, K. Targeting Epigenetic Machinery: Emerging Novel Allosteric Inhibitors. *Pharmacol. Ther.* **2019**, *204*, 107406. [CrossRef] [PubMed]
29. Peixoto, A.; Relvas-Santos, M.; Azevedo, R.; Santos, L.L.; Ferreira, J.A. Protein Glycosylation and Tumor Microenvironment Alterations Driving Cancer Hallmarks. *Front. Oncol.* **2019**, *9*, 380. [CrossRef] [PubMed]
30. Huang, S.-C.; Ng, K.-F.; Chang, I.Y.-F.; Chang, C.-J.; Chao, Y.-C.; Chang, S.-C.; Chen, M.-C.; Yeh, T.-S.; Chen, T.-C. The Clinicopathological Significance of SWI/SNF Alterations in Gastric Cancer Is Associated with the Molecular Subtypes. *PLoS ONE* **2021**, *16*, e0245356. [CrossRef]

31. Takeshima, H.; Niwa, T.; Takahashi, T.; Wakabayashi, M.; Yamashita, S.; Ando, T.; Inagawa, Y.; Taniguchi, H.; Katai, H.; Sugiyama, T.; et al. Frequent Involvement of Chromatin Remodeler Alterations in Gastric Field Cancerization. *Cancer Lett.* **2015**, *357*, 328–338. [CrossRef] [PubMed]
32. Katona, B.W.; Rustgi, A.K. Gastric Cancer Genomics: Advances and Future Directions. *Cell Mol. Gastroenterol. Hepatol.* **2017**, *3*, 211–217. [CrossRef] [PubMed]
33. Li, L.; Li, M.; Jiang, Z.; Wang, X. ARID1A Mutations Are Associated with Increased Immune Activity in Gastrointestinal Cancer. *Cells* **2019**, *8*, 678. [CrossRef] [PubMed]
34. Yamamoto, H.; Watanabe, Y.; Maehata, T.; Morita, R.; Yoshida, Y.; Oikawa, R.; Ishigooka, S.; Ozawa, S.-I.; Matsuo, Y.; Hosoya, K.; et al. An Updated Review of Gastric Cancer in the Next-Generation Sequencing Era: Insights from Bench to Bedside and Vice Versa. *World J. Gastroenterol.* **2014**, *20*, 3927–3937. [CrossRef]

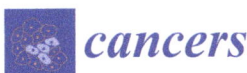

Article

The Unfolded Protein Response Is Associated with Cancer Proliferation and Worse Survival in Hepatocellular Carcinoma

Ankit Patel [1,†], Masanori Oshi [1,2,†], Li Yan [3], Ryusei Matsuyama [2], Itaru Endo [2] and Kazuaki Takabe [1,2,4,5,6,7,*]

1. Department of Surgical Oncology, Roswell Park Comprehensive Cancer Center, Buffalo, NY 14263, USA; ankit.patel@roswellpark.org (A.P.); masa1101oshi@gmail.com (M.O.)
2. Department of Gastroenterological Surgery, Graduate School of Medicine, Yokohama City University, Yokohama 236-0004, Japan; ryusei@yokohama-cu.ac.jp (R.M.); endoit@yokohama-cu.ac.jp (I.E.)
3. Department of Biostatistics & Bioinformatics, Roswell Park Comprehensive Cancer Center, Buffalo, NY 14263, USA; li.yan@roswellpark.org
4. Department of Surgery, Jacobs School of Medicine and Biomedical Sciences, State University of New York, Buffalo, NY 14263, USA
5. Department of Breast Surgery and Oncology, Tokyo Medical University, Tokyo 160-8402, Japan
6. Department of Digestive and General Surgery, Graduate School of Medicine and Dental Sciences, Niigata University, Niigata 951-8520, Japan
7. Department of Breast Surgery, School of Medicine, Fukushima Medical University, Fukushima 960-1295, Japan
* Correspondence: kazuaki.takabe@roswellpark.org; Tel.: +1-716-845-5540; Fax: +1-716-845-1668
† These authors contributed equally to this manuscript.

Simple Summary: We studied the association between the unfolded protein response (UPR) and carcinogenesis, cancer progression, and survival in hepatocellular carcinoma (HCC). We studied 655 HCC patients from 4 independent cohorts using an UPR score. The UPR was enhanced as normal liver became cancerous and as HCC advanced in stage. The UPR was correlated with cancer cell proliferation that was confirmed by multiple parameters. Significantly, a high UPR score was associated with worse patient survival. Interestingly, though UPR was associated with a high mutational load, it was not associated with immune response, immune cell infiltration, or angiogenesis. To our knowledge, this is the first study to investigate the clinical relevance of the unfolded protein response in HCC.

Abstract: Hepatocellular carcinoma is a leading cause of cancer death worldwide. The unfolded protein response (UPR) has been revealed to confer tumorigenic capacity in cancer cells. We hypothesized that a quantifiable score representative of the UPR could be used as a biomarker for cancer progression in HCC. In this study, a total of 655 HCC patients from 4 independent HCC cohorts were studied to examine the relationships between enhancement of the UPR and cancer biology and patient survival in HCC utilizing an UPR score. The UPR correlated with carcinogenic sequence and progression of HCC consistently in two cohorts. Enhanced UPR was associated with the clinical parameters of HCC progression, such as cancer stage and multiple parameters of cell proliferation, including histological grade, mKI67 gene expression, and enrichment of cell proliferation-related gene sets. The UPR was significantly associated with increased mutational load, but not with immune cell infiltration or angiogeneis across independent cohorts. The UPR was consistently associated with worse survival across independent cohorts of HCC. In conclusion, the UPR score may be useful as a biomarker to predict prognosis and to better understand HCC.

Keywords: unfolded protein; hepatocellular cancer; GSVA; unfolded protein score

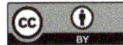

1. Introduction

Primary liver cancer is the sixth most common cancer worldwide with hepatocellular carcinoma (HCC) compromising the majority of cases [1]. Incidence and mortality rates have decreased in high-risk regions in the worlds, yet prognosis remains poor, with an expected 5-year survival rate less than 40% [2]. Improved outcomes may be achieved in the 10–15% of patients in whom surgical resection is possible, but the majority of patients with a nonresectable disease have limited benefit from systemic chemotherapy [3]. A biomarker based on tumor biology can help optimize treatment choices when linked to prognosis.

Cancer cells have the unique ability to evoke adaptive mechanisms to acquire malignant characteristics necessary for cancer progression. Of these mechanisms, known as the "hallmarks of cancer", protein homeostasis as regulated by the Endoplasmic Reticulum (ER) is a recognized process involved in cancer progression [4]. ER stress activates the Unfolded Protein Response (UPR) and has been implicated in a variety of cancers, including HCC. The UPR signal transduction cascade is directly activated as a response to prolonged ER stress conditions including nutrient deprivation, hypoxia, acidosis, drug-induced toxicity, and irradiation. In response to stressors, UPR response plays a major role in regulation of the expression of genes responsible for calcium and redox homeostasis, protein trafficking, ER quality control, autophagy, and lipid synthesis [5]. The UPR is inherently cell protective, aiming to alleviate damage and restore cellular homeostasis via transcriptional induction of specific molecular chaperones [6]. Due to the exposure of chronic stressors, cancer cells learn to adapt to prolonged ER stress by creating pro-survival alterations in the UPR signaling pathway and subsequently drive carcinogenesis [7]. Three major ER stress transducers, *IRE1*, *PERK*, and *ATF6*, are recognized as primary drivers of the UPR [5,8]. The role of protein homeostasis and the UPR in HCC has been studied to highlight of role of a specific UPR signal transducer, IRE1α, in HCC carcinogenesis via a metabolic inflammation mechanism [9]. A downstream regulator of the PERK-dependent branch of the UPR signaling pathway has been recognized to promote tumor cell proliferation via limiting oxidation DNA damage [10].

Hepatocellular carcinogenesis is etiologically linked to viral infection, chemical carcinogens, and other environmental and host factors that cause chronic liver injury. The accumulation of genomic alterations, DNA rearrangements, and chromosomal amplifications initiates the oncogenic progression of a normal hepatocyte to hepatocellular carcinoma [11]. In a related but distinct process from carcinogenesis, cancer progression is defined as the evolution of existing cancer from local regional advancement to metastatic disease, which is often recognized with clinical staging. Given the role of the UPR activation in carcinogenesis, we hypothesized that UPR activation could be recognized with pathological progression, mutational accumulation, clinical stage advancement, and survival in HCC.

Our previous work has reported the utility of scoring the genetic expression profile using gene set variation analysis (GSVA) to understand the relationship between signaling pathways and cancer biology in patients. For example, the G2M checkpoint pathway score identified margin-positive resection in pancreatic cancer [12] and metastasis in estrogen receptor-positive breast cancer patients [13], both resulting in poor survival. The DNA repair pathway was shown to be associated with cell proliferation and worse survival in HCC [14]. Given this background, we hypothesized in this study that the UPR was associated with unique characteristics and worse survival in HCC patients. To test our hypothesis, we analyzed a total of 655 HCC patients from The Cancer Genome Atlas (TCGA) Liver Hepatocellular Carcinoma (TCGA-LIHC; $n = 358$), GSE6764 ($n = 75$), GSE89377 ($n = 107$), and GSE76427 ($n = 115$) cohorts to examine the role of Unfolded Protein Response in clinical outcomes.

2. Materials and Methods

The hepatocellular carcinoma cohorts consisted of the mRNA-sequencing data of 358 hepatocellular carcinoma patients in The Cancer Genome Atlas (TCGA) Liver Hepatocellular Carcinoma cohort (TCGA_LIHC, $n = 358$), which was obtained from the Genomic Data Commons Data Portal (GDC). American Joint Committee on Cancer (AJCC) stage and pathological grade were obtained from GDC. We used the cohorts from Wurmbach et al. (GSE6764; $n = 75$) [15], Eun et al. (GSE89377; $n = 107$) [16], Brandon et al. (GSE56545;

n = 42) [17], and Grinchuk et al. (GSE76427; n = 167) [18] to investigate the association between the DNA repair pathway scores and HCC patients' clinicopathological characteristics and outcomes from the Gene Expression Omnibus (GEO) repository. Pathological classification of the samples in GSE6764 followed the guidelines of the International Working Party [19]. Four pathological HCC stages were defined: (i) Very early HCC (n = 8), which included well-differentiated tumors <2 cm in diameter with no vascular invasion/satellites (size range: 8–20 mm); (ii) early HCC (n = 10), which included tumors measuring <2 cm with microscopic vascular invasion/satellites; well- to moderately differentiated tumors measuring 2–5 cm without vascular invasion/satellites; or 2–3 well-differentiated nodules measuring <3 cm (size range: 3–45 mm); (iii) advanced HCC (n = 7), which included poorly differentiated tumors measuring >2 cm with microvascular invasion/satellites or tumors measuring >5 cm; and (iv) very advanced HCC (n = 10), which included tumors with macrovascular invasion or diffuse liver involvement. All genomic analyses used were log$_2$ transformed normalized transcriptomic data. The average value was used for genes with multiple probes. Given that the TCGA and all GEO cohorts used in this study are de-identified in the public domain, approval from the Institutional Review Board was waived.

The UPR score was used as a surrogate for quantified UPR activity. The activity of UPR was quantified as the degree of enrichment of the "HALLMARK_UNFOLDED_PROTEIN_ RESPONSE" gene set (Table S1 lists all the genes included in this gene set) defined and generated as one of the Hallmark gene set collections of the Molecular Signatures Database (MSigDB) [20] using the gene set variation analysis (GSVA) algorithm [21] in the Bioconductor package (version 3.10). We have previously reported the clinical relevance of multiple signaling pathways and responses using a similar approach [12–14,22–39].

The publicly available software (GSEA version 4.0.3) and the gene set enrichment analysis (GSEA) algorithm [40] was used in this study. Statistical significance was determined to a false discovery rate (FDR) of 0.25 as recommended by the GSEA software (Table S4).

The xCell algorithm [41] was used to calculate the immune cell infiltration in the tumor microenvironment through transcriptomic data. The xCell data were obtained through the xCell website (https://xcell.ucsf.edu/, accessed on 23 February 2021), as we previously reported [22–26].

The score values of the intratumor heterogeneity, single-nucleotide variant (SNV) neoantigens, indel neoantigens, silent mutation, non-silent mutation, leukocyte fraction, lymphocyte infiltration, and interferon (IFN)- response score were calculated and published by Thorsson et al. [42]. Thorsson et al. [42] performed an extensive analysis of TCGA, which includes immune and genomic data from than 10,000 tumors across various cancer types. The study characterizes different immune subtypes by differences in immune cell signatures, extent of neoantigen load, overall cell proliferation, expression of immunomodulatory genes, and prognosis. The results and data analysis offers the structure of our methods.

The median value of the UPR score within cohorts was used to divide the patients into low and high UPR score groups. Statistical significance for comparison analysis between groups was determined to a p-value less than 0.05 by the Kruskal-Wallis test, the Mann-Whitney U test, and two-tail Fisher's exact tests. Tukey-type boxplots showed the median and interquartile level values. R software (R Project for Statistical Computing, Table S4) and Microsoft Excel (Table S4) were used for all data analysis and data plotting.

3. Results

3.1. Unfolded Protein Response (UPR) Was Positively Correlated with Clinical Parameters of Carcinogenesis and Cancer Progression as Well as the AJCC Cancer Stage of HCC Patients

Unfolded Protein Response (UPR) was quantified by the GSVA score of the Molecular Signatures Database (MSigDB) Hallmark gene set using the methodology we previously described [12–14,27–34]. Based on previous basic research studies that have elucidated the role of UPR activation in carcinogenesis [9], we hypothesized that the UPR is enhanced through the step-wise progression of a normal liver into HCC in patients. To test this hypothesis, the UPR score was measured at each stage of histological progression—from normal liver, dysplasia, cirrhosis, low- and high-grade chronic hepatitis, to early and advanced HCC—in the GSE6764 and GSE89377 cohorts. UPR was significantly enhanced in early to advanced HCC compared to normal liver, dysplasia, cirrhosis, and very early HCC in the GSE6764 cohort (Figure 1A; $p < 0.001$). These results were replicated and validated in the GSE89377 cohort where the UPR was significantly enhanced in HCC compared with dysplasia, cirrhosis, and chronic hepatitis (Figure 1A; $p < 0.001$). As a measure of clinical cancer progression, UPR was also noted to be significantly enhanced in tumors with advanced American Joint Committee on Cancer (AJCC) staging (Figure 1B, $p = 0.001$).

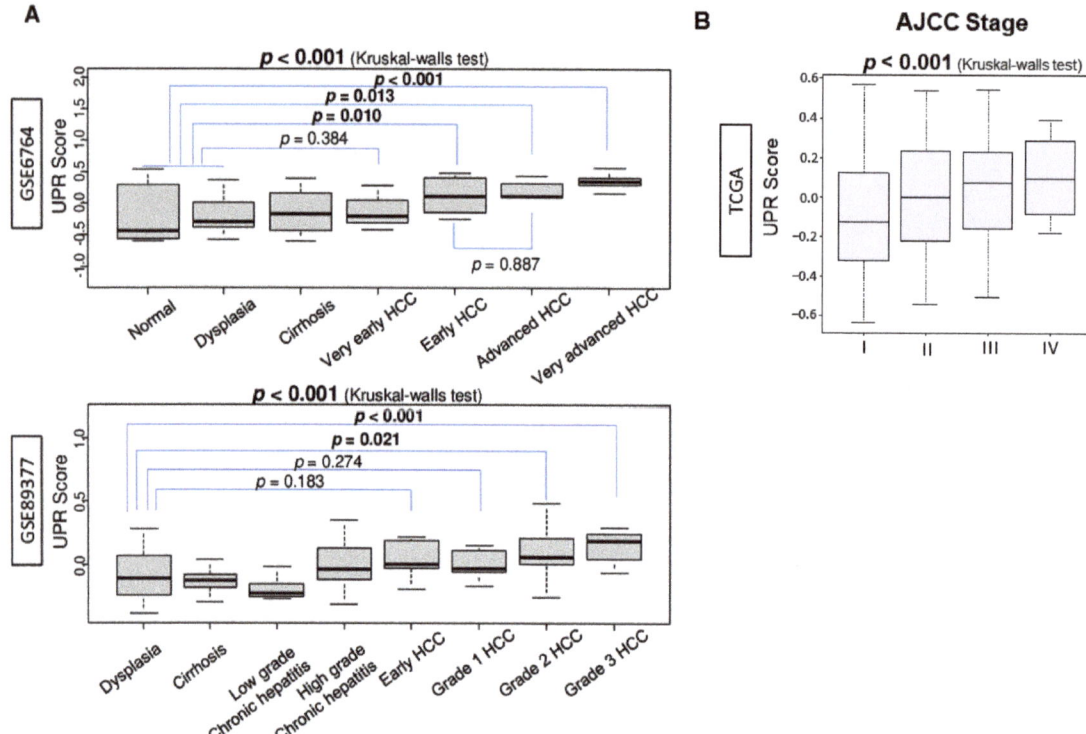

Figure 1. Association between Unfolded Protein Response (UPR) and hepatocarcinogenesis and progression. (**A**) Boxplots of the comparison of the unfolded protein response score by multistep hepatocarcinogenesis, including normal liver tissue ($n = 8$), dysplasia ($n = 17$), cirrhosis ($n = 13$), very early hepatocellular carcinoma (HCC) ($n = 8$), early HCC ($n = 10$), advanced HCC ($n = 7$), and very advanced HCC ($n = 10$) defined by the GSE764 cohort ($n = 75$); and dysplasia ($n = 35$), cirrhosis ($n = 12$), low-grade ($n = 8$) and high-grade ($n = 12$) chronic hepatitis, early HCC ($n = 5$), and grades 1–3 ($n = 9, 12$, and 14, respectively) of HCC defined by the GSE98377 cohort ($n = 107$). The p-value of normal/dysplasia vs. each class of HCC analyzed using the Mann–Whitney U test in the GSE6764 cohort. The p-value of dysplasia vs. each class of HCC analyzed using the Mann–Whitney U test in the in GSE89377 cohort. The overall p-value was calculated using a Kruskal–Wallis test. (**B**) Boxplot of the comparison of the unfolded protein response and the American Joint Committee on Cancer (AJCC) stage I-III ($n = 166, 81$, and 84, respectively) in the TCGA cohort. The overall p-value was calculated using a Kruskal–Wallis test.

3.2. UPR Was Positively Correlated with Multiple Parameters of Cell Proliferation, including Histological Grade, MKI67 Gene Expression and Enrichment of Cell Proliferation-Related Gene Sets by Gene Set Enrichment Assay (GSEA)

Given the finding that UPR was associated with HCC cancer progression, we decided to investigate the association with cancer cell proliferation. We found that UPR was positively correlated with a higher pathological grade as compared to a lower grade HCC tumor in the TCGA cohort (Figure 2A, $p = 0.024$). The expression of *MKI67*, a commonly used marker for cell proliferation in the clinical setting, was found to be significantly different between UPR groups when divided into low and high UPR score groups using the median value as a cut-off. The high UPR group was significantly associated with a high expression level of MKI67. In comparison, the low UPR group was associated with a low expression level of MKI67 (Figure 2C, $p < 0.001$).

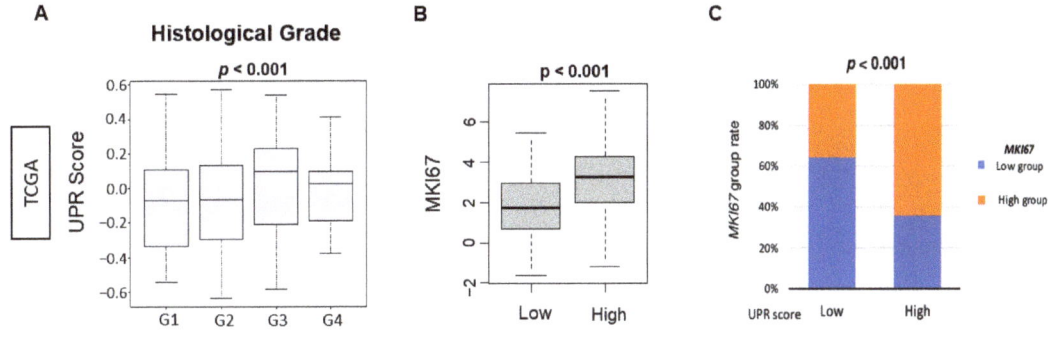

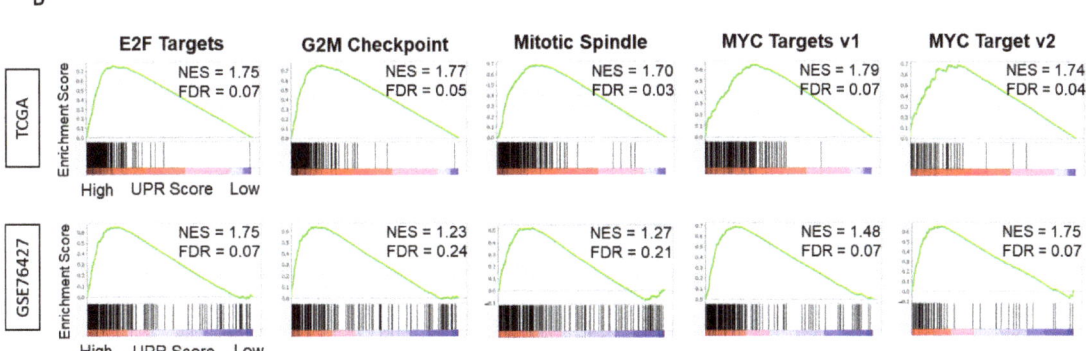

Figure 2. Association between Unfolded Protein Response and histological grade, MKI67 gene expression and cell proliferation-related gene sets. (**A**) Boxplot of the comparison of the unfolded protein response score with histological grade G1- 4 ($n = 53, 168, 121$ and 11, respectively). The *p*-value was calculated using a Kruskal–Wallis test. (**B**) Boxplot of the comparison of the high vs. low unfolded protein response and the MKI67 gene expression (both $n = 179$) in the TCGA cohort. The *p*-value was calculated using the Mann–Whitney U test. (**C**) Bar plot of the comparison of low and high groups of the unfolded protein response score and MKI67 expression. The *p*-value was calculated using Fisher's exact test. (**D**) Gene set enrichment analysis (GSEA) of the Hallmark gene sets by high vs. low unfolded protein response score of HCC in the GSE76427 and TCGA cohorts. Enrichment plots with the normalized enrichment score (NES) and false discovery rate (FDR) for proliferation-related gene sets. An FDR of 0.25 was used to determine statistical significance as recommended by the GSEA software (version 4.1.0, accessed on 27 February 2021) (Table S4).

The MSigDB Hallmark defines six gene sets as cell proliferation-related in GSEA. The UPR high HCC group significantly enriched five cell proliferation-related gene sets, including E2F targets, G2M checkpoint, MYC targets v1, MYC targets v2, and Mitotic spindle consistently in both TCGA and GSE76427 cohorts (Figure 2D, all False Detection Rate (FDR) < 0.25). Reviewed in their entirety, our results indicated that UPR was correlated with multiple measures of cell proliferation consistently, which validates the score as a parameter for cancer proliferation.

3.3. UPR Was Significantly Associated with Increased Mutational Load

As cancer cell proliferation is associated with high mutational rates [36], it was of interest to investigate the relationship between the UPR and mutation rate in HCC. Homologous recombination deficiency is representative of defective DNA repair and is a surrogate marker for increased mutational load. A high UPR score was significantly associated with homologous recombination deficiency, fraction altered, silent mutations, and non-silent mutations (Figure 3A, $p = 0.002$; Figure 3B, $p < 0.001$, $p = 0.027$, $p = 0.030$, respectively). The UPR score was not associated with single-nucleotide variants (SNV) neoantigens, or indel neoantigens (Figure 3B, $p = 0.087$, $p = 0.290$). This study found that a high UPR score was significantly associated with the mutation load.

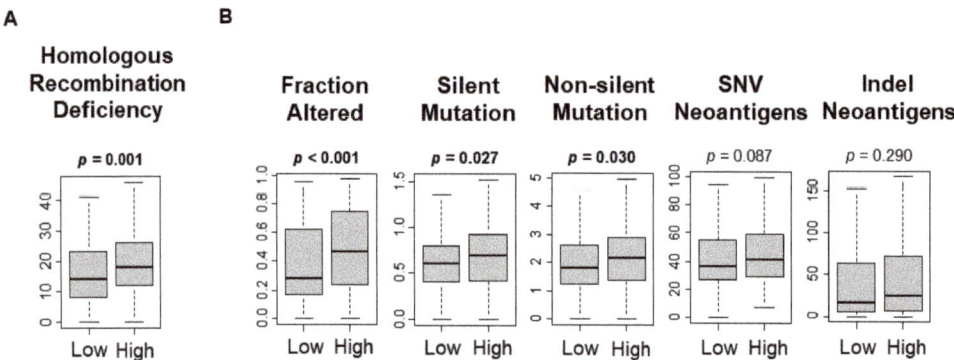

Figure 3. Association between Unfolded Protein Response and mutation-related scores. Boxplots of the comparison of the high vs. low unfolded protein response and (**A**) homologous recombinant defects score; (**B**) fraction altered, silent mutation, non-silent mutation, single-nucleotide variants (SNV) neoantigens, and indel neoantigens. The *p*-value was calculated using the Mann–Whitney U test. Bold format: significant *p* values.

3.4. There Was No Consistently Significant Association between the UPR and Immune Response or Immune Cell Infiltration

A high tumor mutational burden has been suggested to increase neoantigen production that can generate an anti-cancer immune cell infiltration in many types of cancers including HCC [36,43]. Thus, it was of interest to investigate the correlation between UPR and the immune response and immune cell infiltration, since a high mutation rate, but not neoantigens, was associated with high UPR. Although statistically significant (all FDR < 0.25), Normalized Enrichment Scores (NES) were uniformly low in all of the inflammation-related gene sets enriched to high UPR including TNFα signaling, IL6/STAT3 signaling, and complemented in both the TCGA and GSE76427 cohorts (Figure 4A). There was no significant increase in pro-cancer immune cell infiltration as estimated by the xCell algorithm in the UPR high HCC cohort, except for type2 Helper T cells in the TCGA cohort alone (Figure 4B). There was a noted significant increase in infiltration of type1 helper T cells, which are anti-cancer cells, in the TCGA cohort alone (Figure 4B, $p = 0.017$). Low UPR score had a noted increase in M2 macrophages, a pro-cancer immune cell, in the TCGA cohort alone (Figure 4B, $p = 0.029$). Interestingly, with a high degree of mutational variation in the analyzed cohorts and a presumed increase of antigen presentation, there was no consistent immune cell infiltration into the tumor microenvironment of UPR high HCC. There was no correlation between the UPR score and expression of PD-1 or PD-L1 (Figure S1).

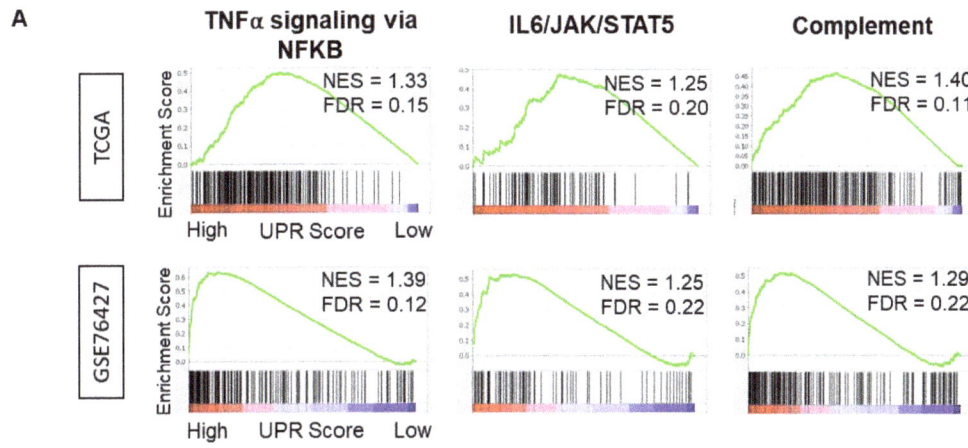

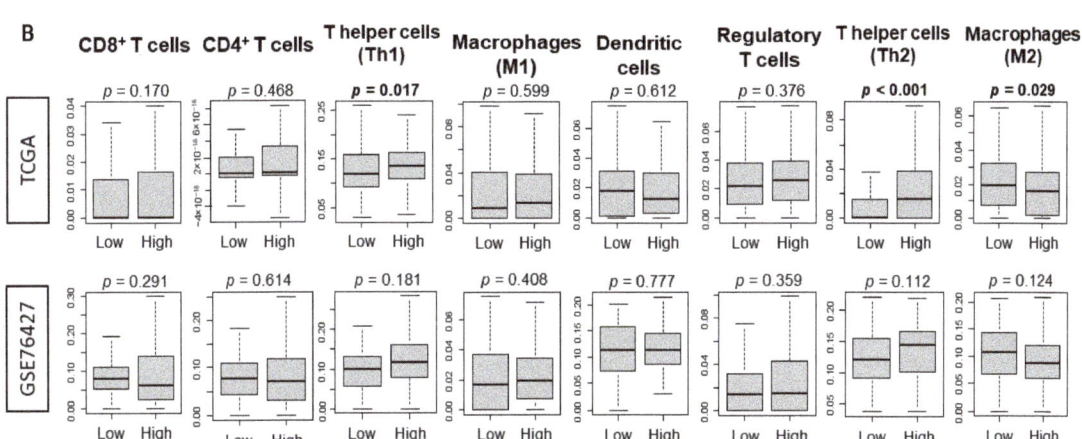

Figure 4. Association between Unfolded Protein Response and inflammation-related gene sets as well as infiltrating immune cells in the TCGA and GSE76427 cohorts. (**A**) Enrichment plots with the normalized enrichment score (NES) and false discovery rate (FDR) for the TNFα signaling via NFKB, IL6/JAK/STAT5, and complement gene sets of the Hallmark gene sets. (**B**) Boxplots of the anti-cancer immune cells including CD8$^+$ T cells, CD4$^+$ T cells, T helper type 1 (Th1) cells, M1 macrophages and dendritic cells; and pro-cancer immune cells including regulatory T cells, T helper type (Th2) cells, and M2 macrophages. The *p*-value was calculated using the Mann-Whitney U test. Bold format: Significant *p* values.

3.5. UPR Was Not Consistently Associated with Angiogeneis across Independent Cohorts of HCC

It was of interest to investigate the association between UPR and angiogenesis because UPR has been shown to mediate angiogenesis through the regulation of transcription factors [44]. The angiogenesis gene set was not enriched to HCC with high UPR in either of the TCGA and GSE76427 cohorts (Figure 5, NES = 1.16 and FDR = 0.268; NES = 1.15 and FDR = 0.306). HCC with high UPR was also associated with a decreased infiltration of lymphatic vessel related cells, including endothelial cells and lymphatic endothelial cells, as well as adipocytes in the TCGA cohort (Figure 5, $p < 0.001$, $p = 0.016$, $p < 0.001$), but this result was not validated in the GSE76427 cohort.

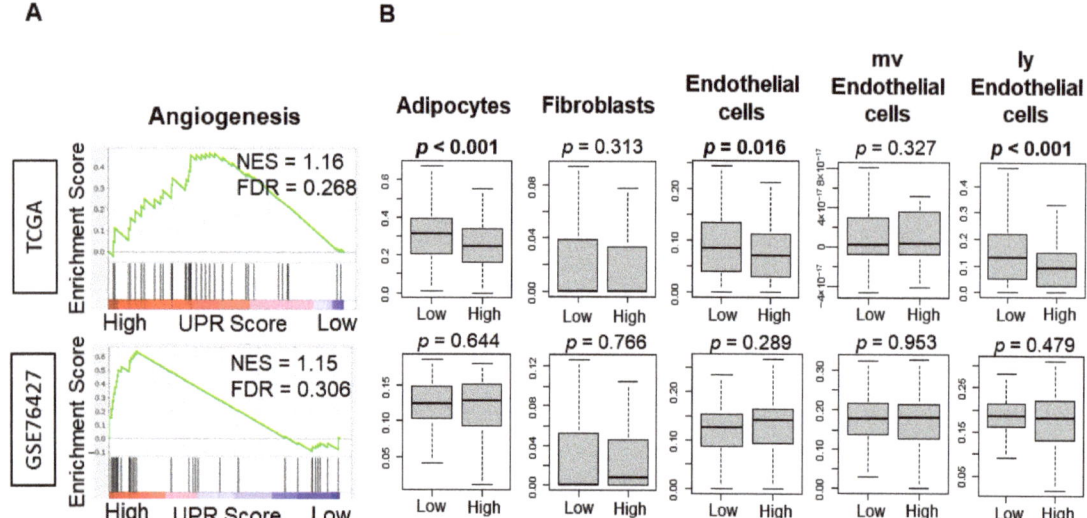

Figure 5. Association between Unfolded Protein Response and angiogenesis in the TCGA and GSE76427 cohorts. (**A**) Enrichment plots with the normalized enrichment score (NES) and false discovery rate (FDR) for the angiogenesis gene sets of the Hallmark gene sets. (**B**) Boxplots of the angiogenesis related gene sets adipocytes, fibroblasts, endothelial cells, mother vessel (mv) endothelial cells, and lymphatic (ly) endothelial cells. The *p*-value was calculated using the Mann–Whitney U test. Bold format: Significant *p* values.

3.6. The Unfolded Protein Response Score Was Consistently Associated with Worse Survival across Independent Cohorts of HCC

As previous studies have reported that enhanced UPR was associated with worse survival in other cancer, most notably in glioblastoma multiform [45,46], it was of interest to investigate a similar relationship with survival in HCC patients. We analyzed the UPR score as related to overall survival (OS), disease-free survival (DFS), risk-free survival (RFS), and disease-specific survival (DSS) in the TCGA, as well as RFS in GSE76427 cohorts. Each cohort was divided into low and high UPS groups using the median value. The high UPS was significantly associated with worse OS, DFS, RFS, and DSS in all cohorts of TCGA, and poor RFS in GSE62452 (Figure 6). In addition, through univariate and multivariate cox regression analysis using OS in the TCGA cohort, the UPR score and AJCC stage were demonstrated to be independent prognostic factors for HCC patients (Table S2). These results suggest that Unfolded Protein score is able to quantify the biological aggressiveness of HCC and has the potential to be used as a prognostic biomarker for survival in HCC. We have previously published that cell proliferation-related scores that are associated with patient survival including MYC [30], G2M checkpoint [12], and E2F target [32] scores in breast cancer.

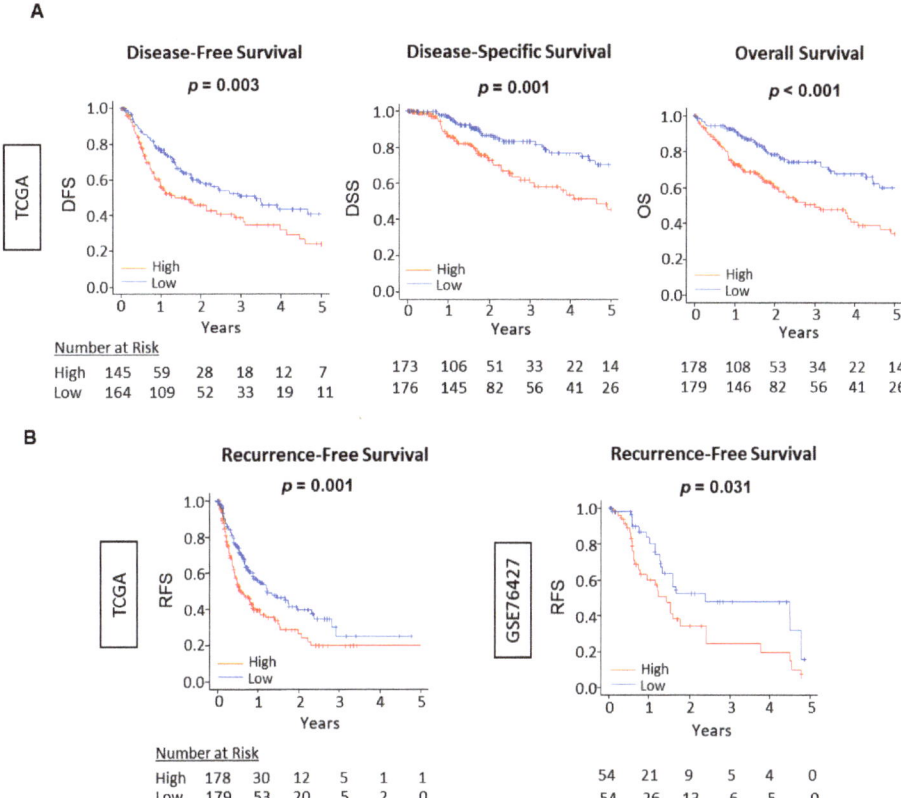

Figure 6. Association between the Unfolded Protein Response and HCC patient survival. (**A**) Kaplan–Meier survival curves comparing the low and high unfolded protein response score in HCC to demonstrate disease-free survival, disease-specific survival, and overall survival in the TCGA cohort (n = 358). (**B**) Kaplan–Meier survival curves comparing the low and high unfolded protein response score in HCC to demonstrate recurrence-free survival in the TCGA and GSE76427 (n = 167) cohorts. We divided the cohort into low and high unfolded protein response score groups using the median value as the cut-off. The p-value was calculated using a log rank test.

We also reported that the G2M checkpoint pathway alone is associated with drug response and survival among cell proliferation-related pathways in pancreatic cancer [12]. However, we have never compared or analyzed which of these scores correlate most with survival in HCC. To this end, we analyzed the clinical benefit of UPR and each cell proliferation-related gene sets, including E2F targets, G2M checkpoints, MYC target v1 and v2, MITOTIC spindle, and MKI67 expression by a Cox Proportional Hazards model. As demonstrated in Supplemental Table S3, the hazard ratio of UPR was the highest among all the biomarkers, which offers it a higher degree of correlation over our previously analyzed cell proliferation-related scores.

4. Discussion

In this study, we looked at the association of the unfolded protein response (UPR), as measured by the UPR Score, with clinical relevance in HCC. Our findings suggested that the UPR was positively correlated with each histological progression in the carcinogenesis and progression of HCC. The UPR high HCC cohort was significantly associated with multiple parameters of cell proliferation including histological grade, *MKI67* gene expression, and enrichment of cell proliferation-related gene sets by GSEA and mutational load. On the contrary, the UPR high HCC cohort was not associated with angiogenesis or increased immune activity. The UPR was also consistently associated with worse survival across independent cohorts of HCC. To our knowledge, this is the first study to investigate the clinical relevance of the unfolded protein response in HCC.

The UPR signaling network operates as a pro-oncogenic mechanism that drives several aspects of cancer progression by increasing cancer cell survival and adapting to intrinsic changes and environmental challenges. Most evidence suggests that the UPR is involved in most hallmarks of cancer, including cell proliferation, immune evasion, angiogenesis, and treatment resistance [4,5]. Chronic environmental stressors, including nutrient deprivation, hypoxia, acidosis, drug-induced toxicity, and irradiation, drives the UPR to adopt a pro-survival mechanism that is co-opted by cancer cells for continued proliferation and survival. These changes are demonstrated in gene expression alteration and changes in protein signal transduction. The role of protein homeostasis and the UPR in HCC has been studied to highlight of role of a specific UPR signal transducer, IRE1α, in HCC carcinogenesis via a metabolic inflammation mechanism [9]. A downstream regulator of the PERK-dependent branch of the UPR signaling pathway has been recognized to promote tumor cell proliferation via limiting oxidation DNA damage [10]. Our findings highlighted a significant correlation between UPR activation through each histological stage in the carcinogenesis of normal liver tissue to hepatocellular cancer. These results offer a clinical observation of the previously defined pre-clinical role of the UPR in carcinogenesis. It is tempting to speculate that this observation offers a translation target for targeted therapy to interrupt hepatocellular carcinogenesis.

Cancer progression is defined as the advancement of existing cancer, from local regional advancement to metastatic disease, which is measured by parameters of clinical staging. Utilizing an in vivo preclinical model, one study noted that cancer failed to progress if a downstream UPR-activated chaperone protein was suppressed, directly demonstrating the role of UPR-related proteins in cancer progression [47]. With the observed preclinical data that elucidates the role of UPR in cancer progression, it can be reasonably assumed that the UPR would be associated with cancer stage. Our study observed the significant enrichment of the UPR in advancing AJCC staging, with high UPR enrichment in stage IV HCC and lower UPR enrichment in stage I HCC.

The UPR is difficult to quantify in the clinical setting. Prior studies have analyzed the actions of three major ER stress transducers, *IRE1*, *PERK*, and *ATF6*, as a measure of the UPR and its adaptive response to ensure cell survival [5,8]. Without gene expression profiling and protein transduction studies, there is a lack of a translational method to quantify the UPR. GSEA allows us to capture genetic activation by the UPR across the transcriptomes of multiple large HCC patient cohorts and create a quantifiable entity in the UPR score. We can then use this score to study its association with common clinical parameters of cancer proliferation and progression. The Hallmark gene sets utilized in this study are widely accepted and recognized as representing well-defined biological processes. The aim of this study was to investigate the clinical relevance of the existing Hallmark Unfolded Protein Response gene set, and not to generate a novel gene set that reflects the UPR. We have previously reported the association of several pathways with clinical outcomes in various cancers [12,13,31,32].

The common histological assessments of grade and *MKI67* expression are used as clinical correlates to recognize degrees of cell proliferation in cancer. A prior study of UPR activation demonstrated that downstream UPR signal transducers were overexpressed more frequently in the higher-grade breast cancers than in lower-grade breast cancers indicating that activation of the UPR can correlate with a clinically more aggressive phenotype [48]. This study observed a similar correlation in that UPR gene set activation was highly enriched with higher grade HCC, and not as highly enriched with lower grade HCC. In addition, the enrichment of cell proliferation gene sets supports the finding of significant UPR association with increased cell proliferation as measured by mKI67 expression.

Neoplastic progression requires several genetic alterations and mutations that allow the cell to ignore growth controls and disable apoptotic signaling. The accumulation of a mutational load is associated with a high rate of proliferation as we have previously observed in breast cancer [36], and so it was interest to investigate if a high mutational load cancer is associated with a high UPR. This study found that a high UPR score was significantly associated with the mutation load. In general, the tumor microenvironment (TME) is manipulated by cancer cells by the release of pro-inflammatory mediators. This results in the recruitment of immune cells, which are involved in angiogenesis, invasion, as well as metastasis [49]. It has been shown that this change in the TME is a form of ER stress that is influenced by sustained activity of IRE1α, a main sensor of the UPR signaling pathway [50]. In addition, in vitro experimental data have shown that macrophages activate UPR when cultured with ER-stressed cancer cells. Furthermore, these macrophages recapitulate, amplify, and expand the proinflammatory response of cancer cells [50]. Thus, we hypothesized that UPR activation would be associated with inflammation in the TME. Interestingly, we did not observe a consistent association between UPR activation and an immune response. In addition, as higher mutational load cancer has been associated with increased neoantigen presentation and subsequent immune cell infiltration [36], this same relationship was not observed in HCC cohorts.

Angiogenesis is crucial to the progression of cancer [31,37–39,51–53]. Rapid tumor growth and inadequate vascularization creates environmental stress that propagates the activation of stress response pathways, include the unfolded protein response. Studies have indicated that cells suffering from insufficient blood supplies experience ER stress and activate the UPR to help cancer cells continue to grow and spread rapidly [54,55]. The UPR has also been shown to play a role in mediating angiogenesis through the regulation of VEGFA transcription factor [44]. Though much pre-clinical evidence points to a correlative relationship, it is conceivable that the activation of the angiogenic and UPR pathways could synergize in some cases and be antagonistic in others [56]. Interestingly, our analysis did not show a consistent relationship between the UPR and angiogenesis across TCGA and GSE76427 cohorts.

This study observed the association of the UPR with clinical parameters of cancer aggressiveness and progression. By extension, it was reasonable to assume that high UPR activation would also be associated with worse survival. Our results indicated a statistically significant and validated correlation with recurrence-free survival across two cohorts of HCC patients. Overall survival was also worse with high UPR activation in the TCGA cohort. Though the aim of the study was not to report a new mechanism of the unfolded protein response in HCC, it does highlight the ability of the UPR score to predict survival in HCC.

The current study has obvious limitations. The uses of databases have an inherent inability to analyze tissue samples directly, thus limiting our ability to perform further comprehensive histological analysis. As we used publicly available cohorts, our results may not reflect the heterogeneity among the patients due to the limited sample size of the databases. Although we believe that the statistical significance is real when the difference exists despite the small sample size, we may not be inclusive of all findings. Another limitation of this study is that is does not accurately reflect the composition of the tumor microenvironment as represented by immunological milieu of the original cancer tissue, which cannot be reliably replicated outside of in vivo experiments. Finally, the cohorts we access do not contain treatment data and it is assumed that the patients underwent standard-of-care treatments. In the future, our result needs validation with prospectively analyzing UPR score in patient samples with treatment data.

5. Conclusions

The unfolded protein response (UPR) was associated with carcinogenesis and progression of HCC, with multiple parameters of cell proliferation, including histological grade, MKI67 gene expression, and cell proliferation-related gene sets, with increased mutational load, but not with immune infiltration nor angiogenesis, and with worse survival across independent cohorts of HCC. Thus, the UPR score may be useful as a biomarker to predict prognosis and to better understand HCC.

Supplementary Materials: The following are available online at https://www.mdpi.com/article/10.3390/cancers13174443/s1, Figure S1: Co-relation curve of PD-1, PDL-1 expressions and UPR score, Table S1: Member genes of the Unfolded protein response score. Table S2: Univariate and multivariate analysis with overall survival in the TCGA cohort. Table S3: Cox regression analysis of cell proliferation-related gene sets, Table S4: List of Software used in analysis.

Author Contributions: Conceptualization, A.P., M.O. and K.T.; methodology and analyses, M.O. and L.Y.; resources, R.M., I.E. and K.T.; writing—original draft preparation, A.P. and M.O.; writing—review and editing, R.M., I.E. and K.T.; supervision, I.E. and K.T.; funding acquisition, I.E and K.T. All authors have read and agreed to the published version of the manuscript.

Funding: This research was funded by US National Institutes of Health/National Cancer Institute grant R01CA160688, R01CA250412, R37CA248018, US Department of Defense BCRP grant W81XWH-19-1-0674, to K.T., and US National Cancer Institute cancer center support grant P30-CA016056 to Roswell Park Comprehensive Cancer Center.

Institutional Review Board Statement: This study was deemed exempt from the Institutional Review Board because all information within the cohorts used in this study is publicly accessible and de-identified.

Informed Consent Statement: Patient consent was waived as all data was obtained from deidentified publicly available databases.

Data Availability Statement: All data was obtained from deidentified publicly available databases, TCGA cohort from the Genomic Data Commons Data Portal (GDC) (https://portal.gdc.cancer.gov/, accessed on 27 August 2021), and GSE6764, GSE89377, GSE56545, and GSE76427 from the Gene Expression Omnibus (GEO) repository (https://www.ncbi.nlm.nih.gov/geo/, accessed on 27 August 2021).

Acknowledgments: K.T. is the Alfiero Foundation Chair of Breast Oncology at Roswell Park Comprehensive Cancer Center.

Conflicts of Interest: The authors declare no conflict of interest.

References

1. Sung, H.; Ferlay, J.; Siegel, R.L.; Laversanne, M.; Soerjomataram, I.; Jemal, A.; Bray, F. Global Cancer Statistics 2020: GLOBOCAN Estimates of Incidence and Mortality Worldwide for 36 Cancers in 185 Countries. *CA Cancer J. Clin.* **2021**, *71*, 209–249. [CrossRef]
2. Connell, L.C.; Harding, J.J.; Abou-Alfa, G.K. Advanced Hepatocellular Cancer: The Current State of Future Research. *Curr. Treat. Options Oncol.* **2016**, *17*, 43. [CrossRef]
3. Llovet, J.M.; Fuster, J.; Bruix, J. Intention-to-treat analysis of surgical treatment for early hepatocellular carcinoma: Resection versus transplantation. *Hepatology* **1999**, *30*, 1434–1440. [CrossRef]
4. Siwecka, N.; Rozpędek, W.; Pytel, D.; Wawrzynkiewicz, A.; Dziki, A.; Dziki, Ł.; Diehl, J.A.; Majsterek, I. Dual role of endoplasmic reticulum stress-mediated unfolded protein response signaling pathway in carcinogenesis. *Int. J. Mol. Sci.* **2019**, *20*, 4354. [CrossRef]
5. Vandewynckel, Y.-P.; Laukens, D.; Geerts, A.; Bogaerts, E.; Paridaens, A.; Verhelst, X.; Janssens, S.; Heindryckx, F.; Van Vlierberghe, H. The paradox of the unfolded protein response in cancer. *Anticancer. Res.* **2013**, *33*, 4683–4694.
6. Kozutsumi, Y.; Segal, M.R.; Normington, K.; Gething, M.-J.; Sambrook, J. The presence of malfolded proteins in the endoplasmic reticulum signals the induction of glucose-regulated proteins. *Nature* **1988**, *332*, 462–464. [CrossRef]
7. Wang, W.-A.; Groenendyk, J.; Michalak, M. Endoplasmic reticulum stress associated responses in cancer. *Biochim. Et Biophys. Acta (BBA)-Mol. Cell Res.* **2014**, *1843*, 2143–2149. [CrossRef]
8. Chakrabarti, A.; Chen, A.W.; Varner, J.D. A review of the mammalian unfolded protein response. *Biotechnol. Bioeng.* **2011**, *108*, 2777–2793. [CrossRef]
9. Wu, Y.; Shan, B.; Dai, J.; Xia, Z.; Cai, J.; Chen, T.; Lv, S.; Feng, Y.; Zheng, L.; Wang, Y.; et al. Dual role for inositol-requiring enzyme 1α in promoting the development of hepatocellular carcinoma during diet-induced obesity in mice. *Hepatology* **2018**, *68*, 533–546. [CrossRef]
10. Bi, M.; Naczki, C.; Koritzinsky, M.; Fels, D.; Blais, J.; Hu, N.; Harding, H.; Novoa, I.; Varia, M.; Raleigh, J.; et al. ER stress-regulated translation increases tolerance to extreme hypoxia and promotes tumor growth. *EMBO J.* **2005**, *24*, 3470–3481. [CrossRef]
11. Ozturk, M. Genetic aspects of hepatocellular carcinogenesis. *Semin. Liver Dis.* **1999**, *19*, 235–242. [CrossRef]

12. Oshi, M.; Newman, S.; Tokumaru, Y.; Yan, L.; Matsuyama, R.; Endo, I.; Katz, M.H.G.; Takabe, K. High G2M Pathway Score Pancreatic Cancer is Associated with Worse Survival, Particularly after Margin-Positive (R1 or R2) Resection. *Cancers* **2020**, *12*, 2871. [CrossRef]
13. Oshi, M.; Takahashi, H.; Tokumaru, Y.; Yan, L.; Rashid, O.M.; Matsuyama, R.; Endo, I.; Takabe, K. G2M Cell Cycle Pathway Score as a Prognostic Biomarker of Metastasis in Estrogen Receptor (ER)-Positive Breast Cancer. *Int. J. Mol. Sci.* **2020**, *21*, 2921. [CrossRef]
14. Oshi, M.; Kim, T.; Tokumaru, Y.; Yan, L.; Matsuyama, R.; Endo, I.; Cherkassky, L.; Takabe, K. Enhanced DNA Repair Pathway is Associated with Cell Proliferation and Worse Survival in Hepatocellular Carcinoma (HCC). *Cancers* **2021**, *13*, 323. [CrossRef]
15. Wurmbach, E.; Chen, Y.-B.; Khitrov, G.; Zhang, W.; Roayaie, S.; Schwartz, M.; Fiel, I.; Thung, S.; Mazzaferro, V.M.; Bruix, J.; et al. Genome-wide molecular profiles of HCV-induced dysplasia and hepatocellular carcinoma. *Hepatology* **2007**, *45*, 938–947. [CrossRef] [PubMed]
16. Eun, J.; Nam, S. *Identifying Novel Drivers of Human Hepatocellular Carcinoma and Revealing Clinical Relevance as Early Diagnostic and Prognostic Biomarker*; The Catholic University of Korea: Seoul, Korea, 2017. Available online: https://www.omicsdi.org/dataset/geo/GSE89377 (accessed on 27 August 2021).
17. Brandon, H.; Shen, D. mRNA Profiling of Hepatocellular Carcinoma (HCC). Gene Expression Omnibus. 2016; GSE56545 (Medimmune). Available online: https://www.ncbi.nlm.nih.gov/geo/query/acc.cgi?acc=GSE56545 (accessed on 27 August 2021).
18. Grinchuk, O.V.; Yenamandra, S.P.; Iyer, R.; Singh, M.; Lee, H.K.; Lim, K.H.; Chow, P.K.; Kuznetsov, V.A. Tumor-adjacent tissue co-expression profile analysis reveals pro-oncogenic ribosomal gene signature for prognosis of resectable hepatocellular carcinoma. *Mol. Oncol.* **2017**, *12*, 89–113. [CrossRef] [PubMed]
19. Wanless, I.R.; Party, I.W. Terminology of nodular hepatocellular lesions. *Hepatology* **1995**, *22*, 983–993.
20. Liberzon, A.; Birger, C.; Thorvaldsdóttir, H.; Ghandi, M.; Mesirov, J.P.; Tamayo, P. The Molecular Signatures Database Hallmark Gene Set Collection. *Cell Syst.* **2015**, *1*, 417–425. [CrossRef]
21. Hänzelmann, S.; Castelo, R.; Guinney, J. GSVA: Gene set variation analysis for microarray and RNA-Seq data. *BMC Bioinform.* **2013**, *14*, 7. [CrossRef] [PubMed]
22. Gandhi, S.; Elkhanany, A.; Oshi, M.; Dai, T.; Opyrchal, M.; Mohammadpour, H.; Repasky, E.A.; Takabe, K. Contribution of Immune Cells to Glucocorticoid Receptor Expression in Breast Cancer. *Int. J. Mol. Sci.* **2020**, *21*, 4635. [CrossRef]
23. Oshi, M.; Asaoka, M.; Tokumaru, Y.; Yan, L.; Matsuyama, R.; Ishikawa, T.; Endo, I.; Takabe, K. CD8 T Cell Score as a Prognostic Biomarker for Triple Negative Breast Cancer. *Int. J. Mol. Sci.* **2020**, *21*, 6968. [CrossRef]
24. Tokumaru, Y.; Oshi, M.; Katsuta, E.; Yan, L.; Huang, J.L.; Nagahashi, M.; Matsuhashi, N.; Futamura, M.; Yoshida, K.; Takabe, K. Intratumoral Adipocyte-High Breast Cancer Enrich for Metastatic and Inflammation-Related Pathways but Associated with Less Cancer Cell Proliferation. *Int. J. Mol. Sci.* **2020**, *21*, 5744. [CrossRef]
25. Oshi, M.; Newman, S.; Murthy, V.; Tokumaru, Y.; Yan, L.; Matsuyama, R.; Endo, I.; Takabe, K. ITPKC as a Prognostic and Predictive Biomarker of Neoadjuvant Chemotherapy for Triple Negative Breast Cancer. *Cancers* **2020**, *12*, 2758. [CrossRef]
26. Oshi, M.; Tokumaru, Y.; Asaoka, M.; Yan, L.; Satyananda, V.; Matsuyama, R.; Matsuhashi, N.; Futamura, M.; Ishikawa, T.; Yoshida, K.; et al. M1 Macrophage and M1/M2 ratio defined by transcriptomic signatures resemble only part of their conventional clinical characteristics in breast cancer. *Sci. Rep.* **2020**, *10*, 1–12. [CrossRef]
27. Chouliaras, K.; Tokumaru, Y.; Asaoka, M.; Oshi, M.; Attwood, K.M.; Yoshida, K.; Ishikawa, T.; Takabe, K. Prevalence and clinical relevance of tumor-associated tissue eosinophilia (TATE) in breast cancer. *Surgery* **2020**, *169*, 1234–1239. [CrossRef]
28. Oshi, M.; Newman, S.; Tokumaru, Y.; Yan, L.; Matsuyama, R.; Endo, I.; Takabe, K. Inflammation Is Associated with Worse Outcome in the Whole Cohort but with Better Outcome in Triple-Negative Subtype of Breast Cancer Patients. *J. Immunol. Res.* **2020**, *2020*, 1–17. [CrossRef]
29. Oshi, M.; Tokumaru, Y.; Angarita, F.A.; Yan, L.; Matsuyama, R.; Endo, I.; Takabe, K. Degree of Early Estrogen Response Predict Survival after Endocrine Therapy in Primary and Metastatic ER-Positive Breast Cancer. *Cancers* **2020**, *12*, 3557. [CrossRef]
30. Schulze, A.; Oshi, M.; Endo, I.; Takabe, K. MYC Targets Scores Are Associated with Cancer Aggressiveness and Poor Survival in ER-Positive Primary and Metastatic Breast Cancer. *Int. J. Mol. Sci.* **2020**, *21*, 8127. [CrossRef]
31. Oshi, M.; Newman, S.; Tokumaru, Y.; Yan, L.; Matsuyama, R.; Endo, I.; Nagahashi, M.; Takabe, K. Intra-Tumoral Angiogenesis Is Associated with Inflammation, Immune Reaction and Metastatic Recurrence in Breast Cancer. *Int. J. Mol. Sci.* **2020**, *21*, 6708. [CrossRef]
32. Oshi, M.; Takahashi, H.; Tokumaru, Y.; Yan, L.; Rashid, O.M.; Nagahashi, M.; Matsuyama, R.; Endo, I.; Takabe, K. The E2F pathway score as a predictive biomarker of response to neoadjuvant therapy in ER+/HER2− breast cancer. *Cells* **2020**, *9*, 1643.
33. Tokumaru, Y.; Oshi, M.; Katsuta, E.; Yan, L.; Satyananda, V.; Matsuhashi, N.; Futamura, M.; Akao, Y.; Yoshida, K.; Takabe, K. KRAS signaling enriched triple negative breast cancer is associated with favorable tumor immune microenvironment and better survival. *Am. J. Cancer Res.* **2020**, *10*, 897–907.
34. Tokumaru, Y.; Oshi, M.; Patel, A.; Tian, W.; Yan, L.; Matsuhashi, N.; Futamura, M.; Yoshida, K.; Takabe, K. Organoids Are Limited in Modeling the Colon Adenoma–Carcinoma Sequence. *Cells* **2021**, *10*, 488. [CrossRef]
35. Oshi, M.; Tokumaru, Y.; Mukhopadhyay, S.; Yan, L.; Matsuyama, R.; Endo, I.; Takabe, K. Annexin A1 Expression Is Associated with Epithelial–Mesenchymal Transition (EMT), Cell Proliferation, Prognosis, and Drug Response in Pancreatic Cancer. *Cells* **2021**, *10*, 653. [CrossRef]

36. Takahashi, H.; Asaoka, M.; Yan, L.; Rashid, O.M.; Oshi, M.; Ishikawa, T.; Nagahashi, M.; Takabe, K. Biologically Aggressive Phenotype and Anti-cancer Immunity Counterbalance in Breast Cancer with High Mutation Rate. *Sci. Rep.* **2020**, *10*, 1–13. [CrossRef]
37. Oshi, M.; Satyananda, V.; Angarita, F.A.; Kim, T.H.; Tokumaru, Y.; Yan, L.; Matsuyama, R.; Endo, I.; Nagahashi, M.; Takabe, K. Angiogenesis is associated with an attenuated tumor microenvironment, aggressive biology, and worse survival in gastric cancer patients. *Am. J. Cancer Res.* **2021**, *11*, 1659–1671. [PubMed]
38. Oshi, M.; Huyser, M.; Le, L.; Tokumaru, Y.; Yan, L.; Matsuyama, R.; Endo, I.; Takabe, K. Abundance of Microvascular Endothelial Cells Is Associated with Response to Chemotherapy and Prognosis in Colorectal Cancer. *Cancers* **2021**, *13*, 1477. [CrossRef] [PubMed]
39. Okano, M.; Oshi, M.; Butash, A.L.; Katsuta, E.; Tachibana, K.; Saito, K.; Okayama, H.; Peng, X.; Yan, L.; Kono, K.; et al. Triple-Negative Breast Cancer with High Levels of Annexin A1 Expression Is Associated with Mast Cell Infiltration, Inflammation, and Angiogenesis. *Int. J. Mol. Sci.* **2019**, *20*, 4197. [CrossRef]
40. Bild, A.; Febbo, P.G. Application of a priori established gene sets to discover biologically important differential expression in microarray data. *Proc. Natl. Acad. Sci. USA* **2005**, *102*, 15278–15279. [CrossRef] [PubMed]
41. Aran, D.; Hu, Z.; Butte, A.J. xCell: Digitally portraying the tissue cellular heterogeneity landscape. *Genome Biol.* **2017**, *18*, 1–14. [CrossRef]
42. Thorsson, V.; Gibbs, D.; Brown, S.D.; Wolf, D.; Bortone, D.S.; Yang, T.-H.O.; Porta-Pardo, E.; Gao, G.F.; Plaisier, C.L.; Eddy, J.A.; et al. The Immune Landscape of Cancer. *Immunity* **2019**, *51*, 411–412. [CrossRef]
43. Chalmers, Z.R.; Connelly, C.F.; Fabrizio, D.; Gay, L.; Ali, S.M.; Ennis, R.; Schrock, A.; Campbell, B.; Shlien, A.; Chmielecki, J.; et al. Analysis of 100,000 human cancer genomes reveals the landscape of tumor mutational burden. *Genome Med.* **2017**, *9*, 1–14. [CrossRef]
44. Ghosh, R.; Lipson, K.L.; Sargent, K.E.; Mercurio, A.M.; Hunt, J.S.; Ron, D.; Urano, F. Transcriptional Regulation of VEGF-A by the Unfolded Protein Response Pathway. *PLoS ONE* **2010**, *5*, e9575. [CrossRef]
45. Lee, A.S. GRP78 Induction in Cancer: Therapeutic and Prognostic Implications: Figure 1. *Cancer Res.* **2007**, *67*, 3496–3499. [CrossRef]
46. Pluquet, O.; Dejeans, N.; Bouchecareilh, M.; Lhomond, S.; Pineau, R.; Higa, A.; Delugin, M.; Combe, C.; Loriot, S.; Cubel, G.; et al. Posttranscriptional Regulation of PER1 Underlies the Oncogenic Function of IREα. *Cancer Res.* **2013**, *73*, 4732–4743. [CrossRef]
47. Jamora, C.; Dennert, G.; Lee, A.S. Inhibition of tumor progression by suppression of stress protein GRP78/BiP induction in fibrosarcoma B/C10ME. *Proc. Natl. Acad. Sci. USA* **1996**, *93*, 7690–7694. [CrossRef]
48. Fernandez, P.M.; Tabbara, S.O.; Jacobs, L.K.; Manning, F.C.R.; Tsangaris, T.N.; Schwartz, A.M.; Kennedy, K.A.; Patierno, S.R. Overexpression of the glucose-regulated stress gene GRP78 in malignant but not benign human breast lesions. *Breast Cancer Res. Treat.* **2000**, *59*, 15–26. [CrossRef]
49. Mantovani, A.; Marchesi, F.; Malesci, A.; Laghi, L.; Allavena, P. Tumour-associated macrophages as treatment targets in oncology. *Nat. Rev. Clin. Oncol.* **2017**, *14*, 399–416. [CrossRef] [PubMed]
50. Mahadevan, N.R.; Rodvold, J.; Sepulveda, H.; Rossi, S.; Drew, A.F.; Zanetti, M. Transmission of endoplasmic reticulum stress and pro-inflammation from tumor cells to myeloid cells. *Proc. Natl. Acad. Sci. USA* **2011**, *108*, 6561–6566. [CrossRef] [PubMed]
51. Aoki, M.; Aoki, H.; Mukhopadhyay, P.; Tsuge, T.; Yamamoto, H.; Matsumoto, N.M.; Toyohara, E.; Okubo, Y.; Ogawa, R.; Takabe, K. Sphingosine-1-Phosphate Facilitates Skin Wound Healing by Increasing Angiogenesis and Inflammatory Cell Recruitment with Less Scar Formation. *Int. J. Mol. Sci.* **2019**, *20*, 3381. [CrossRef] [PubMed]
52. Katsuta, E.; Rashid, O.M.; Takabe, K. Clinical relevance of tumor microenvironment: Immune cells, vessels, and mouse models. *Hum. Cell* **2020**, *33*, 930–937. [CrossRef]
53. Ramanathan, R.; Olex, A.L.; Dozmorov, M.; Bear, H.D.; Fernandez, L.J.; Takabe, K. Angiopoietin pathway gene expression associated with poor breast cancer survival. *Breast Cancer Res. Treat.* **2017**, *162*, 191–198. [CrossRef] [PubMed]
54. Drogat, B.; Auguste, P.; Nguyen, D.T.; Bouchecareilh, M.; Pineau, R.; Nalbantoglu, J.; Kaufman, R.J.; Chevet, E.; Bikfalvi, A.; Moenner, M. IRE1 Signaling Is Essential for Ischemia-Induced Vascular Endothelial Growth Factor-A Expression and Contributes to Angiogenesis and Tumor Growth In vivo. *Cancer Res.* **2007**, *67*, 6700–6707. [CrossRef] [PubMed]
55. Koumenis, C.; Bi, M.; Ye, J.; Feldman, D.; Koong, A.C. Hypoxia and the Unfolded Protein Response. *Methods Enzymol.* **2007**, *435*, 275–293. [CrossRef]
56. Ma, Y.; Hendershot, L.M. The role of the unfolded protein response in tumour development: Friend or foe? *Nat. Rev. Cancer* **2004**, *4*, 966–977. [CrossRef] [PubMed]

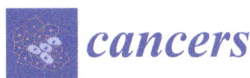

Article

Identification of Blood-Based Biomarkers for the Prediction of the Response to Neoadjuvant Chemoradiation in Rectal Cancer

Delphine Dayde [1], Jillian Gunther [2], Yutaka Hirayama [3], David C. Weksberg [2,4,†], Adam Boutin [5], Gargy Parhy [1], Clemente Aguilar-Bonavides [6], Hong Wang [7,8,†], Hiroyuki Katayama [7], Yuichi Abe [9], Kim-Anh Do [6], Kazuo Hara [10], Takashi Kinoshita [11], Koji Komori [11], Yasuhiro Shimizu [11], Masahiro Tajika [3], Yasumasa Niwa [3], Y. Alan Wang [5], Ronald DePinho [5], Samir Hanash [7], Sunil Krishnan [2,12,†] and Ayumu Taguchi [1,9,13,*]

1. Department of Translational Molecular Pathology, The University of Texas MD Anderson Cancer Center, Houston, TX 77030, USA; delphine.dayde@inserm.fr (D.D.); gparhy@deloitte.com (G.P.)
2. Department of Radiation Oncology, The University of Texas MD Anderson Cancer Center, Houston, TX 77030, USA; JGunther@mdanderson.org (J.G.); weksbergdc@upmc.edu (D.C.W.); Krishnan.Sunil@mayo.edu (S.K.)
3. Department of Endoscopy, Aichi Cancer Center Hospital, Nagoya 464-8681, Japan; yhirayama@aichi-cc.jp (Y.H.); mtajika@aichi-cc.jp (M.T.); yniwa@aichi-cc.jp (Y.N.)
4. UPMC Pinnacle Radiation Oncology, Harrisburg, PA 17109, USA
5. Department of Cancer Biology, The University of Texas MD Anderson Cancer Center, Houston, TX 77030, USA; adam@glympsebio.com (A.B.); yalanwang@mdanderson.org (A.Y.W.); rdepinho@mdanderson.org (R.D.)
6. Department of Biostatistics, The University of Texas MD Anderson Cancer Center, Houston, TX 77030, USA; jaguil21@its.jnj.com (C.A.-B.); kimdo@mdanderson.org (K.-A.D.)
7. Department of Clinical Cancer Prevention, The University of Texas MD Anderson Cancer Center, Houston, TX 77030, USA; wh@cwmda.com (H.W.); HKatayama1@mdanderson.org (H.K.); SHanash@mdanderson.org (S.H.)
8. Hangzhou Cosmos Wisdom Mass Spectrometry Center of Zhejiang University Medical School, Hangzhou 311200, China
9. Division of Molecular Diagnostics, Aichi Cancer Center, Nagoya 464-8681, Japan; y.abe@aichi-cc.jp
10. Department of Gastroenterology, Aichi Cancer Center Hospital, Nagoya 464-8681, Japan; khara@aichi-cc.jp
11. Department of Gastroenterological Surgery, Aichi Cancer Center Hospital, Nagoya 464-8681, Japan; t-kinoshita@aichi-cc.jp (T.K.); kkomori@aichi-cc.jp (K.K.); yshimizu@aichi-cc.jp (Y.S.)
12. Department of Radiation Oncology, Mayo Clinic Florida, Jacksonville, FL 32224, USA
13. Division of Advanced Cancer Diagnostics, Nagoya University Graduate School of Medicine, Nagoya 466-8550, Japan
* Correspondence: a.taguchi@aichi-cc.jp; Tel.: +81-52-764-9884
† Present address.

Simple Summary: Although pathologic complete response (pCR) to neoadjuvant chemoradiation (nCRT) in locally advanced rectal cancer (LARC) is associated with better outcomes, a subset of tumors exhibit resistance to nCRT. Therefore, there is a need of biomarkers to predict the nCRT response and increment efforts for personalized therapeutic options. To this end, we analyzed pretreatment plasma proteome of a mouse model of rectal cancer treated with concurrent chemoradiation, resulting in identification and validation of plasma VEGFR3 as a potential predicting biomarker. In addition, plasma levels of EGFR and COX2, previously validated tissue-based predicting biomarkers, were significantly higher in non-pCR than pCR LARC patients, indicating that EGFR and COX2 can also serve as blood-based biomarkers. The performance of the biomarker panel combining VEGFR3, EGFR, and COX2 were significantly improved compared to that of each marker alone, providing a rationale for further integration and refinement of the biomarker panel and validation in the larger sample sets.

Abstract: The current standard of care for patients with locally advanced rectal cancer (LARC) is neoadjuvant chemoradiation (nCRT) followed by total mesorectal excision surgery. However, the response to nCRT varies among patients and only about 20% of LARC patients achieve a pathologic complete response (pCR) at the time of surgery. Therefore, there is an unmet need for biomarkers that could predict the response to nCRT at an early time point, allowing for the selection of LARC patients

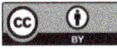

who would or would not benefit from nCRT. To identify blood-based biomarkers for prediction of nCRT response, we performed in-depth quantitative proteomic analysis of pretreatment plasma from mice bearing rectal tumors treated with concurrent chemoradiation, resulting in the quantification of 567 proteins. Among the plasma proteins that increased in mice with residual rectal tumor after chemoradiation compared to mice that achieved regression, we selected three proteins (Vascular endothelial growth factor receptor 3 [VEGFR3], Insulin like growth factor binding protein 4 [IGFBP4], and Cathepsin B [CTSB]) for validation in human plasma samples. In addition, we explored whether four tissue protein biomarkers previously shown to predict response to nCRT (Epidermal growth factor receptor [EGFR], Ki-67, E-cadherin, and Prostaglandin G/H synthase 2 [COX2]) also act as potential blood biomarkers. Using immunoassays for these seven biomarker candidates as well as Carcinoembryonic antigen [CEA] levels on plasma collected before nCRT from 34 patients with LARC (6 pCR and 28 non-pCR), we observed that levels of VEGFR3 ($p = 0.0451$, AUC = 0.720), EGFR ($p = 0.0128$, AUC = 0.679), and COX2 ($p = 0.0397$, AUC = 0.679) were significantly increased in the plasma of non-pCR LARC patients compared to those of pCR LARC patients. The performance of the logistic regression model combining VEGFR3, EGFR, and COX2 was significantly improved compared with the performance of each biomarker, yielding an AUC of 0.869 (sensitivity 43% at 95% specificity). Levels of VEGFR3 and EGFR were significantly decreased 5 to 7 months after tumor resection in plasma from 18 surgically resected rectal cancer patients, suggesting that VEGFR3 and EGFR may emanate from tumors. These findings suggest that circulating VEGFR3 can contribute to the prediction of the nCRT response in LARC patients together with circulating EGFR and COX2.

Keywords: rectal cancer; neoadjuvant chemoradiation; mouse model; proteomics; biomarkers

1. Introduction

The current standard of care for patients with clinical stage II or III locally advanced rectal cancer (LARC), defined as T3–T4 or node-positive non-metastatic disease, is neoadjuvant chemoradiation (nCRT) followed by total mesorectal excision (TME) surgery to improve resectability, anal sphincter preservation, and long-term outcome [1,2]. However, the response to nCRT in LARC varies among patients. After nCRT, about 20% of LARC patients achieve a pathological complete response (pCR), which is associated with favorable 5-year disease-free survival compared to those without complete response (non-pCR) [3,4]. Conversely, while ~40% of LARC patients achieve a wide range of partial responses, a subset (~20%) of tumors exhibit resistance to nCRT, demonstrating either progression or only minimal regression/stable disease [5].

Given the achievement of pCR in a significant proportion of patients undergoing nCRT and the adverse effects of major TME surgery such as perioperative mortality, anastomotic leak, stoma-related complications, and long-term urinary and sexual dysfunction [6–8], there is a growing interest in organ preservation for LARC patients who achieve a clinical complete response (cCR) after nCRT. Since 2004, a series of studies have reported the promising potential of a watch-and-wait strategy to avoid major TME surgery [9–12]. Recent large datasets from meta-analyses and registry studies indicated that 5-year overall survival did not differ between patients treated with a watch-and-wait and those with surgery [13,14], suggesting that the watch-and-wait strategy can be an alternative to TME surgery with low oncological risk. However, the significant limitation of the watch-and-wait strategy is the poor concordance between pCR and cCR, which can result in local regrowth after nCRT [13–15]. Therefore, there is an immense need for biomarkers for safe adoption of the watch-and-wait strategy to predict pCR and identify patients who may potentially avoid surgery after completion of nCRT.

A wide variety of clinical, pathologic, and radiologic factors, including tumor size, differentiation, clinical T and N stages, and tumor regression rates, have been associated with nCRT response [16–19]. Several potential tissue- or blood-based molecular biomarkers to predict the nCRT response, including DNA methylation, protein, miRNA, and cfDNA, have also been described [20–23]. As carcinoembryonic antigen (CEA) is routinely used for disease monitoring in colorectal cancer, the relationship of CEA and the nCRT response has been most widely studied. A recent meta-analysis suggest that pretreatment CEA levels were significantly and inversely correlated with the rate of pCR [24]. However, to date, none of these clinicopathological, radiological, or molecular biomarkers have yet reached the clinic due to inadequate sensitivity and specificity.

In this study, we sought to identify blood-based biomarkers that can differentiate patients who will achieve a pCR versus non-pCR by analyzing the plasma proteome of a mouse model with rectal cancer that recapitulate molecular and biological features of human rectal cancer [25]. This approach allows minimization of extraneous variability and blood sampling at defined pre-therapeutic time points during the course of tumor progression [26]. In addition, we investigated whether previously validated tissue-based biomarkers for nCRT response [20] can also serve as blood-based biomarkers for predicting pCR.

2. Materials and Methods

2.1. Mouse Model

All animal experiments were conducted in accordance with institutional and national guidelines and regulations with approval by the Institutional Animal Care and Use Committee at The University of Texas MD Anderson Cancer Center. At 8 weeks of age, mice were administered with a 4-hydroxytamoxifen (4-OHT) enema (1 mg/mL) and doxycycline [25]. Beginning at 4 weeks post-induction, tumor size was measured as the percentage of tumor occlusion of the lumen by weekly colonoscopy. Once the percentage of tumor occlusion of the lumen reached 50%, intraperitoneal injection of 5-FU (30 mg/kg) and concurrent radiation (5 Gy per fraction) were administered to four mice with rectal tumors for 5 consecutive days, resulting in two mice showing complete tumor regression and two mice with residual tumors. Four control mice at the same age without Cre DNA recombinase were also treated with the same regimen. Five days prior to the treatment, plasma was collected, and Magnetic resonance imaging (MRI) was performed to assess rectal tumors. Mice were euthanized a week after chemoradiation and response to chemoradiation was pathologically evaluated.

2.2. Mass Spectrometry Analysis of Pretreatment Mouse Plasma Samples

An independent pool of pretreatment plasmas from two mice with rectal tumors achieving regression, two mice with residual rectal tumors after chemoradiation, and four control mice were created. Each pool of mouse plasma was subjected to immunodepletion, whereby the top three abundant proteins (albumin, IgG, and transferrin) were removed using an Immunodepletion column (Agilent Technologies, Santa Clara, CA, USA). The remaining low abundant proteins in each sample were treated with 25 mM tris(2-carboxyethyl)phosphine (TCEP) for Cys reduction and subsequently labeled with Iodoacetyl Tandem Mass Tag (IodoTMT) sixplex isobaric label reagent (Thermo Fisher Scientific, Waltham, USA). The mixture of labeled samples was separated by an orthogonal two-dimensional high-performance liquid chromatography (2D-HPLC) system (Shimadzu, Kyoto, Japan) with eight fractions of anion-exchange (Agilent Technologies, Santa Clara, USA) as the first dimension followed by 12 reversed-phase fractions by RPGS reversed-phase column (4.6 mm I.D. × 150 mm, 15 µm, 1000 Å, Column Technology Inc, Fremont, CA, USA) as the second dimension. Collected protein fractions were lyophilized, digested with trypsin, and analyzed by nano LC–high definition MS^E ($HDMS^E$) with Synapt G2Si ion-mobility quadrupole time-of-flight (Q-TOF) mass spectrometry (Waters, Milford, USA).

The 2 h gradient elution was performed in a capillary column (C18, 3 µm 120 Å, 75 µmID × 25 cmL, Column Technology, Inc., Fremont, USA) at 500 nl/min with the mobile phase A 0.1% formic acid (FA) in 2% acetonitrile (ACN) and B 0.1% FA in 98% ACN. The mass spectrometer was operated with a resolving power of at least 20,000 full width at half maximum (FWHM) at m/z 785.843 (+2, Glu1-fibrinopeptide B) nano electrospray ionization (ESI) source with a NanoLockSpray. The lock mass channel was sampled every 60 s.

Accurate LC-HDMS^E data were acquired in an alternating low energy (HDMS) and high energy (HDMS$^{E)}$) mode with mass scan range from m/z 50 to 1800 under a capillary voltage of 2.8 kV, a source temperature of 100 °C, and a cone voltage of 30 V. The spectral acquisition in each mode is 1.0 s with a 0.1 s inter-scan. In HDMS mode, data are collected at a collision energy of 2 eV in both Trap and Transfer cell. In HDMS^E mode, the collision energy is ramped up from 25 to 55 eV in the Transfer cell. The acquired data were processed through ProteinLynx Global Server (PLGS, WATERS, Milford, USA) and searched against the Uniprot mouse database at 4% false discovery rate (FDR). The identified proteins were filtered with ≤ 5 ppm mass accuracy of sequenced peptides. Quantile normalization approach was used to normalize the peak intensities of reporter ions before protein quantification.

2.3. Human Plasma Samples

All human plasma samples were obtained following Institutional Review Board approval and informed consent. Plasma samples were collected from 34 treatment-naïve LARC patients undergoing neoadjuvant chemoradiation (50.4 Gy in 28 daily fractions of 1.8 Gy with concurrent capecitabine (an oral prodrug of 5-fluorouracil)) at the MD Anderson Cancer Center, and used for validation of biomarker candidates (pretreatment LARC set). After completion of chemoradiation, patients underwent surgical excision, and standardized pathological procedures were followed for the assessment of residual disease. An independent set of plasma samples collected at the time of diagnosis and 5 to 7 months after surgery from 18 surgically resected rectal cancer patients at the Aichi Cancer Center was used to assess the association between biomarker candidates and surgical resection (pre-and post-surgery RC set). All patients in the pre- and post-surgery RC set were treated by surgery alone.

2.4. Luminex Assays

Levels of Vascular endothelial growth factor receptor 3 (VEGFR3), Insulin like growth factor binding protein 4 (IGFBP4), Carcinoembryonic antigen (CEA), Epidermal growth factor receptor (EGFR), and E-cadherin were measured using the Luminex kit (HANG2MAG-12K, HIGFBMAG-53K, HCCBP1MAG-58K, and HSCRMAG-32K from Millipore, and EPX010-12315-901 from Life Technologies), according to the manufacturer's instructions. Each sample was assayed in duplicate, and the absorbance was measured with a calibrated Bio-Plex machine (Bio-Plex MAGPIX System, Bio-Rad, Hercules, CA, USA).

2.5. ELISA Assays

Levels of Cathepsin B (CTSB), Ki-67, and Prostaglandin G/H synthase 2 (COX2) were determined using enzyme-linked immunosorbent assay (ELISA) kits (ab119584 from Abcam, Cambridge, UK; DY7617-05 from R&D Systems, Minneapolis, MN, USA; and RAB1034-1KT from Sigma-Aldrich, St. Louis, MO, USA) and according to the manufacturer's protocol. For all ELISA experiments, each sample was assayed in duplicate, and the absorbance was measured with a FLUOstar Omega microplate reader (BMG Labtech, Ortenberg, Germany).

2.6. Statistical Analysis

Categorical data were compared by Fisher's exact test or a chi-square test using Prism 7.05/e software (GraphPad). For all Luminex and ELISA assays, an internal control sample was run in every plate, and each value of the samples was divided by the mean value of the internal control in the same plate to correct the interplate variability. Individual biomarker performance was assessed using the Welch's t-test or the paired t-test. Sensitivity, specificity, and the area under the curve (AUC) were determined by a receiver operating characteristic analysis. The likelihood ratio test was employed to assess the significance of the model based on the biomarker panel combining VEGFR3, EGFR, and COX2.

3. Results

3.1. Proteomic Profiling of Pretreatment Plasmas from a Mouse Model of Rectal Cancer Treated with Chemoradiation

To faithfully recapitulate the development of human locally advanced rectal cancer (LARC), we utilized a genetically engineered mouse model of colorectal cancer, which harbors a Doxycycline (Dox)-inducible oncogenic Kras allele and conditional null alleles of Apc and Trp53 (iKAP) [25]. Approximately 25% of iKAP mice are expected to develop only rectal tumors by colon-specific activation of Cre DNA recombinase with rectal enema of 4-OHT. Occurrence of rectal tumors in Dox-treated iKAP mice was confirmed by endoscopy, MRI, and biopsy (Figure 1A). iKAP mice with rectal tumors and control mice without Cre DNA recombinase received intraperitoneal injection of 5-FU (30 mg/kg) and concurrent radiation (5 Gy per fraction) for 5 consecutive days (Figure 1B). To assess the response to chemoradiation, mice were sacrificed a week after the treatment. Figure 1C depicts macroscopic images of colons of iKAP mice with residual tumors (non-regression) (#1) and with complete tumor regression (Regression) (#2), while rectal tumors of #1 and #2 mice were not distinctively different before chemoradiation (Figure 1A).

To identify plasma proteins that can predict pCR before chemoradiation, plasma samples were collected 5 days prior to chemoradiation from iKAP mice with rectal tumors and control mice (Figure 1B). For mass spectrometry analysis, plasma samples from two Regression mice, two Non-regression mice, and four control mice were respectively pooled. In-depth quantitative proteomic analysis with using tandem mass tags (TMT) labeling resulted in quantification of 567 proteins (393 unique genes). To gain insights into the underlying biological difference of increased plasma proteins in Regression mice and Non-regression mice, we performed a pathway analysis of proteins with more than a two-fold increase in the plasma of either Regression mice or Non-regression mice compared to control mice using WebGestalt (http://www.webgestalt.org/, accessed on 25 March 2020) [27]. Over-Representation Analysis based on KEGG (https://www.genome.jp/kegg/, accessed on 25 March 2020) [28] resulted in identification of 5 and 13 pathways that were significantly associated with increased proteins in the plasma of Regression mice or Non-regression mice compared to control mice, respectively (p values < 0.05, hypergeometric test, and with three or more overlapping proteins) (Figure 2A and Supplementary Table S1). While four pathways commonly identified in the comparison of Regression vs. control and Non-regression vs. control were associated with metabolism, nine pathways that were uniquely identified in the comparison of Non-regression vs. control were associated with the immune system and infectious disease (Complement and coagulation cascades; Antigen processing and presentation; Staphylococcus aureus infection; Pertussis), intracellular transport and catabolism (Lysosome; Phagosome), focal adhesion (Focal adhesion; Proteoglycans in cancer), and the endocrine system (Thyroid hormone synthesis) (Figure 2A,B).

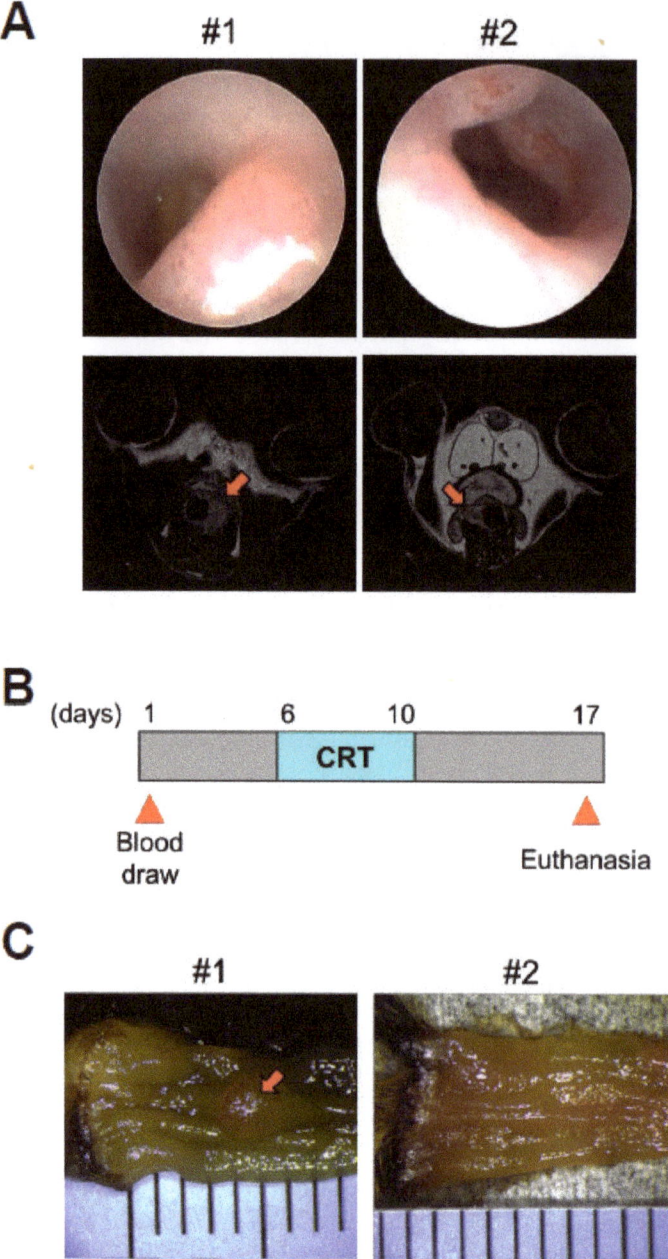

Figure 1. Chemoradiation treatment of iKAP mice with rectal tumors. (**A**). Endoscopic images (top) and MRI scans (bottom) of rectal tumors. Red arrows in MRI scans indicate rectal tumors. (**B**). Outline of the experimental design for intraperitoneal injection of 5-FU and concurrent radiation. (**C**). Macroscopic images of colons of iKAP mice with residual tumor (Non-regression) (#1) and with complete tumor regression (Regression) (#2). A red arrow indicates residual tumors. CRT: chemoradiation.

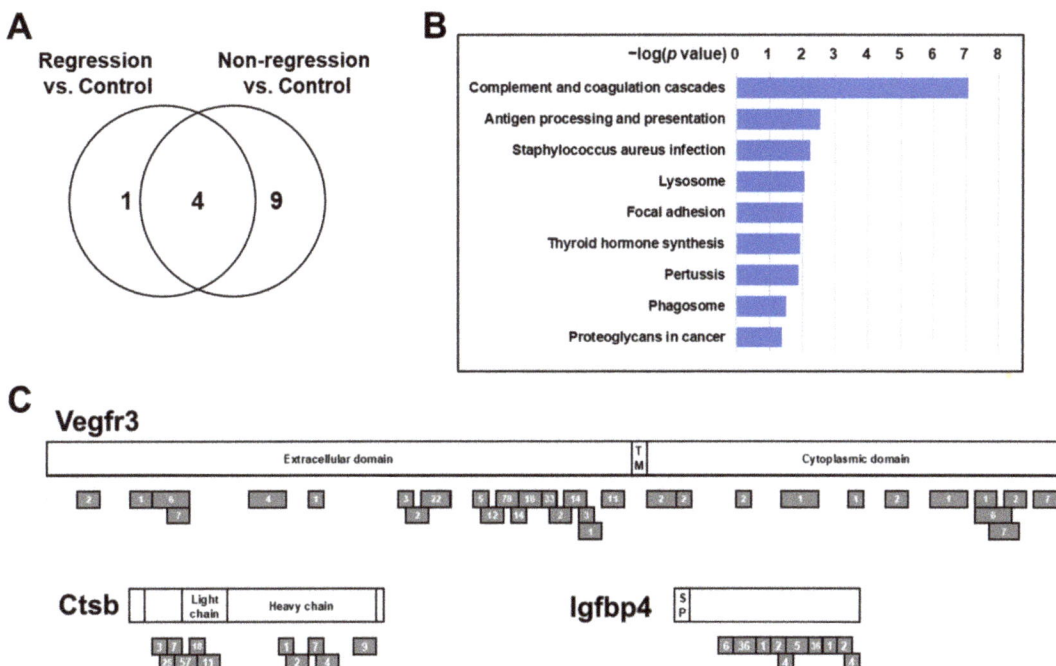

Figure 2. Proteomic analysis of pretreatment plasmas from iKAP mice with complete tumor regression and with residual tumors. (**A**). Venn diagrams of pathways are significantly associated with more than a two-fold increase of proteins in the plasma of Regression mice or Non-regression mice compared to control mice. (**B**). Pathways uniquely identified in the comparison of Non-regression vs. control. p values were calculated by hypergeometric test. (**C**). Schema of mouse Vegfr3, Ctsb, and Igfbp4. Gray bars indicate peptides identified in mouse plasma. Numbers indicate mass spectra counts for each peptide. The amino acid sequences are based on P35917-1 for Vegfr3, P10605-1 for Ctsb, and P47879-1 for Igfbp4.

To determine biomarker candidates for prediction of pCR, we applied the following criteria: (1) the number of quantified peptides ≥ 10, (2) Non-regression/Control ratio > 3, and (3) Non-regression/Regression ratio > 3. Nine proteins passed these criteria (Table 1), and intriguingly, Collagen type I alpha 1 chain (Col1a1), Cathepsin B (Ctsb), and Vascular endothelial growth factor receptor 3 (Vegfr3) were included in the pathways uniquely associated with increased plasma proteins in Non-regression mice (Supplementary Table S1), suggesting a possible biological link between these proteins and rectal tumors resistant to chemoradiation. In addition, Insulin like growth factor binding protein 4 (Igfbp4) is of interest, as it can bind to and modulate the function of Insulin-like growth factor I (Igf1) [29], which is also included in two pathways associated with focal adhesion (Supplementary Table S1). Our mass spectrometry analysis yielded substantial peptide coverage for Vegfr3, Ctsb, and Igfbp4 (Figure 2C and Table 1), and therefore, we selected these three proteins for validation in human plasma samples.

3.2. Validation of Protein Biomarker Candidates in a Set of LARC Plasma Samples

VEGFR3, CTSB, and IGFBP4, as well as Carcinoembryonic antigen (CEA) were assayed in the pretreatment LARC set consisting of plasma samples collected prior to nCRT from 34 patients with LARC. In the pretreatment LARC set, 6 (17.6%) patients achieved pCR (pCR) and 28 (82.4%) patients had residual tumors after nCRT (non-pCR). While non-pCR LARC patients had more advanced T stages, clinical factors did not show a statistically significant difference between pCR and non-pCR LARC patients (Table 2).

Table 1. Plasma proteins increased in Non-regression iKAP mice.

Protein	Total Number of Peptides	Non-Regression/Control Ratio	Non-Regression/Regression Ratio
Igfbp4	38	9.9	3.6
Col1a1	13	8.1	3.7
Prdx6	10	6.4	5.2
Park7	13	4.9	5.0
F13b	138	4.2	3.7
Flna	20	4.1	3.4
Ctsb	44	4.0	3.0
Vegfr3	91	3.8	3.7
Blvrb	14	3.3	4.4

Igfbp4: Insulin like growth factor binding protein 4, Col1a1: Collagen type I alpha 1 chain, Prdx6: Peroxiredoxin-6, Park7: Parkinson disease protein 7, F13b: Coagulation factor XIII B chain, Flna: Filamin-A, Ctsb: Cathepsin B, Vegfr3: Vascular endothelial growth factor receptor 3, Blvrb: Biliverdin reductase B.

Table 2. Subject characteristics in the pretreatment LARC set.

Characteristics	pCR ($n = 6$)	Non-pCR ($n = 28$)	p Value
Gender			
Female	3	13	>0.9999
Male	3	15	
Age (years)			
Mean (range)	56.0 (45–67)	56.5 (28–74)	
<56	3	12	>0.9999
≥56	3	16	
T stage			
T2	3	3	0.0603
T3	3	21	
T4	0	4	
N stage			
N0	0	1	0.2528
N1	6	18	
N2	0	8	
Stage			
IIa	0	1	0.1379
IIIa	3	3	
IIIb	3	22	
IIIc	0	2	
Tumor length (cm)			
<4.5	2	13	0.6722
≥4.5	4	15	
Distance from anal verge (cm)			
<6.5	4	13	0.6562
≥6.5	2	15	

p values were calculated by Fisher's exact test or a chi-square test.

In addition to three selected biomarker candidates, as many potential tissue-based biomarkers have been associated with nCRT response [20], we sought to determine whether tissue-based protein biomarkers in blood also can have the potential to predict pCR. According to prior studies, we selected four proteins, including Epidermal growth factor receptor (EGFR), Ki-67, Prostaglandin G/H synthase 2 (COX2), and E-cadherin, for testing in the pretreatment LARC set.

Plasma levels of VEGFR3, EGFR, and COX2 were significantly higher in non-pCR LARC compared to pCR LARC (VEGFR3: $p = 0.0451$, EGFR: $p = 0.0128$, COX2: $p = 0.0397$, Welch's t-test) (Figure 3A). CEA and other four biomarker candidates were not significantly different between pCR and non-pCR LARC patients (CEA: $p = 0.1940$, CTSB: $p = 0.7894$, IGFBP4: $p = 0.3469$, Ki-67: $p = 0.1547$, E-cadherin: $p = 0.3836$, Welch's t-test).

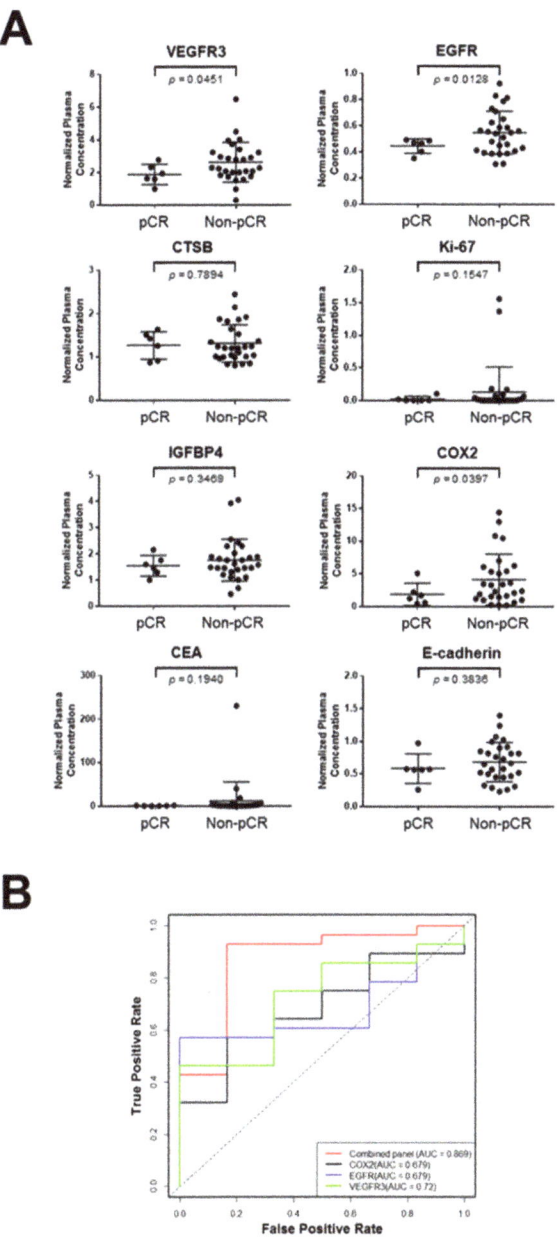

Figure 3. Validation of biomarker candidates in the pretreatment LARC set. (**A**). Levels of VEGFR3, CTSB, IGFBP4, CEA, EGFR, Ki-67, COX2, and E-cadherin in plasmas collected before nCRT from LARC patients who achieved pCR (pCR; n = 6) and LARC patients who had residual tumors after nCRT (non-pCR; n = 28). Horizontal lines indicate mean and standard deviation. p values were calculated using Welch's t-test. (**B**). Receiver operating characteristic curves for VEGFR3, EGFR, COX2, and their combination in the pretreatment LARC set. CEA: Carcinoembryonic antigen, EGFR: Epidermal growth factor receptor, COX2: Prostaglandin G/H synthase 2, AUC: the area under the curve.

We explored whether a combination rather than individual biomarkers allows for better discrimination of pCR and non-CR. The combination of VEGFR3, EGFR, and COX2 using logistic regression yielded an area under the curve (AUC) of 0.869 with a sensitivity of 43% at 95% specificity in the comparison of pCR and non-pCR LARC patients, which was significantly higher than AUC of each marker alone (VEGFR3: AUC = 0.720, p = 0.0152, likelihood ratio test; EGFR: AUC = 0.679, p = 0.0160, likelihood ratio test; COX2: AUC = 0.679, p = 0.0151, likelihood ratio test) in the pretreatment LARC set (Figure 3B).

3.3. Correlation of VEGFR3, EGFR, and COX2 in the Plasma of Rectal Cancer Patients Before and After Surgery

We next determined whether plasma levels of VEGFR3, EGFR, and COX2 are associated with surgical resection of rectal cancer. For this analysis, VEGFR3, EGFR, and COX2 were assayed in an independent set of plasma consisting of samples collected from 18 rectal cancer patients at the time of diagnosis and 5 to 7 months after surgical resection (pre-and post-surgery RC set; Figure 4A). All these rectal cancer patients remained disease-free for five years after surgery. Plasma levels of VEGFR3 and EGFR were significantly decreased after tumor resection (VEGFR3: p = 0.0119, EGFR: p = 0.0058, paired t-test) (Figure 4B). Levels of plasma COX2 did not change significantly after surgery compared to presurgical levels (p = 0.1867, paired t-test).

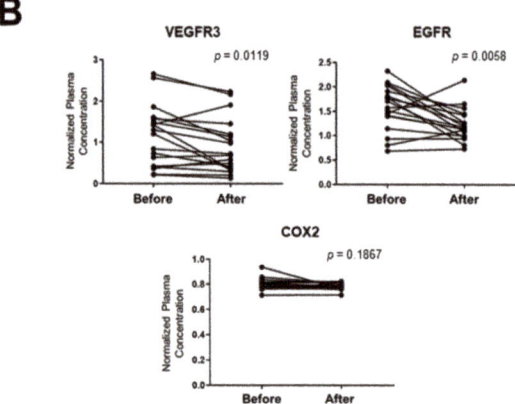

Figure 4. Correlation of plasma VEGFR3, EGFR, and COX2 with surgical resection in patients with rectal cancer. (**A**). Subject characteristics in the pre-and post-surgery RC set. (**B**). Levels of VEGFR3, EGFR, and COX2 in plasmas collected at the time of diagnosis (Before) and 5 to 7 months after surgery (After) from 18 rectal cancer patients. p values were calculated by paired t-tests.

4. Discussion

In this study, we profiled the pretreatment plasma proteome of a mouse model of rectal cancer treated with concurrent chemoradiation to identify potential blood-based biomarkers for predicting pCR in LARC patients. Among plasma protein signatures associated with Non-regression, proteins involved in focal adhesion are of particular interest, as deregulation of integrin-mediated focal adhesion has been shown to lead to therapeutic resistance [30]. We found that levels of Vegfr3, one of the proteins in the "Focal adhesion" pathway, was significantly increased in the pretreatment plasma of Non-regression mice compared to Regression mice and control mice. Increased levels of circulating VEGFR3 were validated in plasma collected prior to nCRT from non-pCR LARC patients compared to pCR LARC patients. We also demonstrated that plasma VEGFR3 levels were significantly decreased after surgical resection of rectal tumors. Yeh et al. recently showed a significant correlation between circulating VEGFR3 levels and expression of VEGFR3 in tumor tissues [31]. These findings suggest that circulating VEGFR3 emanated from tumor tissues. VEGFR3 is crucial for the development and maintenance of blood and lymphatic vascular systems [32]. While VEGFR3 is primarily expressed in lymphatic endothelial cells, VEGFR3 and its main ligand VEGF-C are expressed in tumor cells of various types of cancer, including colorectal cancer [33]. Higher expression of VEGFR3 in tumor tissues has been also associated with advanced TNM stages, the occurrence of metastasis, and poor prognosis in colorectal cancer [31,34]. Recent studies have revealed that activation of VEGF-C/VEGFR3 signaling promotes tumor growth and invasion by disrupting the lymphatic endothelial barrier and by recruiting and inducing immunosuppressive tumor-associated macrophages in colorectal cancer [34,35]. Given the emerging evidence suggesting crucial roles of VEGF-C/VEGFR3 axis in cancer progression, multiple therapeutic strategies for VEGF-C/VEGFR3-targeted therapies, including small molecule VEGFR3 inhibitors, monoclonal antibodies targeting VEGF-C, and neutralizing antibodies or peptides that block VEGFR3 signaling, have been developed [33]. Therefore, while our findings indicated the potential of circulating VEGFR3 as a biomarker for nCRT response, circulating VEGFR3 may also serve as a biomarker for the prediction of prognosis and response to VEGF-C/VEGFR3-targeted therapies.

In this study, we also explored whether tissue-based biomarkers that have been associated with nCRT response can serve as blood-based biomarkers for pCR prediction. Among four tissue-based biomarkers selected for testing, we observed significantly increased levels of circulating EGFR and COX2 in plasmas collected prior to nCRT from non-pCR LARC patients compared to pCR LARC patients.

Several studies have reported the significant association of tissue EGFR expression and response to nCRT in LARC [36]. A recent study indicated that higher expression of EGFR in the nucleus is associated with poor survival in LARC patients treated with nCRT [37]. While we demonstrated for the first time that circulating EGFR could be used as a potential biomarker for predicting pCR in rectal cancer, circulating EGFR has been associated with response to therapy in several types of cancer [38]. Interestingly, Okada et al. demonstrated that downregulation of EGFR in tumor tissue after treatment with anti-EGFR antibodies was significantly correlated with therapeutic response in patients with colorectal cancer [39]. Although a recent meta-analysis indicated the addition of EGFR inhibitors did not improve the efficacy of neoadjuvant therapy in KRAS-wild type LARC patients [40], monitoring circulating EGFR may help determine whether to continue EGFR-targeted therapy or not.

Regarding tissue COX2 expression in LARC, previous studies have reported an association of COX2 overexpression and poor response to nCRT [20]. While we demonstrated that circulating COX2 was significantly increased in the plasma of non-pCR LARC patients compared to pCR LARC patients, surgical resection of rectal tumors did not affect circulating COX2 levels. As COX2 is induced by various inflammation mediators [41], increased levels of circulating COX2 in LARC patients may be due to cancer-associated systemic inflammation or some other physiological stress, such as infection. However, given that development of cancer-associated systemic inflammation is associated with a poorer outcome [42] and that a recent phase II clinical trial of nCRT combining COX2 inhibitor celecoxib in LARC improved efficacy and decreased toxicity [43], it would be interesting to determine whether circulating COX2 levels can predict prognosis and response to nCRT combined with COX2 inhibitors.

The logistic regression model combining circulating VEGFR3, EGFR, and COX2 yielded a significantly higher AUC in differentiating pCR and non-CR compared to that of each marker alone. However, blood contains a wide variety of measurable molecules and cellular materials, including exosomes, tumor-derived DNAs, microRNAs, autoantibodies, and metabolites, making blood a rich resource of biomarkers. Therefore, it is critical to determine the relevance and relative contributions of the different types of biomarkers in the same samples [20], allowing to further refine the biomarker panel with integrating other previously or newly identified biomarkers. In addition, due to a small sample size in the current study, the performance of these three blood-based biomarkers will need to be assessed in larger sample sets, and the biomarker panel will need to be further refined with integrating other previously validated biomarkers.

5. Conclusions

In conclusion, we identified circulating VEGFR3 as a novel biomarker for predicting pCR through proteomic analysis of plasmas from a mouse model of rectal cancer, and further confirmed increased VEGFR3 levels in pretreatment plasmas from non-pCR LARC patients compared to pCR LARC patients. We also demonstrated that levels of circulating EGFR and COX2, known tissue-based biomarkers for nCRT response, were significantly increased in pretreatment plasma of non-pCR LARC patients. Our findings provide a rationale for further studies to safely adopt the watch-and-wait strategy with using blood-based biomarkers in LARC patients.

Supplementary Materials: The following are available online at https://www.mdpi.com/article/10.3390/cancers13143642/s1. Table S1: Significantly associated pathways for more than a two-fold increase of proteins in the plasma of pCR mice or non-pCR mice compared to control mice.

Author Contributions: Conceptualization, S.K. and A.T.; Data curation, H.W., H.K. and S.H.; Formal analysis, C.A.-B. and K.-A.D.; Investigation, D.D., J.G., D.C.W., G.P., Y.A., S.H., S.K. and A.T.; Methodology, D.D., D.C.W. and A.B.; Resources, J.G., Y.H., D.C.W., A.B., K.H., T.K., K.K., Y.S., M.T., Y.N., Y.A.W. and R.D.; Writing—Original Draft, D.D. and A.T.; Writing—review and editing, all authors. All authors have read and agreed to the published version of the manuscript.

Funding: This work was supported in part by the MD Anderson start-up funds, the Aichi Cancer Research Foundation, the Suzuken Memorial Foundation, the Daiwa Securities Health Foundation, and the JSPS KAKENHI Grant Number JP20K09116. K.A.D. was partially supported by a Cancer Center Support Grant NCI Grant P30 CA016672, NIH grants UL1TR003167 and 5R01GM122775, the prostate cancer SPORE P50 CA140388, CPRIT grant RP160693, and the Moon Shots funding at the MD Anderson Cancer Center.

Institutional Review Board Statement: This study was conducted according to the guidelines of the Declaration of Helsinki, and approved by the Institutional Review Board of the University of Texas MD Anderson Cancer Center (PA12-0614) and Aichi Cancer Center (2016-1-310).

Informed Consent Statement: Informed consent was obtained from all subjects involved in the study.

Data Availability Statement: The results of the proteomic analysis of mouse plasmas presented in this study are available upon reasonable request from the corresponding author.

Conflicts of Interest: The authors declare no competing interests to disclose.

References

1. Brenner, H.; Kloor, M.; Pox, C.P. Colorectal cancer. *Lancet* **2014**, *383*, 1490–1502. [CrossRef]
2. Sineshaw, H.M.; Jemal, A.; Thomas, C.R.; Mitin, T. Changes in treatment patterns for patients with locally advanced rectal cancer in the United States over the past decade: An analysis from the National Cancer Data Base. *Cancer* **2016**, *122*, 1996–2003. [CrossRef] [PubMed]
3. Maas, M.; Nelemans, P.J.; Valentini, V.; Das, P.; Rödel, C.; Kuo, L.-J.; Calvo, A.F.; García-Aguilar, J.; Glynne-Jones, R.; Haustermans, K.; et al. Long-term outcome in patients with a pathological complete response after chemoradiation for rectal cancer: A pooled analysis of individual patient data. *Lancet Oncol.* **2010**, *11*, 835–844. [CrossRef]
4. Martin, S.T.; Heneghan, H.; Winter, D.C. Systematic review and meta-analysis of outcomes following pathological complete response to neoadjuvant chemoradiotherapy for rectal cancer. *BJS* **2012**, *99*, 918–928. [CrossRef] [PubMed]
5. Fokas, E.; Liersch, T.; Fietkau, R.; Hohenberger, W.; Beissbarth, T.; Hess, C.; Becker, H.; Ghadimi, M.; Mrak, K.; Merkel, S.; et al. Tumor Regression Grading After Preoperative Chemoradiotherapy for Locally Advanced Rectal Carcinoma Revisited: Updated Results of the CAO/ARO/AIO-94 Trial. *J. Clin. Oncol.* **2014**, *32*, 1554–1562. [CrossRef]
6. Paun, B.C.; Cassie, S.; MacLean, A.R.; Dixon, E.; Buie, W.D. Postoperative Complications Following Surgery for Rectal Cancer. *Ann. Surg.* **2010**, *251*, 807–818. [CrossRef] [PubMed]
7. Hendren, S.K.; O'Connor, B.I.; Liu, M.; Asano, T.; Cohen, Z.; Swallow, C.J.; MacRae, H.M.; Gryfe, R.; McLeod, R.S. Prevalence of Male and Female Sexual Dysfunction Is High Following Surgery for Rectal Cancer. *Ann. Surg.* **2005**, *242*, 212–223. [CrossRef]
8. Lange, M.M.; Maas, C.P.; Marijnen, C.; Wiggers, T.; Rutten, H.J.; Kranenbarg, E.K.; van de Velde, C.J.H. Urinary dysfunction after rectal cancer treatment is mainly caused by surgery. *BJS* **2008**, *95*, 1020–1028. [CrossRef] [PubMed]
9. Habr-Gama, A.; Perez, R.O.; Nadalin, W.; Sabbaga, J.; Ribeiro, U.; e Sousa, A.H.S.; Campos, F.G.; Kiss, D.R.; Gama-Rodrigues, J. Operative Versus Nonoperative Treatment for Stage 0 Distal Rectal Cancer Following Chemoradiation Therapy. *Ann. Surg.* **2004**, *240*, 711–718. [CrossRef]
10. Renehan, A.G.; Malcomson, L.; Emsley, R.; Gollins, S.; Maw, A.; Myint, A.S.; Rooney, P.S.; Susnerwala, S.; Blower, A.; Saunders, M.P.; et al. Watch-and-wait approach versus surgical resection after chemoradiotherapy for patients with rectal cancer (the OnCoRe project): A propensity-score matched cohort analysis. *Lancet Oncol.* **2016**, *17*, 174–183. [CrossRef]
11. Maas, M.; Beets-Tan, R.G.; Lambregts, D.; Lammering, G.; Nelemans, P.J.; Engelen, S.M.; Van Dam, R.M.; Jansen, R.L.; Sosef, M.; Leijtens, J.W.; et al. Wait-and-See Policy for Clinical Complete Responders After Chemoradiation for Rectal Cancer. *J. Clin. Oncol.* **2011**, *29*, 4633–4640. [CrossRef] [PubMed]
12. Habr-Gama, A.; Gama-Rodrigues, J.; Julião, G.P.S.; Proscurshim, I.; Sabbagh, C.; Lynn, P.B.; Perez, R.O. Local Recurrence After Complete Clinical Response and Watch and Wait in Rectal Cancer After Neoadjuvant Chemoradiation: Impact of Salvage Therapy on Local Disease Control. *Int. J. Radiat. Oncol.* **2014**, *88*, 822–828. [CrossRef] [PubMed]
13. Dossa, F.; Chesney, T.R.; Acuna, S.; Baxter, N.N. A watch-and-wait approach for locally advanced rectal cancer after a clinical complete response following neoadjuvant chemoradiation: A systematic review and meta-analysis. *Lancet Gastroenterol. Hepatol.* **2017**, *2*, 501–513. [CrossRef]
14. Van der Valk, M.J.M.; Hilling, D.; Bastiaannet, E.; Kranenbarg, E.M.-K.; Beets, G.L.; Figueiredo, N.; Habr-Gama, A.; Perez, O.R.; Renehan, A.G.; van de Velde, C.J.H.; et al. Long-term outcomes of clinical complete responders after neoadjuvant treatment for rectal cancer in the International Watch & Wait Database (IWWD): An international multicentre registry study. *Lancet* **2018**, *391*, 2537–2545. [CrossRef] [PubMed]
15. Smith, J.J.; Strombom, P.; Chow, O.S.; Roxburgh, C.S.; Lynn, P.; Eaton, A.; Widmar, M.; Ganesh, K.; Yaeger, R.; Cercek, A.; et al. Assessment of a Watch-and-Wait Strategy for Rectal Cancer in Patients With a Complete Response After Neoadjuvant Therapy. *JAMA Oncol.* **2019**, *5*, e185896. [CrossRef] [PubMed]
16. Ryan, E.J.; Warrier, S.K.; Lynch, A.C.; Ramsay, R.; Phillips, W.; Heriot, A.G. Predicting pathological complete response to neoadjuvant chemoradiotherapy in locally advanced rectal cancer: A systematic review. *Color. Dis.* **2016**, *18*, 234–246. [CrossRef]
17. Huh, J.W.; Kim, H.R.; Kim, Y.J. Clinical Prediction of Pathological Complete Response After Preoperative Chemoradiotherapy for Rectal Cancer. *Dis. Colon Rectum* **2013**, *56*, 698–703. [CrossRef]
18. Bitterman, D.S.; Salgado, L.R.; Moore, H.G.; Sanfilippo, N.J.; Gu, P.; Hatzaras, I.; Du, K.L. Predictors of Complete Response and Disease Recurrence Following Chemoradiation for Rectal Cancer. *Front. Oncol.* **2015**, *5*. [CrossRef]
19. Al-Sukhni, E.; Attwood, K.; Mattson, D.M.; Gabriel, E.; Nurkin, S.J. Predictors of Pathologic Complete Response Following Neoadjuvant Chemoradiotherapy for Rectal Cancer. *Ann. Surg. Oncol.* **2015**, *23*, 1177–1186. [CrossRef]
20. Dayde, D.; Tanaka, I.; Jain, R.; Tai, M.C.; Taguchi, A. Predictive and Prognostic Molecular Biomarkers for Response to Neoadjuvant Chemoradiation in Rectal Cancer. *Int. J. Mol. Sci.* **2017**, *18*, 573. [CrossRef] [PubMed]
21. Massihnia, D.; Pizzutilo, E.G.; Amatu, A.; Tosi, F.; Ghezzi, S.; Bencardino, K.; Di Masi, P.; Righetti, E.; Patelli, G.; Scaglione, F.; et al. Liquid biopsy for rectal cancer: A systematic review. *Cancer Treat. Rev.* **2019**, *79*, 101893. [CrossRef]
22. Machackova, T.; Prochazka, V.; Kala, Z.; Slaby, O. Translational Potential of MicroRNAs for Preoperative Staging and Prediction of Chemoradiotherapy Response in Rectal Cancer. *Cancers* **2019**, *11*, 1545. [CrossRef] [PubMed]
23. Barchitta, M.; Maugeri, A.; Destri, G.L.; Basile, G.; Agodi, A. Epigenetic Biomarkers in Colorectal Cancer Patients Receiving Adjuvant or Neoadjuvant Therapy: A Systematic Review of Epidemiological Studies. *Int. J. Mol. Sci.* **2019**, *20*, 3842. [CrossRef] [PubMed]

24. Colloca, G.; Venturino, A.; Vitucci, P. Pre-treatment carcinoembryonic antigen and outcome of patients with rectal cancer receiving neo-adjuvant chemo-radiation and surgical resection: A systematic review and meta-analysis. *Med Oncol.* **2017**, *34*. [CrossRef] [PubMed]
25. Boutin, A.T.; Liao, W.-T.; Wang, M.; Hwang, S.S.; Karpinets, T.V.; Cheung, H.; Chu, G.C.; Jiang, S.; Hu, J.; Chang, K.; et al. Oncogenic Kras drives invasion and maintains metastases in colorectal cancer. *Genes Dev.* **2017**, *31*, 370–382. [CrossRef]
26. Hanash, S.M.; Taguchi, A. Mouse to Human Blood-Based Cancer Biomarker Discovery Strategies. *Cold Spring Harb. Protoc.* **2013**, *2014*, 144–149. [CrossRef]
27. Liao, Y.; Wang, J.; Jaehnig, E.J.; Shi, Z.; Zhang, B. WebGestalt 2019: Gene set analysis toolkit with revamped UIs and APIs. *Nucleic Acids Res.* **2019**, *47*, W199–W205. [CrossRef]
28. Kanehisa, M.; Furumichi, M.; Tanabe, M.; Sato, Y.; Morishima, K.; Kanehisa, M.; Furumichi, M.; Tanabe, M.; Sato, Y.; Morishima, K. KEGG: New perspectives on genomes, pathways, diseases and drugs. *Nucleic Acids Res.* **2016**, *45*, D353–D361. [CrossRef]
29. Bethel, C.R.; Vitullo, J.C.; Miller, E.R.; Aron, D.C. Molecular cloning of mouse insulin-like growth factor binding protein 4 (IGFBP4) cDNA and expression of a fusion protein with IGF-binding activity. *Biochem. Mol. Boil. Int.* **1994**, *34*, 385–392.
30. Cooper, J.; Giancotti, F.G. Integrin Signaling in Cancer: Mechanotransduction, Stemness, Epithelial Plasticity, and Therapeutic Resistance. *Cancer Cell* **2019**, *35*, 347–367. [CrossRef] [PubMed]
31. Yeh, C.-C.; Shih, L.-J.; Chang, J.-L.; Tsuei, Y.-W.; Wu, C.-C.; Hsiao, C.-W.; Chuu, C.-P.; Kao, Y.-H. Synchronous vascular endothelial growth factor protein profiles in both tissue and serum identify metastasis and poor survival in colorectal cancer. *Sci. Rep.* **2019**, *9*, 4228. [CrossRef]
32. Olsson, A.-K.; Dimberg, A.; Kreuger, J.; Claesson-Welsh, L. VEGF receptor signalling? in control of vascular function. *Nat. Rev. Mol. Cell Biol.* **2006**, *7*, 359–371. [CrossRef] [PubMed]
33. Hsu, M.-C.; Pan, M.-R.; Hung, W.-C. Two Birds, One Stone: Double Hits on Tumor Growth and Lymphangiogenesis by Targeting Vascular Endothelial Growth Factor Receptor. *Cells* **2019**, *8*, 270. [CrossRef] [PubMed]
34. Tacconi, C.; Ungaro, F.; Correale, C.; Arena, V.; Massimino, L.; Detmar, M.; Spinelli, A.; Carvello, M.; Mazzone, M.; Oliveira, A.I.; et al. Activation of the VEGFC/VEGFR3 Pathway Induces Tumor Immune Escape in Colorectal Cancer. *Cancer Res.* **2019**, *79*, 4196–4210. [CrossRef] [PubMed]
35. Tacconi, C.; Correale, C.; Gandelli, A.; Spinelli, A.; Dejana, E.; D'Alessio, S.; Danese, S. Vascular Endothelial Growth Factor C Disrupts the Endothelial Lymphatic Barrier to Promote Colorectal Cancer Invasion. *Gastroenterology* **2015**, *148*, 1438–1451. [CrossRef]
36. Spolverato, G.; Pucciarelli, S.; Bertorelle, R.; De Rossi, A.; Nitti, D.; Spolverato, G.; Pucciarelli, S.; Bertorelle, R.; De Rossi, A.; Nitti, D. Predictive Factors of the Response of Rectal Cancer to Neoadjuvant Radiochemotherapy. *Cancers* **2011**, *3*, 2176–2194. [CrossRef] [PubMed]
37. Yang, C.; Lin, L.; Lin, Y.; Tian, Y.; Lin, C.; Sheu, M.; Li, C.; Tai, M. Higher nuclear EGFR expression is a better predictor of survival in rectal cancer patients following neoadjuvant chemoradiotherapy than cytoplasmic EGFR expression. *Oncol. Lett.* **2018**, *17*, 1551–1558. [CrossRef] [PubMed]
38. Maramotti, S.; Paci, M.; Manzotti, G.; Rapicetta, C.; Gugnoni, M.; Galeone, C.; Cesario, A.; Lococo, F. Soluble Epidermal Growth Factor Receptors (sEGFRs) in Cancer: Biological Aspects and Clinical Relevance. *Int. J. Mol. Sci.* **2016**, *17*, 593. [CrossRef] [PubMed]
39. Okada, Y.; Kimura, T.; Nakagawa, T.; Fukuya, A.; Goji, T.; Fujimoto, S.; Muguruma, N.; Tsuji, Y.; Okahisa, T.; Takayama, T.; et al. EGFR Downregulation after Anti-EGFR Therapy Predicts the Antitumor Effect in Colorectal Cancer. *Mol. Cancer Res.* **2017**, *15*, 1445–1454. [CrossRef]
40. Zhong, X.; Zhou, Y.; Cui, W.; Su, X.; Guo, Z.; Hidasa, I.; Li, Q.; Wang, Z.; Song, Y.; Zhong, X.; et al. The Addition of EGFR Inhibitors in Neoadjuvant Therapy for KRAS-Wild Type Locally Advanced Rectal Cancer Patients: A Systematic Review and Meta-Analysis. *Front. Pharmacol.* **2020**, *11*. [CrossRef]
41. Smith, W.L.; DeWitt, D.L.; Garavito, R.M. Cyclooxygenases: Structural, Cellular, and Molecular Biology. *Annu. Rev. Biochem.* **2000**, *69*, 145–182. [CrossRef] [PubMed]
42. Roxburgh, C.S.D.; McMillan, D.C. Cancer and systemic inflammation: Treat the tumour and treat the host. *Br. J. Cancer* **2014**, *110*, 1409–1412. [CrossRef] [PubMed]
43. Araujo-Mino, E.P.; Patt, Y.Z.; Murray-Krezan, C.; Hanson, J.A.; Bansal, P.; Liem, B.J.; Rajput, A.; Fekrazad, M.H.; Heywood, G.; Lee, F.C. Phase II Trial Using a Combination of Oxaliplatin, Capecitabine, and Celecoxib with Concurrent Radiation for Newly Diagnosed Resectable Rectal Cancer. *Oncology* **2017**, *23*, 2-e5. [CrossRef] [PubMed]

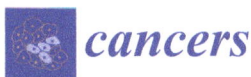

Article

Prognostic Significance of CXCR4 in Colorectal Cancer: An Updated Meta-Analysis and Critical Appraisal

Alessandro Ottaiano [1,*,†], Mariachiara Santorsola [1,†], Paola Del Prete [1], Francesco Perri [1], Stefania Scala [1], Michele Caraglia [2,3] and Guglielmo Nasti [1]

[1] Istituto Nazionale Tumori di Napoli, IRCCS "G. Pascale", via M. Semmola, 80131 Naples, Italy; mariachiara.santorsola@istitutotumori.na.it (M.S.); p.delprete@istitutotumori.na.it (P.D.P.); f.perri@istitutotumori.na.it (F.P.); s.scala@istitutotumori.na.it (S.S.); g.nasti@istitutotumori.na.it (G.N.)
[2] BiogemScarl, Laboratory of Precision and Molecular Oncology, ContradaCamporeale, 83031 ArianoIrpino, Italy; michele.caraglia@unicampania.it
[3] Department of Precision Medicine, University of Campania "L. Vanvitelli", Via L. De Crecchio, 7, 80138 Naples, Italy
* Correspondence: a.ottaiano@istitutotumori.na.it; Tel.: +39-081-5903510
† Co-first authors.

Simple Summary: C-X-C chemokine receptor type 4 (CXCR4), a G-protein-coupled receptor, has been demonstrated to stimulate proliferation and invasiveness of many different tumors, including colorectal cancer. Through in vitro evidence, overexpression of CXCR4 has been identified as a negative prognostic factor in colorectal cancer. The identification of prognostic biomarkers can improve the prediction of disease evolution and disease characterization, and guide treatment efforts. This systematic review with a meta-analysis was conducted to pool hazard ratios from prognostic studies on CXCR4, provide an updated estimate of prognostic power of CXCR4, and analyze modalities of evaluating and reporting CXCR4 expression.

Abstract: *Background:* This study was conducted to provide an updated estimate of the prognostic power of C-X-C chemokine receptor type 4 (CXCR4) in colorectal cancer (CRC), and analyze modalities of evaluating and reporting its expression. *Methods:* A systematic review with meta-analysis was performed and described according to the Preferred Reporting Items for Systematic Reviews and Meta-Analyses statement. Studies were identified through PubMed and Google Scholar. The pooled hazard ratios (HRs) for overall survival (OS) or progression-free survival (PFS) with 95% confidence interval (CI) were estimated with the random-effect model. *Results:* Sixteen studies were selected covering a period from 2005 to 2020. An immunohistochemical evaluation of CXCR4 was performed in all studies. Only in three studies assessment of mRNA through RT–PCR was correlated with prognosis; in the remaining studies, the authors identified prognostic categories based on immunohistochemical expression. In pooled analyses, significant associations were found between positive or high or strong expression of CXCR4 and T stage ≥ 3 ($P = 0.0001$), and positive or high or strong expression of CXCR4 and left side primary tumor localization ($P = 0.0186$). The pooled HR for OS was 2.09 (95% CI: 1.30–2.88) in favor of high CXCR4 expression; for PFS, it was 1.42 (95% CI: 1.13–1.71) in favor of high CXCR4 expression. *Conclusion:* High CXCR4 expression is clearly associated with increased risk of death and progression in CRC. However, strong methodologic heterogeneity in CXCR4 assessment hinders direct translation into clinical practice; thus, a consensus to streamline detection and scoring of CXCR4 expression in CRC is indicated.

Keywords: CXCR4; colorectal cancer; prognosis; overall survival

1. Introduction

C-X-C chemokine receptor type 4 (CXCR4) belongs to the G-protein-coupled receptor superfamily, and it is expressed in a wide variety of cells, predominantly of hematopoietic origin. It binds to C-X-C motif chemokine ligand 1 (CXCL12), also called stromal cell-derived factor-1α (SDF-1α) and mediates a potent chemotactic stimulus [1]. In embryos, it has a major role in processes of neurogenesis, influencing the migration of neurons from neuroprogenitor cells [2]; in adults, one of the most important biological roles of the CXCR4/SDF-1α axis is the regulation of hematopoietic stem cell homing to the bone marrow [3]. However, CXCR4 has been demonstrated to stimulate proliferation and invasiveness of many different tumors including prostate [4], breast [5], lung [6–8], melanoma [9,10], glioblastoma [11,12], lymphoma [13,14], and colorectal cancer [15,16]. Through in vitro evidence, overexpression of CXCR4 has been identified as a negative prognostic factor in many different neoplasms [17–20].

Colorectal cancer (CRC) is the third most common cause of cancer-related deaths worldwide. Survival rates at five years strictly depend on the stage at diagnosis, varying from 90% of American Joint Committeeon Cancer 8th Edition (AJCC) stages I-II to 10% of stage IV [21]. The survival rate of Stage III patients is about 40% and it has been improved in recent years with the administration of adjuvant chemotherapy [22]. The survival of metastatic colorectal cancer (mCRC) patients significantly improved in recent years with the introduction of target-oriented drugs and a better selection of patients based on biologic/molecular characteristics (*KRAS/NRAS/BRAF* mutations, MSI, HER-2 overexpression, and other molecular markers) [23]. The identification of new prognostic cancer biomarkers is important because it can improve the prediction of disease evolution, enhance disease characterization, and guide treatment efforts. CXCR4 expression is considered a prognostic marker in CRC. However, patients' risk stratification requires rigorous scientific validation. We previously reported that CXCR4 is able to predict progression-free (PFS) [24] and overall survival (OS) [25] in CRC.

This study was conducted to pool hazard ratios from prognostic studies on CXCR4, provide an updated estimate of prognostic power of CXCR4, and analyze modalities of evaluating and reporting CXCR4 expression.

2. Materials and Methods

2.1. Search Strategy

This meta-analysis was performed and described according to the Preferred Reporting Items for Systematic Reviews and Meta-Analyses (PRISMA) statement [26]. Two-hundred seventy-three studies were identified through PubMed and Google Scholar searching with the following key words algorithm: "colorectal cancer" OR "colorectal tumor" OR "colorectal carcinoma" AND "CXCR4" OR "cxc chemokine receptor type 4" AND "prognosis" OR "disease free survival" OR "progression" OR "survival" (last update on 16 December 2020).

2.2. Study Eligibility

A flowchart summarizing the criteria for studies selection and exclusion is reported in Figure 1. Abstracts of studies in English language that were initially identified were examined to exclude those not reporting prognostic information. Thereafter, all full texts were retrieved and analyzed. Studies were included in the final analysis if they (1) reported prognostic data (association with PFS or OS) about the expression of CXCR4 in CRC patients, (2) reported hazard ratios (HRs) with 95% confidence intervals (CIs), and, (3) had a sample size >30 patients. All the studies presented a score > 6 at the Newcastle–Ottawa Scale for methodology quality assessment [27]. Articles reporting the prognostic role of concomitant biomarker expression (i.e., CXCR4/SDF-1α, CXCR4/CD133, etc.) were excluded.

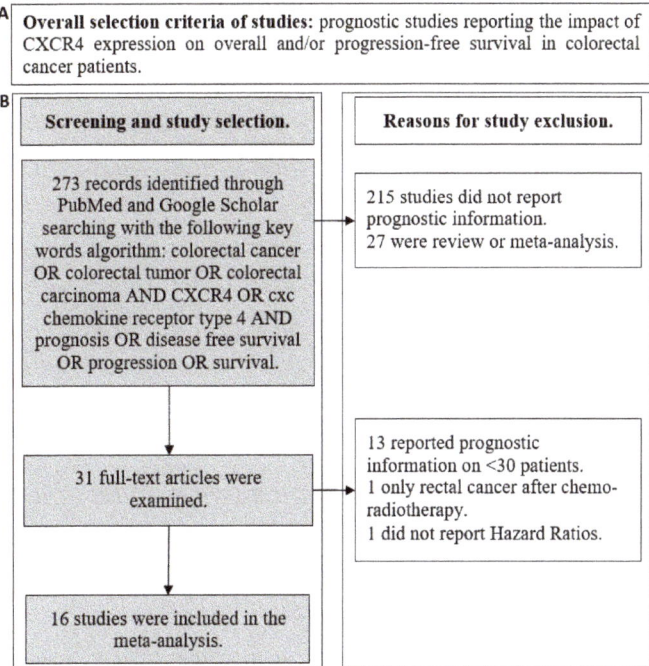

Figure 1. Overall selection criteria for study selection (**A**). Detailed flowchart reporting the criteria for study selection and exclusion (**B**).

2.3. Data Extraction

The following data were extracted by four investigators for each publication: first author; year of publication; accrual time; number of patients; methods for CXCR4 assessment (including details on IHC scores and eventual fresh tissue evaluation); information about morphologic localization of immunohistochemical CXCR4 expression; eventual presence of ancillary studies; information on study design; association with clinico-pathological variables (age, sex, lymph-nodes involvement, stage, T, side, clinical response, and *KRAS* mutational status); information on follow-up; HRs of progression and/or death with 95% CIs. Criticisms and/or discordances were discussed between all authors to reach a consensus.

2.4. Hazard Ratio Interpretation

A hazard ratio of 1.0 indicates an identical risk (event probability (EP)) between high and low CXCR4-expressing groups (EP CXCR4 high/EP CXCR4 low). An HR greater than 1.0 indicates that a high CXCR4-expressing group at the numerator has an increased risk of death or progression. When a study reported an HR with low CXCR4 in the numerator (CXCR4 low vs. high), the HR and CI were recalculated (the calculated $HR_{CXC4\ high\ vs.\ low}$ was $1/HR_{CXC4\ low\ vs.\ high}$) according to Altman et al. [28] in order to harmonize the comparison trajectory (CXCR4 high vs. CXCR4 low).

2.5. Statistical Analysis

The present meta-analysis was performed in order to assess the prognostic impact of CXCR4 expression in terms of OS and PFS in CRC. The secondary end-points were the analysis of the association between CXCR4 and clinico-pathologic variables, and the description of methods and scores used to assess it. Given the significant heterogeneity (see above) among the selected studies, the analysis was performed with the random-effects model. It aims to provide a more conservative estimate of the pooled HR and it is the preferred model when heterogeneity is present. Under the random-effects model, the true effects are assumed to vary between studies, and the summary effect is the weighted average of the effects reported in the different studies [29]. Meta-analysis is depicted in classical forest plots, with point estimates, 95% CIs for each HR, and a final pooled HR.

Heterogeneity was evaluated through I^2, that is, the percentage of observed total variation across studies due to real heterogeneity rather than chance. It is calculated as $I^2 = 100\% \times (Q - DF)/Q$, where Q is Cochran's heterogeneity statistic and DF is the degrees of freedom. Negative values of I^2 are set to be equal to zero so that I^2 lies between 0% and 100%. A value of 0% indicates no observed heterogeneity, and larger values show increasing heterogeneity [30]. The risk of publication bias was also evaluated with funnel plot analysis and Egger's test [31]. The latter is a test for the Y intercept = 0 from a linear regression of normalized effect estimate (estimate divided by its standard error) against precision (reciprocal of the standard error of the estimate). $P < 0.005$ indicates a significant publication bias.

Associations between CXCR4 expression and clinico-pathological variables were evaluated with the chi-square test.

Analyses were performed with the MedCalc Statistical Software (MedCalc® Statistical Software version 19.6, MedCalc Software Ltd., Ostend, Belgium; https://www.medcalc.org (accessed on 19 December 2020).

3. Results

3.1. Study Characteristics

Sixteen studies were selected covering a period from 2005 to 2020 [24,25,32–45]. The accrual time varied from a minimum of 3 to 14 years. The number of enrolled patients ranged from 31 to 684. Only four studies reported ancillary data including evaluation of CXCR4-related biologic pathways. All studies were retrospective and had a Newcastle–Ottawa Scale score ≥ 6 (Table S1). Most articles described the prognostic power of CXCR4 in stages I-IV or stage IV disease (11/16). The reporting of association with clinico-pathological characteristics was heterogeneous (lymph-nodal status: 13/16; T status: 7/16; side: 5/16); however, very few studies reported data about association with clinical response (1/16) or KRAS status (2/16) (Table S2).

3.2. CXCR4 Expression Methodology

The methodology to assess CXCR4 expression is crucial to identifying prognostic categories and adequately interpreting results. Therefore, we performed a detailed analysis of technical modalities of CXCR4 evaluation (Table 1). Immunohistochemical evaluation of CXCR4 was performed in all studies. Evaluation of fresh tumor tissue was performed only by Kim et al. In eight studies, an mRNA assessment was added (through RT-PCR or FISH). In only three studies assessment of mRNA through RT-PCR was correlated with prognosis; in the remaining studies, the authors identified prognostic categories based on immunohistochemical expression. Ten studies differentiated nuclear versus cytoplasmic CXCR4 expression. Only one study referred to membrane CXCR4 expression. Modalities of building expression scores (number of categories, number of positive cells, and inclusion of staining intensity) were heterogeneous. A detailed description is reported in Table 1.

Table 1. Description of CXCR4 assessment methodology among selected studies.

First Author	Methods	Fresh Tissue Evaluation	Detection Correlated with TTO	Differential Nuclear, Cytoplasmic, Membrane IHC Staining	IHC Distribution Correlated with Prognosis	Scores	No. of Positive Cells for Expression Evaluation	Inclusion of "Staining Intensity"
Kim J.	IHC, RT-PCR	Yes	RT-PCR	NA	NA	Low vs. High	mRNA median CXCR4 expression	No
Ottaiano A.	IHC	No	IHC	Yes	Overall expression	Neg/Low vs. High	≤50% vs. >50%	No
Yoshitake N.	IHC, Western Blot	No	IHC	Yes	Overall expression	Neg vs. Pos	No CXCR4 immunoreactivity vs others	No
Speetjens F.M.	RT-PCR	No	RT-PCR	NA	NA	Low vs. High	mRNA median CXCR4 expression	No
Speetjens F.M.	IHC	No	IHC	Yes	Nuclear expression	Weak vs. Strong	Examples are included in the work	Yes. Absent, faint cytoplasmic, moderate cytoplasmic and slight membranous, strong cytoplasmic and strong membranous
Ingold B.	IHC	No	IHC	No	Overall expression	0, 1+, 2+, 3+	NA	Yes. Weak, medium, strong, very strong
Wang S.C.	IHC, RT-PCR	No	IHC	Yes	Nuclear expression	0, 1+, 2+, 3+	0; <30%; 30-50%; >50%	No
Yopp A.C.	IHC	No	IHC	Yes	Overall expression	Neg vs. Pos	≤10% vs. >10%	No
Sakai N.	IHC, fluorescence microscopy	No	IHC	Cyto	Cytoplasm	Low vs. High	NA	Yes. Relative to the staining intensity of hepatocytes

Table 1. Cont.

First Author	Methods	Fresh Tissue Evaluation	Detection Correlated with TTO	Differential Nuclear, Cytoplasmic, Membrane IHC Staining	IHC Distribution Correlated with Prognosis	Scores	No. of Positive Cells for Expression Evaluation	Inclusion of "Staining Intensity"
Sakai N.	IHC, fluorescence microscopy	No	IHC	Nucleus	Nuclear	Neg vs. Pos	NA	Yes Relative to the staining intensity of hepatocytes
Du C.	IHC	No	IHC	Not Specified	Overall expression	0, 1+, 2+; Low 3+: High	<1%; 1–50% (1+ and 2+); >50%	Yes Negative, weak, strong
Gao Y.	IHC, RT-PCR	No	IHC	No	Overall expression	Sporadic, focal, diffuse	<10%, ≥11<50%, ≥50%	Yes Negative, weak, moderate, strong
Stanisavljevic L. (cohort 1)	IHC, ISH	No	IHC	Yes	Nuclear expression	Low vs. High	0–20%, >20%	No
Stanisavljevic L. (cohort 2)	IHC	No	IHC	Yes	Nuclear expression	Low vs. High	0–20%, >20%	No
D'Alterio C.	IHC, RT-PCR	No	IHC	Yes	Overall expression	Negative/Low vs. High	0–50%, >50%	No
Wu W.	IHC, RT-PCR	No	RT-PCR	NA	NA	Low vs. High	mRNA median CXCR4 expression	No
Weixler B.	IHC	No	IHC	No	Overall expression	Histoscores (a continuous variable)	(% of positive cells)x (staining intensity)	Yes Negative, 0; weak, 1; moderate, 2; strong, 3
Xu C.	IHC, RT-PCR	No	IHC	No	Membrane	0, 1, 2, 3, 4	0%, 1–25%, 26–50%, 51–75%, >75%	Yes No staining, weak, moderate, strong
Ottaiano A.	IHC, RT-PCR	No	IHC	Yes	Overall expression	Neg/Low vs. High	≥0≤50%, >50%	No

IHC: Immunohistochemistry; ISH: In situ hybridization; mRNA: messenger ribonucleic acid; NA: not applicable; Neg: negative; Pos: positive; RT-PCR: reverse transcriptase-polymerase chain reaction; TTO: time to outcome.

3.3. Association between CXCR4 Expression and Clinico-Pathological Characteristics of Colorectal Cancer Patients

Exploration of association between a potential biomarker in cancer and patients' clinico-pathological characteristics is important to generate hypotheses on its biologic role, to improve disease extent prediction, and to prevent biases in subsequent prognostic analyses. Table 2 reports a detailed description of the clinico-pathological characteristics of the patients and tumors according to CXCR4 expression in the selected studies. In a pooled analysis, significant associations were found between positive or high or strong expression of CXCR4 and T stage ≥ 3 (cancer growing outside the muscularis propria) ($P = 0.0001$), and positive or high or strong expression of CXCR4 and left-side primary tumor localization ($P = 0.0186$) (Table S3).

Table 2. Clinico-pathological characteristics according to CXCR4 expression.

Author	Year	CXCR4 Scores	Age		Sex		T		Side		Lymph nodes	
			Young	Old	Male	Female	≤2	≥3	Left	Right	Involved	Not Involved
Kim J.	2005	Low 44			23	21	18	9	-	-	8	36
		High 48			22	26	11	19	-	-	8	40
Ottaiano A.	2006	Neg 16	<70:10	≥70:6	6	10	5	11	-	-	0	15
		Low 25	<70:13	≥70:12	15	10	13	12	-	-	8	18
		High 31	<70:21	≥70:10	17	14	11	20	-	-	7	24
Yoshitake N.	2008	Negative 13	-	-	10	3	-	-	-	-	7	6
		Positive 47	-	-	31	16	-	-	-	-	38	9
Speetjens F.M.	2009	Low 35	<68.5:20	>68.5:15	16	19	-	-	17	18	12	23
		High 35	<68.5:15	>68.5:20	19	16	-	-	17	18	11	24
Speetjens F.M.	2009	Strong 43	<69.7:21	>69.7:22	21	22	-	-	22	21	15	28
		Weak 15	<69.7:8	>69.7:7	7	8	-	-	5	10	4	11
Ingold B.	2009	Negative 267	≤65:115	>65:152	145	122	46	206	-	-	133	119
		Positive 135	≤65:51	>65:84	69	66	23	108	-	-	72	59
Wang SC.	2010	Negative 245	-	-	180	65	138	107	186	59	142	141
		Positive 143	-	-	89	54	47	96	99	44	101	158
Yopp A.C.	2012	Negative 28	≤60:11	>60:17	13	15	-	-	-	-	-	-
		Positive 47	≤60:21	>60:26	38	9	-	-	-	-	-	-
Sakai N.	2012	Low 56 (cytoplasm)	<60:26	≥60:30	36	20	-	-	-	-	-	-
		High 36 (cytoplasm)	<60:10	≥60:26	22	14	-	-	-	-	-	-
Du C.	2014	Low 89	<65:39	≥65:50	51	38	16	73	47	42	6	83
		High 56	<65:19	≥65:37	33	23	9	47	29	27	4	52
Gao Y.	2014	Negative 512	<55:243	≥55:269	292	220	-	-	-	-	201	311
		Positive 208	<55:89	≥55:119	120	88	-	-	-	-	138	70
Stanisavljevic L.	2015	Low 78	-	-	45	33	3	75	-	-	-	-
		High 186	-	-	93	93	10	176	-	-	-	-
Stanisavljevic L.	2015	Low 35	-	-	20	15	6	29	-	-	-	-
		High 190	-	-	110	80	28	162	-	-	-	-
D'Alterio C.	2016	Negative/Low 10	-	-	-	-	-	-	-	-	-	-
		High 21	-	-	-	-	-	-	-	-	-	-
Wu W.	2016	Low 40	-	-	-	-	-	-	-	-	-	-
		High 40	-	-	-	-	-	-	-	-	-	-
Weixler B.	2017	Low 289	-	-	145	144	51	230	205	82	142	141
		High 267	-	-	117	150	60	204	190	77	101	158
Xu C.	2018	Low 26	<60:21	≥60:5	16	10	4	22	-	-	1	25
		High 22	<60:20	≥60:4	18	4	5	17	-	-	5	17
Ottaiano A.	2020	Negative/Low 26	≤65:12	>65:14	17	9	-	-	19	7	-	-
		High 52	≤65:20	>65:32	27	25	-	-	26	26	-	-

3.4. Time to Outcome According to CXCR4 Expression

The primary endpoint of this meta-analysis was to provide a pooled and updated estimate of the prognostic value of CXCR4 expression in CRC. Data regarding timeto outcome (OS and/or PFS) were extracted and are reported in Table 3. Three studies reported both OS and PFS, five reported PFS, and eight reported OS.

Funnel plots for the HRs of OS and PFS were asymmetric (Figure 2A,B) with a significant I^2 test for OS ($P < 0.001$). Egger's test was significant for both OS ($P = 0.04$) and PFS ($P = 0.03$). The meta-analysis was performed with the random-effects model in order to obtain a more conservative and reliable estimate of the pooled HR, and no attempts were made to conduct a subgroup meta-analysis. A forest plot of treatment effect on OS is shown in Figure 3A. The pooled HR was 2.09 (95% CI: 1.30–2.88) in favor of high CXCR4 expression. The effect on PFS is shown in Figure 3B where the pooled HR is 1.42 (95% CI: 1.13–1.71) in favor of high CXCR4 expression.

Table 3. Follow-up, time to outcome, and hazard ratios of progression and/or death in selected studies.

Author	Year	Median Follow-Up (Months)	Median PFS (Months)	HR	CI	P	Median OS (Months)	HR	CI	P
Kim J.	2005	28	NR	1.35	1.09–1.68	0.0065	High 9; Low 23	2.53	1.19–5.40	0.016
Ottaiano A.	2006	23	NR	3.01	0.88–5.21	0.0991	NR			
Yoshitake N.	2008						NR	5.08	0.65–40.00	0.123
Speetjens F.M.	2009	NR	NR	2	1.1–3.7	0.03	NR	1.8	1–3.6	0.07
Speetjens F.M.	2009	NR	NR	2.6	1–6.2	0.04	NR	3.7	1.35–11	0.02
Ingold B.	2009	32					NR	2.87	1.31–6.29	0.009
Wang SC.	2010	61	5 years DFS rate: High 70%; Low 55%	1.23	0.7–2.18	0.458				
Yopp A.C.	2012	68	(Nuc CXCR4) Pos. 15 vs Neg. 73	2.2	1.2–4.2	0.012				
Sakai N.*	2012	38					3 years OS rate: High 67%; Low 78%	Cyto: 0.43	Cyto: 0.18–1.02	Cyto: 0.056
Sakai N.*	2012	38					3 years OS rate: Pos 93%; Neg 67%	Nuc: 4.05	Nuc: 1.19–13.8	Nuc: 0.025
Du C.*	2014	68.5	5 years DFS rate: High 76.8%; Low 84.3%	0.81	0.36–1.8	0.618				
Gao Y.	2014						NR	1.3	1.38–1.85	0.001
Stanisavljevic L.*	2015	Min from 3–5 years	5 years DFS rate: High 65%; Low 85%	0.42	0.22–0.78	0.006				
Stanisavljevic L.*	2015	Min from 3–5 years	High 82%; Low 89%	0.89	0.31–2.61	0.838				
D'Alterio C.*	2016	28	High 14 vs. Neg/Low 46	3.405	1.70–17.33	0.004	High 28; Neg/Low 46	0.079	0.062–0.480	0.0008
Wu W.	2016	Max 60					NR	5.38	2.42–9.13	0.002
Weixler B.	2017	NR					5 years OS rate: High 48%; Low 48%	0.99	0.99–1.0	0.322
Xu C.*	2018	NR					High 51; Low 54	0.188	0.03–0.75	0.020
Ottaiano A.	2020	53					High 19; Neg/Low 31	3.18	2.01–5.02	0.0312

* HR was transformed in forest plot (see Methods). CI: confidence interval; Cyto: cytoplasmic; DFS: disease-free survival; HR: hazard ratio; Neg: negative; NR: not reported; Nuc: nuclear; OS: overall survival.

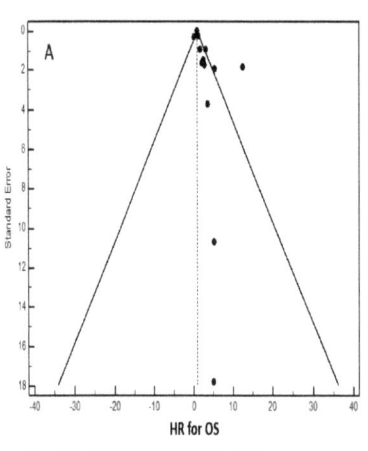
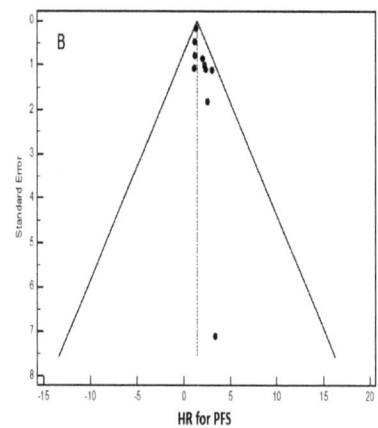

I² (inconsistency)=81.16%; 95%CI=68.82-88.62; P<0.001
Publication bias by Egger's test: Intercept: 1.28; 95%CI: 0.005-2.56; P=0.04

I² (inconsistency)=0.00%; 95%CI=0.00-29.08; P= 0.85
Publication bias by Egger's test: Intercept: 0.62; 95% CI: 0.03-1.20; P=0.03

Figure 2. Funnel plots of selected studies for overall survival (OS) (**A**) and progression-free survival (PFS) (**B**).

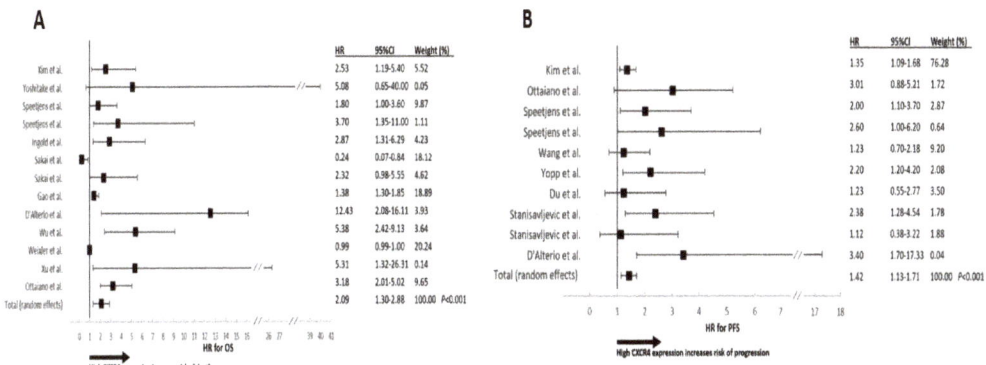

Figure 3. Forest plots for OS(**A**) and PFS(**B**) according to CXCR4 expression. Studies are reported by author's first name, HRs, 95% CIs and percent of the weighted effects (see Methods). The pooled effect is reported in the last line.

4. Discussion

Identification and validation of predictive and/or prognostic biomarkers in CRC have revolutionized the management of the disease (*BRAF*, *K-*, *N-RAS*, and MSI), and others will also be used in the near future in clinical practice (HER2 and PD-1/PD-L1) [23]. Given relevant biologic reasons, CXCR4 has been explored for many years as a potential prognostic marker in CRC. Our group and others previously reported that CXCR4 expression predicted PFS and OS in CRC [24,25,32–45]. In the present study, we aimed to provide a more accurate and updated estimate of the prognostic power of CXCR4 considering some contradictory results, the maturity of available data, and the intense interest around the role of CXCR4 in modulating the metastatic behavior of CRC.

The search of articles was systematic, and the selection primarily based on a few characteristics indirectly related to the overall quality of the articles (>30 patients enrolled, HRs and CXCR4 expression methods clearly reported, and evaluation of CXCR4 before any treatment).

We found that high CXCR4 expression is clearly associated with increased risk of death and progression (HR OS: 2.09; 95% CI: 1.30–2.88 and HR PFS: 1.42; 95% CI: 1.13–1.71). However, the following major issue deserves to be evidenced and discussed: a strong methodologic heterogeneity in CXCR4 assessment was identified. Table 1 shows a wide heterogeneity in CXCR4 assessment methodology regarding techniques, scores, and categories. Some studies evaluated the membrane or nuclear expression values; however, the evaluation of the total expression value can provide an objective determination of the level of expression of CXCR4. CXCR4 nuclear localization is an atypical compartmentalization of the receptor, likely linked to its still unknown functions, and an IHC determination not sensitive enough to specifically detect the subcellular localization of a molecule, especially in paraffin-embedded tissue can be affected by artifacts and by cell space overlapping. The use of antibodies standardized for IHC studies should be recommended, and standard methods of expression evaluation scores, including the apparent subcellular localization, should be developed with an appropriate consensus between pathologists. Western blotting analysis of protein expression should be avoided because it is a qualitative method that does not distinguish the cell subtype source of the assessed protein and does not assure that the protein has been extracted by cancer cells or other tumor microenvironment cells. qRT-PCR is a quantitative technique, but it requires a strict standardization of the procedure, the selection of the tumor area by a pathologist, and the extraction of RNA from tumor tissues that are often paraffin-embedded, with the consequent decrease in the RNA sample quality. It is likely that the best procedure would be a world-standardized IHC procedure performed with an automated test. Therefore, this methodological issue in CXCR4 assessment, along with the physiologic heterogeneity in treatments, a downsized sample size (nine studies enrolled <100 patients), and the retrospective nature of all studies are responsible for the large HR confidence intervals in some studies. Finally, the evidence of a publication bias makes these heterogeneities even more relevant. In this regard, we cannot rule out the hypothesis that selection of the studies we applied could have been influenced by this publication bias. Moreover, all selected studies were retrospective. Therefore, their nature is intrinsically biased by mostly unknown and uncontrolled clinical (patients' location, selection, treatments, etc.) and methodological (techniques, reagents, methods, etc.) biases. Based on these considerations, our group is planning the first prospective evaluation of CXCR4 in both primary and/or metastatic tissues (resected metastases or biopsies) in order to predict the time to relapse after surgery and the response to therapy/subsequent prognosis in CRC. Assessment of CXCR4 will be performed through IHC according to a previously published homogeneous evaluation method (negative, low, high) [24,25]. The hypothesis of the study is based on the following statistical assumptions: (i) HR for high expression of CXCR4 of 2.09 (vs. negative/low), (ii) test power of 80%, (iii) alpha value of the I-type error of 5%, and (iv) median survival of 18 months (in unselected mCRC patients). The survival curves will be depicted with the Kaplan–Meier method, and the statistical significance verified with a two-tailed log-rank test. The final sample will be 200 patients.

5. Conclusions

For the first time, we showed a detailed and critical analysis of technical approaches applied to assess CXCR4 in CRC, finding a wide diversity in the modalities of assessment and the reporting of the receptor expression. This strong methodological heterogeneity hinders direct translation into clinical practice, suggesting that CXCR4 assessment should be revised and harmonized. Based on this, a consensus among experts to harmonize detection and scoring of CXCR4 expression in CRC should be reached; the present work may represent a critical starting point to discussions about methodological issues regarding the assessment of CXCR4 in CRC as a prognostic factor.

Supplementary Materials: The following are available online at https://www.mdpi.com/article/cancers13133284/s1. Table S1: Study characteristics I, Table S2: Study characteristics II, Table S3: Pooled analysis of CXCR4 expression according to clinico-pathological characteristics.

Author Contributions: Conceptualization, A.O. and M.S.; methodology, A.O. and M.S.; software, A.O.; validation, M.C., G.N., and F.P.; formal analysis, A.O. and P.D.P.; investigation, A.O., M.S., P.D.P., and G.N.; resources, G.N.; data curation, A.O.; writing—original draft preparation, A.O. and M.C.; writing—review and editing, S.S., M.S., and G.N.; supervision, G.N. All authors have read and agreed to the published version of the manuscript.

Funding: This research received no external funding.

Institutional Review Board Statement: Not applicable.

Informed Consent Statement: Not applicable.

Data Availability Statement: The data presented in this study are available on request from the corresponding author.

Acknowledgments: We are grateful for Alessandra Trocino, Librarian at Istituto Nazionale Tumori di Napoli, IRCCS "G. Pascale", Italy, for bibliographic assistance. We thank Daniela Capobianco, Istituto Nazionale Tumori di Napoli, IRCCS "G. Pascale", Italy, for assistance with data management.

Conflicts of Interest: The authors declare no conflict of interest.

References

1. Kucia, M.; Jankowski, K.; Reca, R.; Wysoczynski, M.; Bandura, L.; Allendorf, D.J.; Zhang, J.; Ratajczak, J.; Ratajczak, M.Z. CXCR4-SDF-1 signalling, locomotion, chemotaxis and adhesion. *J. Mol. Histol.* **2004**, *35*, 233–245. [CrossRef]
2. Hwang, H.M.; Ku, R.Y.; Hashimoto-Torii, K. Prenatal environment that affects neuronal migration. *Front. Cell. Dev. Biol.* **2019**, *7*, 138. [CrossRef]
3. Kawaguchi, N.; Zhang, T.T.; Nakanishi, T. Involvement of CXCR4 in Normal and Abnormal Development. *Cells* **2019**, *8*, 185. [CrossRef] [PubMed]
4. Taichman, R.S.; Cooper, C.; Keller, E.T.; Pienta, K.J.; Taichman, N.S.; McCauley, L.K. Use of the stromal cell-derived factor-1/CXCR4 pathway in prostate cancer metastasis to bone. *Cancer Res.* **2002**, *62*, 1832–1837. [PubMed]
5. Müller, A.; Homey, B.; Soto, H.; Ge, N.; Catron, D.; Buchanan, M.E.; McClanahan, T.; Murphy, E.; Yuan, W.; Wagner, S.N.; et al. Involvement of chemokine receptors in breast cancer metastasis. *Nature* **2001**, *41*, 50–56. [CrossRef] [PubMed]
6. Kijima, T.; Maulik, G.; Ma, P.C.; Tibaldi, E.V.; Turner, R.E.; Rollins, B.; Sattler, M.; Johnson, B.E.; Salgia, R. Regulation of cellular proliferation, cytoskeletal function, and signal transduction through CXCR4 and c-Kit in small cell lung cancer cells. *Cancer Res.* **2002**, *62*, 6304–6311. [PubMed]
7. Burger, M.; Glodek, A.; Hartmann, T.; Schmitt-Gräff, A.; Silberstein, L.E.; Fujii, N.; Kipps, T.J.; Burger., J.A. Functional expression of CXCR4 (CD184) on small-cell lung cancer cells mediates migration, integrin activation, and adhesion to stromal cells. *Oncogene* **2003**, *22*, 8093–8101. [CrossRef]
8. Hartmann, T.N.; Burger, J.A.; Glodek, A.; Fujii, N.; Burger, M. CXCR4 chemokine receptor and integrin signaling co-operate in mediating adhesion and chemoresistance in small cell lung cancer (SCLC) cells. *Oncogene* **2005**, *24*, 4462–4471. [CrossRef]
9. Bartolomé, R.A.; Gálvez, B.G.; Longo, N.; Baleux, F.; Van Muijen, G.N.; Sánchez-Mateos, P.; Arroyo, A.G.; Teixidó, J. Stromal cell-derived factor-1alpha promotes melanoma cell invasion across basement membranes involving stimulation of membrane-type 1 matrix metalloproteinase and Rho GTPase activities. *Cancer Res.* **2004**, *64*, 2534–2543. [CrossRef]
10. Scala, S.; Giuliano, P.; Ascierto, P.A.; Ieranò, C.; Franco, R.; Napolitano, M.; Ottaiano, A.; Lombardi, M.L.; Luongo, M.; Simeone, E.; et al. Human melanoma metastases express functional CXCR4. *Clin. Cancer Res.* **2006**, *12*, 2427–2433. [CrossRef]
11. Barbero, S.; Bonavia, R.; Bajetto, A.; Porcile, C.; Pirani, P.; Ravetti, J.L.; Zona, G.L.; Spaziante, R.; Florio, T.; Schettini, G. Stromal cell-derived factor 1alpha stimulates human glioblastoma cell growth through the activation of both extracellular signal-regulated kinases 1/2 and Akt. *Cancer Res.* **2003**, *63*, 1969–1974. [PubMed]
12. Rubin, J.B.; Kung, A.L.; Klein, R.S.; Chan, J.A.; Sun, Y.; Schmidt, K.; Kieran, M.W.; Luster, A.D.; Segal, R.A. A small-molecule antagonist of CXCR4 inhibits intracranial growth of primary brain tumors. *Proc. Natl. Acad. Sci. USA* **2003**, *100*, 13513–13518. [CrossRef] [PubMed]
13. Corcione, A.; Ottonello, L.; Tortolina, G.; Facchetti, P.; Airoldi, I.; Guglielmino, R.; Dadati, P.; Truini, M.; Sozzani, S.; Dallegri, F.; et al. Stromal cell-derived factor-1 as a chemoattractant for follicular center lymphoma B cells. *J. Natl. Cancer Inst.* **2000**, *92*, 628–635. [CrossRef] [PubMed]
14. Bertolini, F.; Dell'Agnola, C.; Mancuso, P.; Rabascio, C.; Burlini, A.; Monestiroli, S.; Gobbi, A.; Pruneri, G.; Martinelli, G. CXCR4 neutralization, a novel therapeutic approach for non-Hodgkin's lymphoma. *Cancer Res.* **2002**, *62*, 3106–3112.
15. Zeelenberg, I.S.; Ruuls-Van Stalle, L.; Roos, E. The chemokine receptor CXCR4 is required for outgrowth of colon carcinoma micrometastases. *Cancer Res.* **2003**, *63*, 3833–3839.
16. Ottaiano, A.; Di Palma, A.; Napolitano, M.; Pisano, C.; Pignata, S.; Tatangelo, F.; Botti, G.; Acquaviva, A.M.; Castello, G.; Ascierto, P.A.; et al. Inhibitory effects of anti-CXCR4 antibodies on human colon cancer cells. *Cancer Immunol. Immunother.* **2005**, *54*, 781–791. [CrossRef]
17. Jiang, Q.; Sun, Y.; Liu, X. CXCR4 as a prognostic biomarker in gastrointestinal cancer: A meta-analysis. *Biomarkers* **2019**, *24*, 510–516. [CrossRef]
18. Chen, Q.; Zhong, T. The association of CXCR4 expression with clinicopathological significance and potential drug target in prostate cancer: A meta-analysis and literature review. *Drug. Des. Devel. Ther.* **2015**, *9*, 5115–5122. [CrossRef]
19. Zhao, H.; Guo, L.; Zhao, H.; Zhao, J.; Weng, H.; Zhao, B. CXCR4 over-expression and survival in cancer: A system review and meta-analysis. *Oncotarget* **2015**, *6*, 5022–5040. [CrossRef]
20. Zhang, Z.; Ni, C.; Chen, W.; Wu, P.; Wang, Z.; Yin, J.; Junhua, Y.; Jian, H.; Fuming, Q. Expression of CXCR4 and breast cancer prognosis: A systematic review and meta-analysis. *BMC Cancer* **2014**, *14*, 49. [CrossRef]
21. Ferlay, J.; Colombet, M.; Soerjomataram, I.; Mathers, C.; Parkin, D.M.; Piñeros, M.; Znaor, A.; Bray, F. Estimating the global cancer incidence and mortality in 2018: GLOBOCAN sources and methods. *Int. J. Cancer* **2019**, *144*, 1941–1953. [CrossRef]
22. Iveson, T. Adjuvant chemotherapy in colon cancer: State of the art and future perspectives. *Cur. Opin. Oncol.* **2020**, *32*, 370–376. [CrossRef] [PubMed]
23. Nappi, A.; Berretta, M.; Romano, C.; Tafuto, S.; Cassata, A.; Casaretti, R.; Silvestro, L.; Divitiis, C.; Alessandrini, L.; Fiorica, F.; et al. Metastatic Colorectal Cancer: Role of Target Therapies and Future Perspectives. *Curr. Cancer Drug Targets* **2018**, *18*, 421–429. [CrossRef] [PubMed]
24. Ottaiano, A.; Franco, R.; Aiello Talamanca, A.; Liguori, G.; Tatangelo, F.; Delrio, P.; Nasti, G.; Barletta, E.; Facchini, G.; Daniele, B.; et al. Overexpression of both CXC chemokine receptor 4 and vascular endothelial growth factor proteins predicts early distant relapse in stage II-III colorectal cancer patients. *Clin. Cancer Res.* **2006**, *12*, 2795–2803. [CrossRef] [PubMed]

25. Ottaiano, A.; Scala, S.; Normanno, N.; Botti, G.; Tatangelo, F.; Di Mauro, A.; Capozzi, M.; Facchini, S.; Tafuto, S.; Nasti, G. Prognostic and Predictive Role of CXC Chemokine Receptor 4 in Metastatic Colorectal Cancer Patients. *Appl. Immunohistochem. Mol. Morphol.* **2020**, *28*, 755–760. [CrossRef]
26. Liberati, A.; Altman, D.G.; Tetzlaff, J.; Mulrow, C.; Gotzsche, P.C.; Ioannidis, J.P.; Clarke, M.; Devereaux, P.J.; Kleijnen, J.; Moher, D. The PRISMA statement for reporting systematic reviews and meta-analyses of studies that evaluate health care interventions: Explanation and elaboration. *PLoS Med.* **2009**, *6*, e1000100. [CrossRef] [PubMed]
27. Stang, A. Critical evaluation of the Newcastle-Ottawa scale for the assessment of the quality of nonrandomized studies in meta-analyses. *Eur. J. Epidemiol.* **2010**, *25*, 603–605. [CrossRef]
28. Altman, D.G.; Machin, D.; Bryant, T.N.; Gardner, M.J. (Eds.) *Statistics with Confidence*, 2nd ed.; BMJ USA: London, UK, 2000.
29. DerSimonian, R.; Laird, N. Meta-analysis in clinical trials. *Control Clin. Trials.* **1986**, *7*, 177–188. [CrossRef]
30. Higgins, J.P.; Thompson, S.G.; Deeks, J.J.; Altman, D.G. Measuring inconsistency in meta-analyses. *BMJ* **2003**, *327*, 557–560. [CrossRef]
31. Egger, M.; Smith, G.D.; Schneider, M.; Minder, C. Bias in meta-analysis detected by a simple, graphical test. *BMJ* **1997**, *315*, 629–634. [CrossRef]
32. Kim, J.; Takeuchi, H.; Lam, S.T.; Turner, R.R.; Wang, H.J.; Kuo, C.; Foshag, L.; Bilchik, A.J.; Hoon, D.S. Chemokine receptor CXCR4 expression in colorectal cancer patients increases the risk for recurrence and for poor survival. *J. Clin. Oncol.* **2005**, *23*, 2744–2753. [CrossRef]
33. Yoshitake, N.; Fukui, H.; Yamagishi, H.; Sekikawa, A.; Fujii, S.; Tomita, S.; Ichikawa, K.; Imura, J.; Hiraishi, H.; Fujimori, T. Expression of SDF-1 alpha and nuclear CXCR4 predicts lymph node metastasis in colorectal cancer. *Br. J. Cancer* **2008**, *98*, 1682–1689. [CrossRef]
34. Speetjens, F.M.; Liefers, G.J.; Korbee, C.J.; Mesker, W.E.; Van de Velde, C.J.; Van Vlierberghe, R.L.; Morreau, H.; Tollenaar, R.A.; Kuppen, P.J. Nuclear localization of CXCR4 determines prognosis for colorectal cancer patients. *Cancer Microenviron.* **2009**, *2*, 1–7. [CrossRef]
35. Ingold, B.; Schulz, S.; Budczies, J.; Neumann, U.; Ebert, M.P.; Weichert, W.; Röcken, C. The role of vascular CXCR4 expression in colorectal carcinoma. *Histopathology* **2009**, *55*, 576–586. [CrossRef]
36. Wang, S.C.; Lin, J.K.; Wang, H.S.; Yang, S.H.; Li, A.F.; Chang, S.C. Nuclear expression of CXCR4 is associated with advanced colorectal cancer. *Int. J. Colorectal. Dis.* **2010**, *25*, 1185–1191. [CrossRef] [PubMed]
37. Yopp, A.C.; Shia, J.; Butte, J.M.; Allen, P.J.; Fong, Y.; Jarnagin, W.R.; De Matteo, R.P.; D'Angelica, M.I. CXCR4 expression predicts patient outcome and recurrence patterns after hepatic resection for colorectal liver metastases. *Ann. Surg. Oncol.* **2012**, *19*, S339–S346. [CrossRef]
38. Sakai, N.; Yoshidome, H.; Shida, T.; Kimura, F.; Shimizu, H.; Ohtsuka, M.; Takeuchi, D.; Sakakibara, M.; Miyazaki, M. CXCR4/CXCL12 expression profile is associated with tumor microenvironment and clinical outcome of liver metastases of colorectal cancer. *Clin. Exp. Metastasis* **2012**, *29*, 101–110. [CrossRef] [PubMed]
39. Du, C.; Yao, Y.; Xue, W.; Zhu, W.G.; Peng, Y.; Gu, J. The expression of chemokine receptors CXCR3 and CXCR4 in predicting postoperative tumour progression in stages I-II colon cancer: A retrospective study. *BMJ Open* **2014**, *4*, e005012. [CrossRef] [PubMed]
40. Gao, Y.; Li, C.; Nie, M.; Lu, Y.; Lin, S.; Yuan, P.; Sun, X. CXCR4 as a novel predictive biomarker for metastasis and poor prognosis in colorectal cancer. *Tumour. Biol.* **2014**, *35*, 4171–4175. [CrossRef] [PubMed]
41. Stanisavljević, L.; Aßmus, J.; Storli, K.E.; Leh, S.M.; Dahl, O.; Myklebust, M.P. CXCR4, CXCL12 and the relative CXCL12-CXCR4 expression as prognostic factors in colon cancer. *Tumour. Biol.* **2016**, *37*, 7441–7452. [CrossRef] [PubMed]
42. D'Alterio, C.; Nasti, G.; Polimeno, M.; Ottaiano, A.; Conson, M.; Circelli, L.; Botti, G.; Scognamiglio, G.; Santagata, S.; De Divitiis, C.; et al. CXCR4-CXCL12-CXCR7, TLR2-TLR4, and PD-1/PD-L1 in colorectal cancer liver metastases from neoadjuvant-treated patients. *Oncoimmunology* **2016**, *5*, e1254313. [CrossRef] [PubMed]
43. Wu, W.; Cao, J.; Ji, Z.; Wang, J.; Jiang, T.; Ding, H. Co-expression of Lgr5 and CXCR4 characterizes cancer stem-like cells of colorectal cancer. *Oncotarget* **2016**, *7*, 81144–81155. [CrossRef] [PubMed]
44. Weixler, B.; Renetseder, F.; Facile, I.; Tosti, N.; Cremonesi, E.; Tampakis, A.; Delko, T.; Eppenberger-Castori, S.; Tzankov, A.; Iezzi, G.; et al. Phosphorylated CXCR4 expression has a positive prognostic impact in colorectal cancer. *Cell. Oncol.* **2017**, *40*, 609–619. [CrossRef] [PubMed]
45. Xu, C.; Zheng, L.; Li, D.; Chen, G.; Gu, J.; Chen, J.; Yao, Q. CXCR4 overexpression is correlated with poor prognosis in colorectal cancer. *Life Sci.* **2018**, *208*, 333–340. [CrossRef] [PubMed]

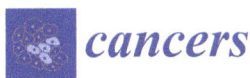

Article

Detection of Hepatocellular Carcinoma in a High-Risk Population by a Mass Spectrometry-Based Test

Devalingam Mahalingam [1,2,3,*], Leonidas Chelis [4,5], Imran Nizamuddin [2], Sunyoung S. Lee [6,7], Stylianos Kakolyris [4], Glenn Halff [3], Ken Washburn [3,8], Kristopher Attwood [6], Ibnshamsah Fahad [5], Julia Grigorieva [9], Senait Asmellash [9], Krista Meyer [9], Carlos Oliveira [9], Heinrich Roder [9], Joanna Roder [9] and Renuka Iyer [6]

[1] Robert H. Lurie Comprehensive Cancer Center of Northwestern University, Northwestern University, Chicago, IL 60611, USA
[2] Department of Medicine, Feinberg School of Medicine, Northwestern University, Chicago, IL 60611, USA; imran.nizamuddin@northwestern.edu
[3] Long School of Medicine, University of Texas Health Science Center at San Antonio, San Antonio, TX 78229, USA; halff@uthscsa.edu (G.H.); ken.washburn@osumc.edu (K.W.)
[4] Department of Medical Oncology, Democritus University of Thrace, 68100 Alexandroupolis, Greece; leonidas.chelis@kfsh.med.sa (L.C.); skakol@her.forthnet.gr (S.K.)
[5] Adult Oncology Department, King Fahad Specialist Hospital Dammam, Dammam 32253, Saudi Arabia; fahad.ibnshamsah@kfsh.med.sa
[6] Department of Medical Oncology, Roswell Park Comprehensive Cancer Center, Buffalo, NY 14203, USA; sslee1@mdanderson.org (S.S.L.); attwood3@buffalo.edu (K.A.); renuka.iyer@roswellpark.org (R.I.)
[7] Department of Gastrointestinal (GI) Medical Oncology, The University of Texas MD Anderson Cancer Center, Houston, TX 77030, USA
[8] Department of Surgery, The Ohio State University Wexner Medical Center, Columbus, OH 43210, USA
[9] Biodesix Inc., Boulder, CO 80301, USA; julia.grigorieva@biodesix.com (J.G.); senait.asmellash@biodesix.com (S.A.); krista.meyer@biodesix.com (K.M.); carlos.oliveira@biodesix.com (C.O.); heinrich.roder@biodesix.com (H.R.); joanna.roder@biodesix.com (J.R.)
* Correspondence: mahalingam@northwestern.edu

Simple Summary: Liver cancer is one of the most common causes of cancer worldwide, but unfortunately, current technology has a limited ability to detect it early in high-risk patients. This study investigates a machine learning algorithm based on protein levels in the blood that can be used to help with diagnosis. The test shows promising results, especially in patients with smaller tumors and compared to current blood detection tests. This research suggests an important role in the future for machine learning algorithm-based blood detection tests.

Abstract: Hepatocellular carcinoma (HCC) is one of the fastest growing causes of cancer-related death. Guidelines recommend obtaining a screening ultrasound with or without alpha-fetoprotein (AFP) every 6 months in at-risk adults. AFP as a screening biomarker is plagued by low sensitivity/specificity, prompting interest in discovering alternatives. Mass spectrometry-based techniques are promising in their ability to identify potential biomarkers. This study aimed to use machine learning utilizing spectral data and AFP to create a model for early detection. Serum samples were collected from three separate cohorts, and data were compiled to make Development, Internal Validation, and Independent Validation sets. AFP levels were measured, and Deep MALDI® analysis was used to generate mass spectra. Spectral data were input into the VeriStrat® classification algorithm. Machine learning techniques then classified each sample as "Cancer" or "No Cancer". Sensitivity and specificity of the test were >80% to detect HCC. High specificity of the test was independent of cause and severity of underlying disease. When compared to AFP, there was improved cancer detection for all tumor sizes, especially small lesions. Overall, a machine learning algorithm incorporating mass spectral data and AFP values from serum samples offers a novel approach to diagnose HCC. Given the small sample size of the Independent Validation set, a further independent, prospective study is warranted.

Citation: Mahalingam, D.; Chelis, L.; Nizamuddin, I.; Lee, S.S.; Kakolyris, S.; Halff, G.; Washburn, K.; Attwood, K.; Fahad, I.; Grigorieva, J.; et al. Detection of Hepatocellular Carcinoma in a High-Risk Population by a Mass Spectrometry-Based Test. *Cancers* **2021**, *13*, 3109. https://doi.org/10.3390/cancers13133109

Academic Editor: Takaya Shimura

Received: 26 May 2021
Accepted: 14 June 2021
Published: 22 June 2021

Publisher's Note: MDPI stays neutral with regard to jurisdictional claims in published maps and institutional affiliations.

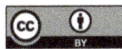

Copyright: © 2021 by the authors. Licensee MDPI, Basel, Switzerland. This article is an open access article distributed under the terms and conditions of the Creative Commons Attribution (CC BY) license (https://creativecommons.org/licenses/by/4.0/).

Keywords: cancer screening; cirrhosis; AFP; machine learning; MALDI-TOF; proteomics

1. Introduction

Primary liver cancer results in a significant global burden of disease, with studies reporting it as the sixth most common cause of cancer and fourth most common cause of cancer-related death worldwide in 2018. Hepatocellular carcinoma (HCC) makes up 75% to 85% of all primary liver cancers [1]. While reports have suggested a decrease in incidence of HCC in Asia due to vaccination and treatment programs for viral hepatitis, HCC is the fastest growing cause of cancer-related deaths in the United States [2]. Chronic liver disease of any etiology remains the most significant risk factor, with 80% to 90% of new HCC cases occurring in this population [3]. Surveillance programs have been developed for earlier detection and mortality reduction. Current AASLD guidelines recommend surveillance in adults with cirrhosis and high-risk patients without cirrhosis using ultrasound with or without alpha-fetoprotein (AFP) assessment at six-month intervals [4]. Unfortunately, screening ultrasound may be of limited use among select populations secondary to body habitus, obesity, early HCC disease, and operator experience [5]. In such cases, biomarkers may supplement ultrasound in the detection of early disease. However, the sensitivity and specificity of AFP is barely satisfactory, necessitating the discovery of circulating biomarkers with a higher diagnostic value [6]. In fact, neither European nor American guidelines include quantification of serum AFP for HCC diagnosis, despite estimated improvement of 6% to 8% in detection rate. Reasons for its suboptimal performance include lack of sensitivity for detecting hepatocellular carcinoma in early stages and large numbers of false-positive results [7].

Several candidate biomarkers are being studied for HCC diagnosis, with des-gamma-carboxy prothrombin (DCP), lens cullinaris agglutin-reactive AFP (AFP-L3), osteopontin, and midkine, amongst others, the most advanced in development. Nevertheless, significant challenges exist, largely stemming from HCC molecular heterogeneity [8]. Furthermore, many of these biomarkers continue to be plagued with low sensitivity, especially when used without AFP [9]. Certain biomarkers, such as DCP and AFP-L3, are markers of advanced tumoral stage, thus preventing their use for early cancer detection [10,11]. Recognizing that HCC tumor biology is highly heterogeneous, composites of biomarkers and clinical factors associated with risk of HCC have been investigated for early detection of HCC. One such panel, the GALAD score, uses objective measures of gender, age, AFP, AFP-L3, and DCP [12]. The sensitivity/specificity of GALAD at a fixed cutoff of -0.63 has ranged from 92%/90%, 71%/96%, and 88%/89% in cohorts from the UK, Japan, and Germany [13] to 79%/79% in a cohort from the USA [14].

Recently developed mass spectrometry-based techniques, such as proteomics, lipidomics, and metabolomics, represent promising tools for the discovery and identification of proteins, peptides, lipids, and metabolites associated with various diseases [15]. Among various mass spectrometric techniques, matrix-assisted laser desorption/ionization time-of-flight (MALDI-TOF) mass spectrometry is a high-throughput technology capable of generating a molecular fingerprint. Thus, it has provided a powerful tool for discovery of biomarkers in different kinds of cancers, including HCC [16–18]. However, traditionally matrix-assisted laser desorption/ionization (MALDI)-based studies have been hampered by lack of sensitivity. A new approach, the Deep MALDI® method, which averages over many more laser shots than conventional methods, allows for a deeper probing of the serum proteome [19]. Machine learning (ML) techniques have been applied to combine MALDI mass spectral (MS) data with clinical data to generate molecular diagnostic tests predictive of outcomes for cancer therapy [20,21].

Herein, we propose using this technology for test development and blinded validation on three independent sample sets from healthy volunteers, patients with known cirrhosis without HCC, and patients with HCC. The main goal of the study is to identify a signature of early HCC among patients with cirrhosis or high-risk patients with chronic liver disease. We focus on the assessment of test performance in the patients with the smallest lesions, where early detection and intervention is most important.

2. Materials and Methods

2.1. Patient Cohorts

Two patient cohorts were used for test development and initial validation: a cohort of 100 pre-transplant patients (48 HCC and 52 cirrhosis) from University of Texas Health Sciences Center San Antonio (UTHSCSA) and a cohort of 193 patients (110 HCC and 83 cirrhosis) from Democritus University of Thrace, Greece (Greek). A third cohort of 156 patients (97 HCC and 59 healthy volunteers) from Roswell Park Comprehensive Cancer Center (Roswell) was used for blinded, independent validation of the test. Serum samples had been collected from patients in the UTHSCSA cohort at time of liver transplant. Blood collection protocols were approved by the respective institutional review committees, and patient consent was obtained. The study conformed to ethical guidelines of the 1975 Declaration of Helsinki.

Of the UTHSCSA cohort containing 100 patients, 48 patients had HCC and 52 patients had liver disease without HCC. Patients undergoing liver transplant for HCC generally had much better liver function than those with other liver diseases. The predominant liver disease etiologies across all 100 patients were alcohol-related cirrhosis and hepatitis C. The Greek cohort consisted of 110 patients with HCC and 83 patients with liver disease without HCC. Within this cohort, 68% of patients had hepatitis B. The Roswell cohort consisted of 97 patients with HCC and 59 healthy volunteers without HCC, totaling 156 patients.

As there were differences in liver function and liver disease etiology between the two cohorts used for test development, the UTHSCSA and Greek cohorts were combined, split, and stratified by presence/absence of HCC to create a Development set and an Internal Validation set (Figure 1). All test development work was carried out using data from only the Development set. Patient characteristics for all three cohorts and the Development set and the Internal Validation set are provided in Table 1.

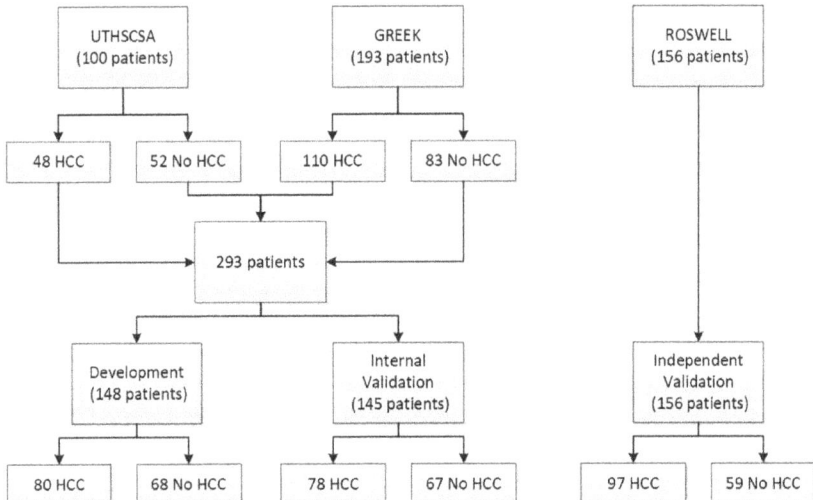

Figure 1. Consort diagram.

Table 1. Patient characteristics by cohort and set.

Patient Characteristic		UTHSCSA		Greek		Roswell		Development		Internal Validation	
		HCC (n = 48)	No HCC (n = 52)	HCC (n = 110)	No HCC (n = 83)	HCC (n = 97)	No HCC (n = 59)	HCC (n = 80)	No HCC (n = 68)	HCC (n = 78)	No HCC (n = 67)
Age	median	59.5	56	69	54	63	62	67	54.5	66	57
	range	50-85	40-67	44-82	28-80	38-89	38-87	44-82	30-74	47-85	28-80
Gender	male, n (%)	32 (67)	25 (48)	92 (84)	60 (72)	84 (87)	40 (68)	63 (79)	42 (62)	61 (78)	43 (64)
	female, n (%)	16 (33)	27 (52)	18 (16)	23 (28)	13 (13)	19 (32)	17 (21)	26 (38)	17 (22)	24 (36)
MELD	median	14	25	10	NA	11	NA	11	25	11	25
	range	7-37	13-47	6-26	NA	6-38	NA	6-34	16-42	7-37	13-47
	NA, n (%)	13 (27)	0 (0)	2 (2)	83 (100)	14 (14)	59 (100)	7 (9)	42 (62)	8 (10)	41 (61)
Child-Pugh	A, n (%)	30 (63)	6 (12)	72 (65)	74 (89)	53 (55)	NA	35 (44)	38 (56)	37 (47)	36 (54)
	B, n (%)	16 (33)	38 (73)	27 (25)	7 (8)	24 (25)	NA	16 (20)	3 (4)	11 (14)	4 (6)
	C, n (%)	2 (4)	8 (15)	11 (10)	2 (2)	6 (6)	NA	5 (6)	1 (1)	6 (8)	1 (1)
	NA, n (%)	0 (0)	0 (0)	0 (0)	0 (0)	14 (14)	NA	24 (30)	26 (38)	24 (31)	26 (39)
BCLC status	A, n (%)	48 (100)	NA	3 (3)	NA	29 (30)	NA	26 (33)	NA	25 (32)	NA
	B, n (%)	0 (0)	NA	15 (14)	NA	12 (12)	NA	9 (11)	NA	6 (8)	NA
	C, n (%)	0 (0)	NA	73 (66)	NA	41 (42)	NA	35 (44)	NA	38 (49)	NA
	D, n (%)	0 (0)	NA	19 (17)	NA	15 (15)	NA	10 (13)	NA	9 (12)	NA
Liver disease origin	HBV, n (%)	4 (8)	1 (2)	72 * (65)	59 (71)	3 (3)	3 (5)	41 (51)	NA	35 * (45)	31
	HCV, n (%)	28 (58)	21 (40)	10 * (9)	7 (8)	26 (27)	13 (22)	18 (23)	NA	20 * (26)	13
	Other/NA, n (%)	17 (35)	30 (58)	29 (26)	17 (20)	68 (70)	43 (73)	21 (26)	NA	24 (35)	23
Serum AFP (ng/mL)	median	4.7	1.6	37.0	2.0	4.0	2.6	16.8	1.8	25.0	2.1
	minimum	<0.8	<0.8	1.1	0.8	<1.5	<1.5	<1.5	<1.5	<0.8	<0.8
	maximum	≥10,000	15.0	≥10,000	115	≥10,000	11.5	≥10,000	20.0	≥10,000	115
Lesion size (cm)	<3, n (%)	13 (27)	NA	1 (1)	NA	5 (5)	NA	8 (10)	NA	6 (8)	NA
	≥3 and <5, n (%)	21 (44)	NA	13 (12)	NA	18 (19)	NA	16 (20)	NA	18 (23)	NA
	≥5 and <7, n (%)	4 (8)	NA	18 (16)	NA	14 (14)	NA	12 (15)	NA	10 (13)	NA
	≥7 and <10, n (%)	3 (6)	NA	12 (11)	NA	26 (27)	NA	7 (9)	NA	8 (10)	NA
	≥10 and <15, n (%)	2 (4)	NA	21 (19)	NA	16 (16)	NA	12 (15)	NA	11 (14)	NA
	≥15, n (%)	2 (4)	NA	7 (6)	NA	3 (3)	NA	4 (5)	NA	5 (6)	NA
	NA, n (%)	3 (6)	NA	38 (34)	NA	15 (15)	NA	21 (26)	NA	20 (26)	NA

* One patient had both hepatitis B and hepatitis C; Abbreviations: not available (NA), hepatocellular carcinoma (HCC), Model for End-Stage Liver Disease (MELD), Barcelona-Clinic Liver Cancer (BCLC), alpha-fetoprotein (AFP), hepatitis B virus (HBV), hepatitis C virus (HCV).

2.2. Methods

2.2.1. Sample Collection and Storage

Serum samples were stored at −80 °C and were shipped frozen in batches to the Biodesix laboratory (Biodesix, Boulder, CO, USA) for MS generation and AFP measurement.

2.2.2. Mass Spectral Acquisition

In total, 3 µL aliquots of each experimental sample were sufficient for generation of mass spectra. To simulate sample collection procedures practical for clinical use with sample shipment at ambient temperature, serum samples were spotted onto cellulose serum cards (Therapak, Claremont, CA, USA), allowed to dry, and then re-eluted. Spectra were obtained using a MALDI-TOF mass spectrometer (Ultraflextreme, Bruker, Billerica, MA, USA). The Deep MALDI® method was used, providing data over a greater dynamic range than standard MALDI approaches [19]. Eight hundred shot spectra were collected from 63 pre-defined positions per MALDI spot (63 × 800 × 3 spots per sample), for a total of 151,200 laser shots per sample. Spectra were collected from the UTHSCSA cohort in November 2013, the cohort of 16 patients with no liver disease in July 2014, the Greek cohort in March 2015, and the Roswell cohort in February 2018.

2.2.3. Mass Spectral Processing

All spectra were aligned (Table S1) and spectra failing quality control metrics were discarded. At random, 140 spectra for each sample were selected and averaged to create one average spectrum (from 112,000 laser shots) per sample. Average spectra then underwent processing to make them comparable between samples (Figure S1). This involved background subtraction, normalization (Table S2, Table S5), batch correction using spectral data from reference samples, and alignment (Table S3). Full details of sample preparation and spectral processing methods are provided in Supplementary Text S1.

Three hundred mass spectral features were defined (Table S4). Each MS feature is defined as a mass/charge region and the value of a MS feature is the integrated intensity of the processed, average spectrum within this mass/charge region. MS feature values were calculated for each processed averaged spectrum for each sample.

2.2.4. AFP Measurement

Serum AFP levels were measured for each sample using the DAFP00 ELISA kit (R&D Systems, Minneapolis, MN, USA) following manufacturer instructions as described in Supplementary Text S1 by ELISA Tech (Aurora, CO, USA).

2.2.5. Application of an Existing MS-Based Serum Proteomic Test

The classification algorithm from a pre-existing serum proteomic test (the VeriStrat® test, Biodesix, CO, USA) was applied to the generated mass spectra [16]. This test produces a binary classification of Good or Poor and has been demonstrated to have prognostic and predictive utility in advanced non-small cell lung cancer [22]. It has been observed that Poor classifications are rarely observed in patients without cancer [23].

2.2.6. Development of the HCC Detection Test

1. Machine Learning Approach

Test development was carried out using machine learning with a dropout regularized combination (the Diagnostic Cortex® system, Biodesix., Boulder, CO, USA) approach [24]. This method was designed to allow reliable estimates of test performance from relatively small development sets in the setting where there are more measured attributes than samples. Briefly, the Development set was divided into a training set and test set. The 300 MS features and AFP were used as attributes to classify the samples into "Cancer" or "No Cancer" groups. Many simple, k-nearest neighbor, atomic classifiers were constructed with the training set using subsets of the attributes. Atomic classifiers not showing any ability to correctly classify the training set samples were discarded during a filtering step.

The remaining atomic classifiers were combined using dropout regularized logistic regression to yield one master classifier. This was repeated for many splits of the Development set into training and test sets, and an ensemble average was created to generate a final score for each sample. As each sample was held in the test set for multiple training/test split stratifications, reliable classification estimates could be obtained for all samples in the Development set by ensemble averaging only test set data (out-of-bag estimation). Application of a threshold to the resulting score yielded a binary classification of "Cancer" or "No Cancer" for each sample. The family of tests produced from varying the threshold value was assessed using receiver operating characteristic (ROC) methods. A final test was produced by choice of a particular threshold best suiting clinical need in terms of its associated sensitivity and specificity.

2. Test Development

As it has been observed that patients with serum samples classified as Poor by the VeriStrat® classification algorithm or with very high AFP are very likely to have cancer, patients meeting these criteria ($n = 40$) were assigned a "Cancer" classification. Data for the remaining samples ($n = 108$) in the Development set were then used within the machine learning platform for training of a classifier able to identify patients with or without HCC, based on their serum AFP and values of the 100 mass spectral features showing the greatest potential for classification (Table S6). Figure 2 shows a heatmap of the 100 MS features used within the classification algorithm for the 108 samples used in classifier development, grouped according to "Cancer" vs. "No Cancer". A list of the feature definitions of the 100 MS features and assessment of the univariate associations of the features with presence or absence of HCC is contained in the Supplementary Text S1. It is noteworthy that no single feature provided outstanding classification alone. We observed that some pairs of features, which individually had relatively poor classification power, provided much better classification as an interaction (i.e., product of the two), indicating the multivariate nature of the test.

Imbalances between the liver function of patients with HCC and without HCC were observed in our cohorts, as evidenced by MELD and Child–Pugh scores. This was particularly apparent in the UTHSCSA cohort. Samples were collected at the time of transplant or resection. Hence, patients without HCC eligible for a liver transplant had very advanced liver disease with associated poor liver function, while patients undergoing transplant or resection for early stage HCC had better liver function, typical of the population at risk for HCC (Table 1). Liver function is easily assessable from measurements of the serum proteome, and serum mass spectra for patients with poor liver function display many differences from those for patients with better liver function. Hence, our data were partially confounded. The dropout regularized combination approach of test development is well-suited to mitigate such confounding effects [24]. In addition to requiring that atomic classifiers had a minimal level of performance classifying the training set, we required that they also were able to classify spectra from serum of healthy patients to the "No Cancer" group. More details on machine learning classifier development are provided in Supplementary Text S1.

All test parameters, including the threshold for the binary result of "Cancer" or "No Cancer" were set using only samples from the Development set and locked prior to all validation.

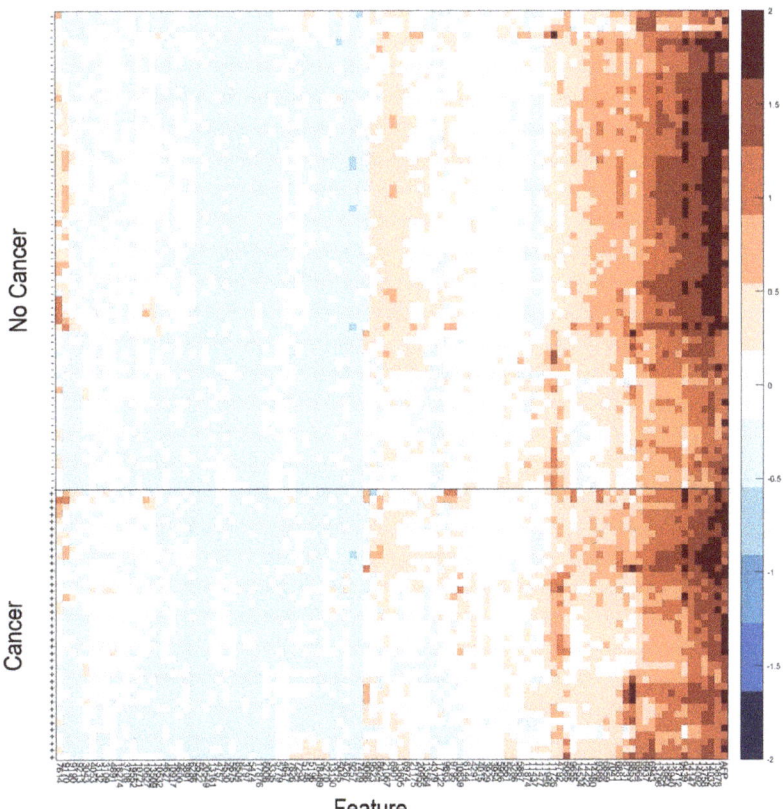

Figure 2. Heatmap of the natural logarithm of serum AFP and the MS features used for classification for the 108 samples used in classifier development. + indicates samples from patients with HCC; -indicates samples from patients without HCC. Features and samples are hierarchically clustered.

2.2.7. Application of the HCC Detection Test to Validation Samples

The HCC detection test was applied to any sample not used in its development following the schema of Figure 3.

First, mass spectra were acquired from the serum sample, and serum AFP was assessed following the protocols outlined above and in Supplementary Text S1. The VeriStrat classification algorithm was then applied to the generated mass spectra and samples yielding a Poor classification were assigned a "Cancer" classification. Samples with serum AFP determined as equal to or exceeding 100 ng/mL were also assigned a "Cancer" classification. Samples not yielding a VeriStrat Poor classification and with AFP < 100 ng/mL were then classified as "Cancer" or "No Cancer" by the machine learning classifier, based on their MS feature values and serum AFP measurement. Quality control metrics were applied to the MS data, so that only samples generating mass spectra of sufficient quality and not exhibiting evidence of sample contamination or degradation received a valid test classification.

2.2.8. Independent Validation

Independent validation was performed using the fully locked test. Mass spectra were generated from samples in the Roswell validation set more than 2 years after collection of spectra used in test development and were classified blinded to all clinical data.

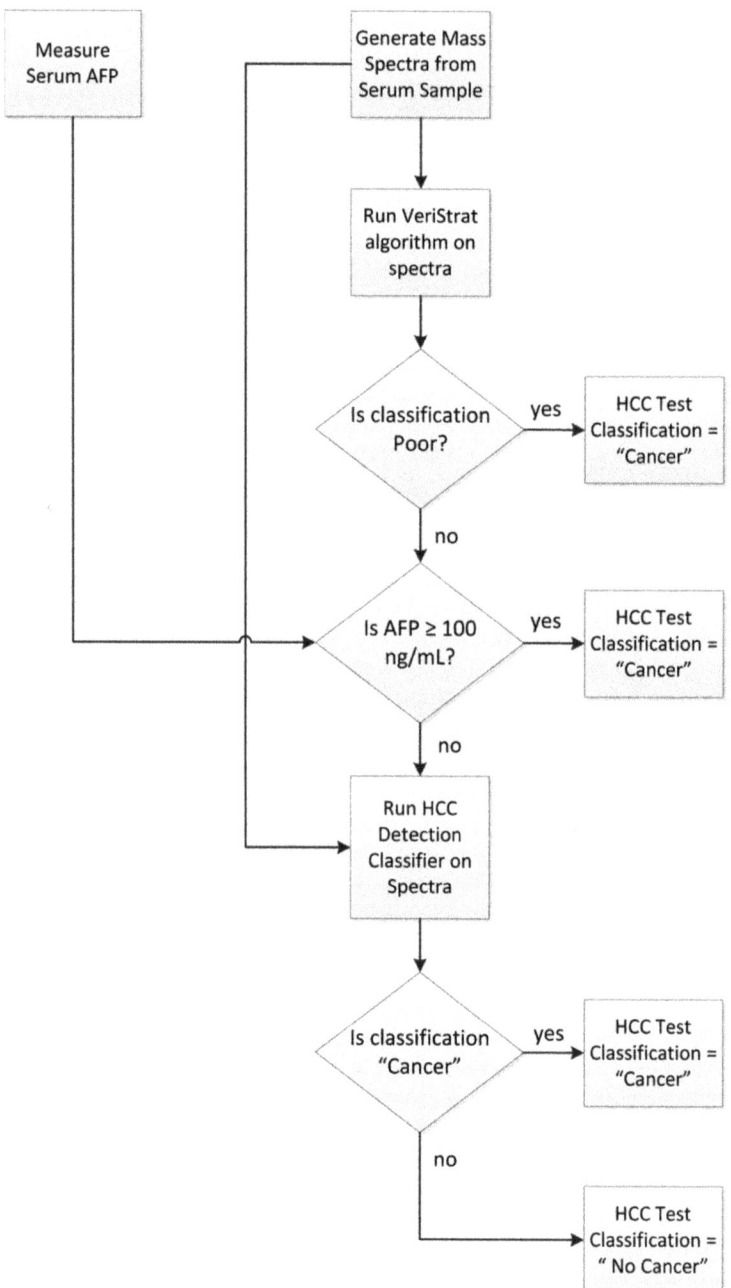

Figure 3. Classification algorithm for the HCC Detection Test.

2.2.9. Statistical Methods

Analyses were performed using SAS 9.3 (SAS, Cary, NC, USA) and PRISM (GraphPad, La Jolla, CA, USA). The area under the curve obtained from the test of Figure 3 was compared with that obtained from AFP alone using the method of DeLong. Test performance was assessed using sensitivity, specificity, and accuracy of detection of HCC within patient subgroups.

3. Results

Analysis of the spectra from the Development set accurately classified 66 of 80 (83% sensitivity) HCC specimens and 57 of 68 (84% specificity) non-HCC specimens. Of the Internal Validation set, 63 of 78 (81% sensitivity) HCC specimens and 53 of 67 (79% specificity) non-HCC specimens were accurately classified. Finally, of the Independent Validation set, 85 of 97 (88% sensitivity) HCC specimens and 59 of 59 (100% specificity) non-HCC specimens were accurately classified.

To compare the classification power of the family of tests obtained by varying the threshold applied to the HCC test classifier with that of serum AFP level, ROC plots were constructed. The ROC plots for the Development, Internal Validation, and Independent Validation sets for AFP alone and the tests using mass spectrometry data and AFP are shown in Figure 4. P values for comparison of the area under the curves (AUCs) between the test and the AFP classification are shown on the right.

The similarity of AUCs between the Development and Internal Validation sets indicates excellent generalization of classification performance. Increased performance in the Independent Validation set is likely due to the differences in population. The test showed significantly better performance than univariate AFP level in both Internal and Independent Validation sets. In the Independent Validation set, at sensitivity of 88%, the test specificity exceeded that of univariate AFP by 20%. At perfect specificity, the test sensitivity exceeded that of univariate AFP by 13%.

Diagnostic performance of the commonly used cut-off for AFP of 20 ng/mL typically produces sensitivities in the range of 41–65% and specificities of 80–90%, depending on patient population [25,26]. In our study, detection of HCC by the 20 ng/mL cut-off (marked on the ROC curves in Figure 4) resulted in sensitivities of 49%, 54%, and 71% in the Development, Internal Validation, and Independent Validation sets, respectively, which is markedly inferior to the results of the test. Specificity of using AFP cut-off as a biomarker was high: 99%, 99%, and 100% in the respective cohorts.

Accuracy of test classification for patients with and without cancer in each of the cohorts overall and in clinical subgroups defined by liver function, origin of the disease, and lesion size is shown in Table 2.

Table 2. Accuracy of the test overall and by clinical subgroups depending on liver function and origin of the disease.

Cohort		Development (n = 148)		Internal Validation (n = 145)		Independent Validation (n = 156)	
		HCC (n = 80)	No HCC (n = 68)	HCC (n = 78)	No HCC (n = 67)	HCC (n = 97)	No HCC (n = 59)
Overall, n (%)		66/80 (83)	57/68 (84)	63/78 (81)	53/67 (79)	85/97 (88)	59/59 (100)
Child–Pugh	A, n (%)	28/35 (80)	35/38 (92)	30/37 (81)	34/36 (94)	unknown	N/A
	B, n (%)	16/16 (100)	3/3 (100)	11/11 (100)	2/4 (50)	unknown	N/A
	C, n (%)	5/5 (100)	1/1 (100)	6/6 (100)	1/1 (100)	unknown	N/A
	NA, n (%)	17/24 (71)	18/26 (69)	16/24 (67)	16/26 (62)	unknown	N/A
Liver Disease Origin *	HBV, n (%)	36/41 (88)	28/29 (97)	31/35 (89)	29/31 (94)	3/3 (100)	N/A
	HCV, n (%)	14/18 (78)	10/15 (67)	18/20 (90)	8/13 (62)	26/26 (100)	N/A
	Other/NA, n (%)	20/26 (77)	21/26 (81)	18/27 (67)	18/26 (69)	56/68 (82)	N/A

* One patient had both hepatitis B and hepatitis C; Abbreviations: not available (N/A).

The test demonstrated high specificity, independent of cause and severity of underlying liver disease in the Internal Validation set. The test also showed excellent specificity in the Independent Validation set, indicating that the utility is not restricted to patients with impaired liver function or advanced liver disease. The results for HCC patients depending on cancer stage and lesion size confirm high sensitivity of the test for early stages and small tumors (Table 3).

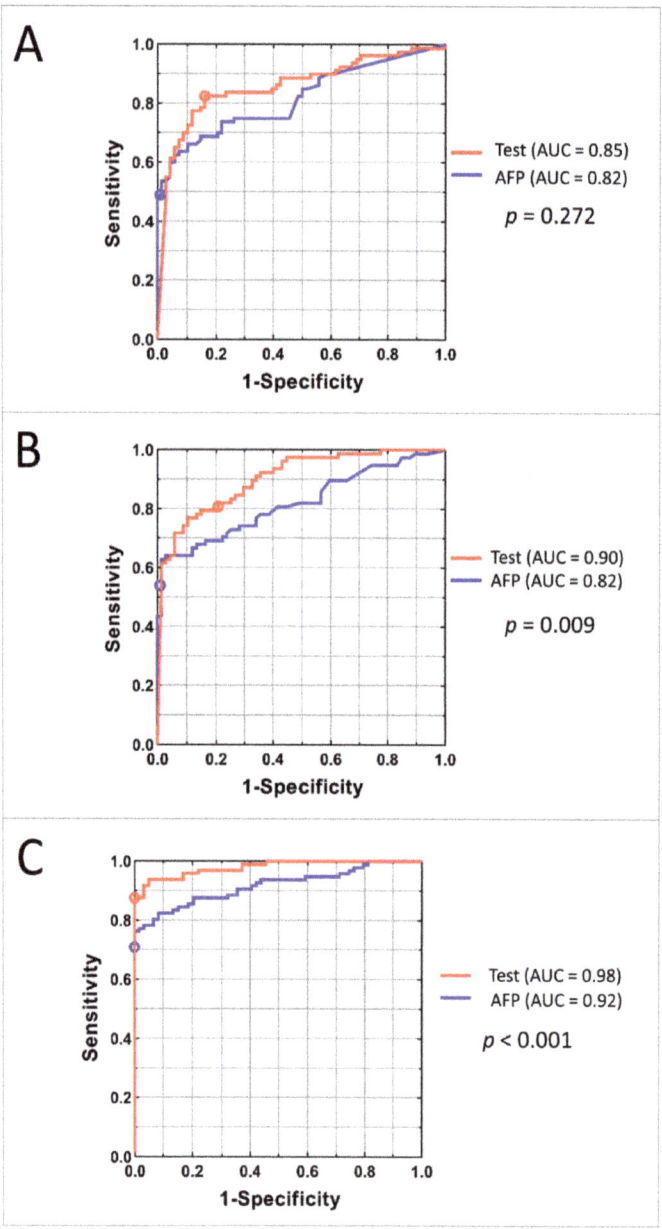

Figure 4. AUC curves for Development (**A**), Internal Validation (**B**), and Independent Validation (**C**) sets. Red line represents the family of tests obtained by adjusting the cutoff of the classifier; the red circle shows the results for the test with specified cutoff. Blue line corresponds to the classification using AFP concentration; blue circle shows the results for the AFP cut-off 20 ng/mL.

Table 3. Sensitivity of the test in HCC subgroups depending on tumor size and BCLC status.

Category		Cohort		
		Development (n = 80)	Internal Validation (n = 78)	Independent Validation (n = 97)
BCLC status	A, n (%)	19/26 (73)	16/25 (64)	unknown
	B, n (%)	4/9 (44)	3/6 (50)	unknown
	C, n (%)	33/35 (94)	35/38 (92)	unknown
	D, n (%)	10/10 (100)	9/9 (100)	unknown
Lesion size (cm)	<3, n (%)	6/8 (75)	4/6 (67)	5/5 (100)
	≥3 and <5, n (%)	12/16 (75)	11/18 (61)	17/18 (94)
	≥5 and <7, n (%)	10/12 (83)	9/10 (90)	11/14 (79)
	≥7 and <10, n (%)	5/7 (71)	5/8 (63)	21/26 (81)
	≥10 and <15, n (%)	10/12 (83)	10/11 (91)	16/16 (100)
	≥15, n (%)	4/4 (100)	5/5 (100)	3/3 (100)
	NA, n (%)	19/21 (90)	19/20 (95)	12/15 (80)

Figure 5 illustrates the sensitivity of the test in the combined Development/Internal Validation sets and in the Independent Validation set depending on tumor size in comparison with the detection by applying the 20 ng/mL AFP concentration cut-off.

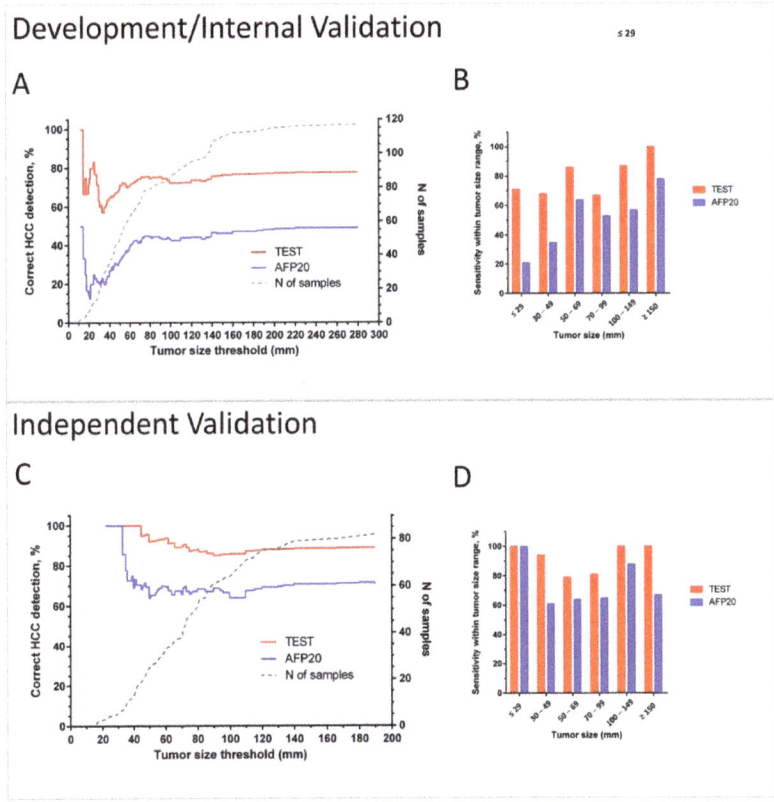

Figure 5. Sensitivity of HCC detection by the test and by AFP using cut-off 20 ng/mL (AFP20) in cancer patients. Plots A and C show in red (Test) and blue (AFP20) lines % of correct identifications of HCC for patients with tumors up to the threshold tumor size in the combined Development/Internal Validation set (**A**) and in the Independent Validation set (**C**). Dotted grey line (corresponding to the right Y-axis) shows the number of patients with tumors up to the threshold size. Bar charts B and D show sensitivity within the selected tumor size ranges in the Development/Internal Validation set (**B**) and in the Independent Validation set (**D**).

Cumulative plots (Figure 5A,C) and bar charts of sensitivity for groups within selected tumor size ranges (Figure 5B,D) show that the test has improved cancer detection compared to AFP for all tumor sizes and independently of the chosen tumor size threshold. The advantage of the test is especially pronounced in diagnosis of small lesions. It detected 69% of HCC cases in BCLC A overall, 71% lesions <3 cm in combined Development and Internal Validation sets, and 100% of tumors <3 cm in the Independent Validation set. The test also correctly diagnosed 75% and 76% of grade I and II tumors, as well as 75% and 86% of HCC in stage I and II patients in the Independent Validation set (see Table S7).

4. Discussion

MALDI-TOF has been a promising tool for the identification of serum biomarkers in many cancers [27]. This technology has been applied to identify proteins, peptides, and metabolites related to gastrointestinal, lung, prostate, renal, breast, ovarian and hematological cancers [27–29]. Furthermore, it has been combined with ML to create algorithms for both diagnosis and patient stratification for cancer therapy [20,21,30]. The utility of ML algorithms for detection of HCC or staging of chronic liver disease has also been explored [31–33], although independent validation of the results is generally not yet available. Many such studies have relied on spectra generated from liver specimens, which are difficult to acquire [32–34]. Thus, HCC detection tests utilizing serum markers, as in this current study, have great potential for accessible use in the clinical setting.

Our current work set out to identify a robust signature of early HCC among high-risk patients with chronic liver disease or cirrhosis and assess its performance in blinded validation using serum samples from healthy volunteers, patients with known cirrhosis, and patients with HCC. Our model incorporates both AFP measurements and MS-based proteomics in a ML algorithm. Overall, the HCC detection test had greater sensitivity and specificity compared to AFP alone and showed significantly better performance than AFP alone in both Internal and Independent Validation sets. Even with differences in patient demographics, test performance was consistent across Development, Internal Validation, and Independent Validation sets. This is despite the collection of the retrospective sample sets under independent protocols, at different institutions and geographic regions, and with the samples run over a period of several years. These observations point toward the generalizability of the ML-based test and the stability and reproducibility of the MS data obtained. The test was able to detect HCC with a sensitivity of 81% or greater at specificity of 79% or above in all three cohorts. In the Independent Validation set, at a sensitivity of 88%, the test specificity exceeded that of univariate AFP by 20%. It is noteworthy that test specificity was high even though the cancer-free subjects in each cohort represented clearly different populations in all three cohorts (liver transplant candidates in the UTHSCSA cohort, high prevalence of hepatitis B in the Greek cohort, and subjects with healthy livers in the Roswell cohort). Moreover, test sensitivity was high across liver disease etiology, including hepatitis B and hepatitis C.

According to a systematic review, AFP with a cut-off value of 20 ng/mL (AFP20) had a sensitivity and specificity of 49% to 71% and 49% to 86%, respectively [6]. However, this analysis included mainly Asian studies with tumor size < 5 cm. In comparison, AFP20 sensitivity in this current study was 49% to 71%, in line with two recently analyzed US cohorts [14], while we found higher specificity in our cohorts of 99% to 100%. At a cutoff of -0.63, GALAD score has demonstrated sensitivity/specificity of 92%/90% in a UK cohort [13] and 79%/79% in a US cohort [14], the EDRN multicenter cohort of 545 subjects. Differences in cohorts make comparison of test performance across studies extremely difficult. Unfortunately, AFP-L3 and DCP levels were not available for our patients, precluding a direct comparison of the performance of our test with GALAD scores. Future studies designed to assess these biomarkers in addition to our HCC detection test would be necessary to reliably establish relative performance and whether MS data can provide information that could supplement these scores.

Early diagnosis of HCC, when resection or intervention may still be possible, is crucial, given that the overall prognosis is dismal, with a 5-year survival rate of less than 10%. By the time of diagnosis, only 20% to 30% of patients are eligible for curative therapy, e.g., with transplantation, surgical resection, or local ablative processes [35]. In our study, the HCC detection test was able to recognize early stages of HCC. Notably, it detected 69% of HCC cases in BCLC A overall, 71% lesions <3 cm in combined Development and Internal Validation sets, and 100% of tumors <3 cm in the Independent Validation set. While AFP20 had similar performance for the smallest tumors in our Independent Validation set, its performance was markedly worse in the Development/Internal Validation, and our test detection rates were much higher than those reported for traditional univariate biomarkers, such as AFP, AFP-L3, and DCP, when used for early detection [6].

Moreover, our test was performed both in cirrhotic and non-cirrhotic patients, demonstrating excellent specificity both for Internal and Independent Validation sets regardless of the underlying liver impairment status. While diagnosis of HCC for cirrhotic patients can be established by imaging criteria using LI-RADS classification [36], diagnosis is more difficult in non-cirrhotic patients given that the LI-RADS score cannot be applied and tissue biopsy is mandatory to establish the diagnosis. Therefore, in the future, after prospective validation, our test may help in establishing HCC diagnosis for non-cirrhotic patients without the need for an invasive tissue biopsy procedure.

While the results of our study are promising, there are several weaknesses. First, the study was retrospective, which introduces possibilities for confounding, and some demographic data from all cohorts were incomplete. Liver function was dramatically different between the patients with HCC in the UTHSCSA and Greek cohorts, which led to these cohorts being combined and then split in two to generate a suitable Development set. The Independent Validation set included only 156 patients, and the subjects without HCC were not representative of patients at high risk of developing HCC. A larger scale validation in patients at high risk of developing HCC would be helpful to ensure generalizability of the results in the most relevant population. Second, in our study, AFP performed surprisingly well in detection of hepatocellular carcinoma, with AFP20 demonstrating very high specificity. Even though AFP had AUCs ranging from 0.82 to 0.92 (Figure 4), we still observed significant differences in AUCs between AFP alone and the HCC detection test. While the high specificity of AFP in the Independent Validation set may be due to it consisting of healthy volunteers, the reason for the good performance of AFP in the other cohorts is not readily apparent. Ongoing validation with larger sample sizes and a range of control populations is needed. Lastly, as in most other studies, the number of patients with early stage cancer in our cohorts was small, making it hard to accurately assess test sensitivity in this population, where improved detection could be most beneficial.

Ultimately, the goal of this study was to use high-throughput MS-based techniques to discover a serum signature for early HCC detection. The high-throughput nature of MALDI mass spectrometry and the use of cards to allow ambient temperature shipment of dried serum make the test practical in a clinical setting. Indeed, the VeriStrat MALDI-based MS test, as used in clinical practice for assessment of patients with NSCLC, uses overnight ambient shipping of dried blood-based samples to a centralized laboratory. However, given that the signature is composed of unidentified features, clinicians would need to become comfortable with relying on a result determined by the relative expression levels of certain proteins without recognizing any obvious mechanistic basis. Nevertheless, this limitation also applies to several biomarker profiles, including the GALAD score, as well as other MS-based approaches. Future studies may further explore combining other protein biomarkers and patient characteristics with AFP and Deep MALDI mass spectral data using ML methods. New approaches to explainability of machine learning algorithms, protein identification of the most important MS features used for classification, and translational studies comparing patients correctly or incorrectly classified by the test may be useful to increase physician trust in the test.

Future studies may further explore combining other protein biomarkers and patient characteristics, such as age, gender, and liver disease etiology, with AFP and Deep MALDI mass spectral data using modern machine learning methods. Incorporating MS data into existing, validated serological models (i.e., GALAD scores) may further contribute to accurate diagnosis. A prospective trial in high-risk populations, including increased numbers of patients with early stage disease, is necessary for further validation, comparison with the GALAD score and other novel HCC detection tests, as well as determination of clinical utility.

5. Conclusions

In summary, the results for our HCC detection test are positive, with impressive sensitivity and specificity, especially on the Independent Validation set with blinded validation. The test was able to identify small tumors in early stages, comparing favorably to currently used biomarker panels. Lastly, the test was conducted on human serum, greatly improving accessibility compared to HCC detection tests requiring liver biopsy samples. Nevertheless, work remains to be carried out prior to adoption of the test in clinical practice. A prospective trial in high-risk populations is necessary for further validation, comparison with other validated scores, and assessment of generalizability and clinical utility.

Supplementary Materials: The following are available online at https://www.mdpi.com/article/10.3390/cancers13133109/s1, Text S1, Table S1: Points in m/z used to align the raster spectra, Table S2: Normalization windows used in pre-processing the spectra, lower and upper m/z boundaries, Table S3: Alignment points used to align the Deep MALDI average spectra, Table S4: Definitions of mass spectral features, Table S5: m/z windows used in the final feature value normalization, Table S6: Features used in classification (rounded to nearest Dalton for MS features) with measures of their univariate association with presence/absence of HCC in the classifier development set of patients (n = 108, no VeriStrat Poor classification and AFP < 100 ng/mL), Table S7: Accuracy of detection of HCC in Independent Validation (n = 97) by grade and stage, Figure S1: Spectra generated from serum from a patient with HCC (in red) and a patient without HCC (in blue).

Author Contributions: D.M.—conceptualization, formal analysis, methodology, writing (original draft, review and editing), resources, investigation/data curation, supervision; L.C.—formal analysis, resources, writing (original draft, review and editing), investigation/data curation, supervision; I.N.—writing (original draft, review and editing), investigation/data curation; S.S.L.—formal analysis, writing (review and editing), investigation/data curation; S.K.—formal analysis, writing (review and editing); G.H.—resources, writing (review and editing), investigation/data curation; K.W.—resources, writing (review and editing), investigation/data curation; K.A.—formal analysis, writing (review and editing); I.F.—writing (review and editing); J.G.—writing (original draft, review and editing); S.A.—formal analysis, methodology, writing (review and editing); K.M.—formal analysis, methodology, writing (review and editing); C.O.—formal analysis, methodology, writing (review and editing); H.R.—conceptualization, formal analysis, methodology, writing (original draft, review and editing), resources, investigation/data curation, supervision; J.R.—conceptualization, formal analysis, methodology, writing (original draft, review and editing), resources, investigation/data curation, supervision; R.I.—formal analysis, resources, writing (original draft, review and editing), investigation/data curation, supervision. All authors have read and agreed to the published version of the manuscript.

Funding: This research received no external funding. The APC was funded by Biodesix, Inc. (Boulder, CO, USA).

Institutional Review Board Statement: The study was conducted according to the guidelines of the Declaration of Helsinki, and approved by the Institutional Review Board of Roswell Park Comprehensive Cancer Center (protocol number I285616 and date of approval 28 March 2016) and the Institutional Review Board of UT Health San Antonio (protocol number 20070181HR and date of approval 11 December 2017).

Informed Consent Statement: Informed consent was obtained from all subjects involved in the study.

Data Availability Statement: The data that support the findings of this study are available from the corresponding author, D.M., upon reasonable request.

Acknowledgments: AFP measurements were carried out by Jay Westcott at ELISA Tech (Aurora, CO, USA).

Conflicts of Interest: L.C., I.N., S.L., S.K., G.H., K.W., K.A., I.F. and R.I. have no conflicts of interest to declare. D.M. is an advisory board member for Amgen, Eisai, Exelixis, and Bristol Myers Squibb. S.A., H.R., J.R. are employees of Biodesix and hold stock and/or stock options in Biodesix. J.G. and K.M. hold stock and/or stock options in Biodesix. H.R., J.R., D.M. and C.O. are inventors on a related patent assigned to Biodesix (United States patent US 2019; 10,217,620 Office USPaT (ed). USA, Biodesix, 2019). K.M., C.O., J.G. were employees of Biodesix.

References

1. Bray, F.; Ferlay, J.; Soerjomataram, I.; Siegel, R.L.; Torre, L.A.; Jemal, A. Global cancer statistics 2018: GLOBOCAN estimates of incidence and mortality worldwide for 36 cancers in 185 countries. *CA Cancer J. Clin.* **2018**, *68*, 394–424. [CrossRef]
2. El-Serag, H.B. Epidemiology of viral hepatitis and hepatocellular carcinoma. *Gastroenterology* **2012**, *142*, 1264–1273.e1261. [CrossRef]
3. Fattovich, G.; Stroffolini, T.; Zagni, I.; Donato, F. Hepatocellular carcinoma in cirrhosis: Incidence and risk factors. *Gastroenterology* **2004**, *127*, S35–S50. [CrossRef]
4. Marrero, J.A.; Kulik, L.M.; Sirlin, C.B.; Zhu, A.X.; Finn, R.S.; Abecassis, M.M.; Roberts, L.R.; Heimbach, J.K. Diagnosis, Staging, and Management of Hepatocellular Carcinoma: 2018 Practice Guidance by the American Association for the Study of Liver Diseases. *Hepatology* **2018**, *68*, 723–750. [CrossRef]
5. Singal, A.G.; Pillai, A.; Tiro, J. Early detection, curative treatment, and survival rates for hepatocellular carcinoma surveillance in patients with cirrhosis: A meta-analysis. *PLoS Med.* **2014**, *11*, e1001624. [CrossRef]
6. Tateishi, R.; Yoshida, H.; Matsuyama, Y.; Mine, N.; Kondo, Y.; Omata, M. Diagnostic accuracy of tumor markers for hepatocellular carcinoma: A systematic review. *Hepatol. Int.* **2008**, *2*, 17–30. [CrossRef]
7. European Association for the Study of the Liver. Electronic address, e.e.e.; European Association for the Study of the, L. EASL Clinical Practice Guidelines: Management of hepatocellular carcinoma. *J. Hepatol.* **2018**, *69*, 182–236. [CrossRef]
8. Sengupta, S.; Parikh, N.D. Biomarker development for hepatocellular carcinoma early detection: Current and future perspectives. *Hepatic Oncol.* **2017**, *4*, 111–122. [CrossRef]
9. De Stefano, F.; Chacon, E.; Turcios, L.; Marti, F.; Gedaly, R. Novel biomarkers in hepatocellular carcinoma. *Dig. Liver Dis.* **2018**, *50*, 1115–1123. [CrossRef]
10. Koike, Y.; Shiratori, Y.; Sato, S.; Obi, S.; Teratani, T.; Imamura, M.; Yoshida, H.; Shiina, S.; Omata, M. Des-gamma-carboxy prothrombin as a useful predisposing factor for the development of portal venous invasion in patients with hepatocellular carcinoma: A prospective analysis of 227 patients. *Cancer* **2001**, *91*, 561–569. [CrossRef]
11. Sterling, R.K.; Jeffers, L.; Gordon, F.; Sherman, M.; Venook, A.P.; Reddy, K.R.; Satomura, S.; Schwartz, M.E. Clinical utility of AFP-L3% measurement in North American patients with HCV-related cirrhosis. *Am. J. Gastroenterol.* **2007**, *102*, 2196–2205. [CrossRef]
12. Johnson, P.J.; Pirrie, S.J.; Cox, T.F.; Berhane, S.; Teng, M.; Palmer, D.; Morse, J.; Hull, D.; Patman, G.; Kagebayashi, C.; et al. The detection of hepatocellular carcinoma using a prospectively developed and validated model based on serological biomarkers. *Cancer Epidemiol. Biomark. Prev.* **2014**, *23*, 144–153. [CrossRef]
13. Berhane, S.; Toyoda, H.; Tada, T.; Kumada, T.; Kagebayashi, C.; Satomura, S.; Schweitzer, N.; Vogel, A.; Manns, M.P.; Benckert, J.; et al. Role of the GALAD and BALAD-2 Serologic Models in Diagnosis of Hepatocellular Carcinoma and Prediction of Survival in Patients. *Clin. Gastroenterol. Hepatol.* **2016**, *14*, 875–886.e6. [CrossRef] [PubMed]
14. Yang, J.D.; Addissie, B.D.; Mara, K.C.; Harmsen, W.S.; Dai, J.; Zhang, N.; Wongjarupong, N.; Ali, H.M.; Ali, H.A.; Hassan, F.A.; et al. GALAD Score for Hepatocellular Carcinoma Detection in Comparison with Liver Ultrasound and Proposal of GALADUS Score. *Cancer Epidemiol. Biomark. Prev.* **2019**, *28*, 531–538. [CrossRef]
15. Aebersold, R.; Mann, M. Mass spectrometry-based proteomics. *Nature* **2003**, *422*, 198–207. [CrossRef]
16. Taguchi, F.; Solomon, B.; Gregorc, V.; Roder, H.; Gray, R.; Kasahara, K.; Nishio, M.; Brahmer, J.; Spreafico, A.; Ludovini, V.; et al. Mass spectrometry to classify non-small-cell lung cancer patients for clinical outcome after treatment with epidermal growth factor receptor tyrosine kinase inhibitors: A multicohort cross-institutional study. *J. Natl. Cancer Inst.* **2007**, *99*, 838–846. [CrossRef]
17. van Adrichem, J.H.; Bornsen, K.O.; Conzelmann, H.; Gass, M.A.; Eppenberger, H.; Kresbach, G.M.; Ehrat, M.; Leist, C.H. Investigation of protein patterns in mammalian cells and culture supernatants by matrix-assisted laser desorption/ionization mass spectrometry. *Anal. Chem.* **1998**, *70*, 923–930. [CrossRef]
18. Zinkin, N.T.; Grall, F.; Bhaskar, K.; Otu, H.H.; Spentzos, D.; Kalmowitz, B.; Wells, M.; Guerrero, M.; Asara, J.M.; Libermann, T.A.; et al. Serum proteomics and biomarkers in hepatocellular carcinoma and chronic liver disease. *Clin. Cancer Res.* **2008**, *14*, 470–477. [CrossRef]
19. Tsypin, M.; Asmellash, S.; Meyer, K.; Touchet, B.; Roder, H. Extending the information content of the MALDI analysis of biological fluids via multi-million shot analysis. *PLoS ONE* **2019**, *14*, e0226012. [CrossRef]

20. Muller, M.; Hummelink, K.; Hurkmans, D.P.; Niemeijer, A.-L.N.; Monkhorst, K.; Roder, J.; Oliveira, C.; Roder, H.; Aerts, J.G.; Smit, E.F. A Serum Protein Classifier Identifying Patients with Advanced Non–Small Cell Lung Cancer Who Derive Clinical Benefit from Treatment with Immune Checkpoint Inhibitors. *Clin. Cancer Res.* **2020**, *26*, 5188. [CrossRef]
21. Weber, J.S.; Sznol, M.; Sullivan, R.J.; Blackmon, S.; Boland, G.; Kluger, H.M.; Halaban, R.; Bacchiocchi, A.; Ascierto, P.A.; Capone, M.; et al. A Serum Protein Signature Associated with Outcome after Anti-PD-1 Therapy in Metastatic Melanoma. *Cancer Immunol. Res.* **2018**, *6*, 79–86. [CrossRef]
22. Fidler, M.J.; Fhied, C.L.; Roder, J.; Basu, S.; Sayidine, S.; Fughhi, I.; Pool, M.; Batus, M.; Bonomi, P.; Borgia, J.A. The serum-based VeriStrat® test is associated with proinflammatory reactants and clinical outcome in non-small cell lung cancer patients. *BMC Cancer* **2018**, *18*, 310. [CrossRef] [PubMed]
23. Molina-Pinelo, S.; Pastor, M.D.; Paz-Ares, L. VeriStrat: A prognostic and/or predictive biomarker for advanced lung cancer patients? *Expert Rev. Respir. Med.* **2014**, *8*, 1–4. [CrossRef]
24. Roder, J.; Oliveira, C.; Net, L.; Tsypin, M.; Linstid, B.; Roder, H. A dropout-regularized classifier development approach optimized for precision medicine test discovery from omics data. *BMC Bioinf.* **2019**, *20*, 325. [CrossRef] [PubMed]
25. Chen, H.; Zhang, Y.; Li, S.; Li, N.; Chen, Y.; Zhang, B.; Qu, C.; Ding, H.; Huang, J.; Dai, M. Direct comparison of five serum biomarkers in early diagnosis of hepatocellular carcinoma. *Cancer Manag. Res.* **2018**, *10*, 1947–1958. [CrossRef]
26. Farinati, F.; Marino, D.; De Giorgio, M.; Baldan, A.; Cantarini, M.; Cursaro, C.; Rapaccini, G.; Del Poggio, P.; Di Nolfo, M.A.; Benvegnù, L.; et al. Diagnostic and prognostic role of alpha-fetoprotein in hepatocellular carcinoma: Both or neither? *Am. J. Gastroenterol.* **2006**, *101*, 524–532. [CrossRef]
27. Karpova, M.A.; Moshkovskii, S.A.; Toropygin, I.Y.; Archakov, A.I. Cancer-specific MALDI-TOF profiles of blood serum and plasma: Biological meaning and perspectives. *J. Proteom.* **2010**, *73*, 537–551. [CrossRef]
28. Rodrigo, M.A.; Zitka, O.; Krizkova, S.; Moulick, A.; Adam, V.; Kizek, R. MALDI-TOF MS as evolving cancer diagnostic tool: A review. *J. Pharm. Biomed. Anal.* **2014**, *95*, 245–255. [CrossRef]
29. Swiatly, A.; Horala, A.; Hajduk, J.; Matysiak, J.; Nowak-Markwitz, E.; Kokot, Z.J. MALDI-TOF-MS analysis in discovery and identification of serum proteomic patterns of ovarian cancer. *BMC Cancer* **2017**, *17*, 472. [CrossRef]
30. Wu, S.; Xu, K.; Chen, G.; Zhang, J.; Liu, Z.; Xie, X. Identification of serum biomarkers for ovarian cancer using MALDI-TOF-MS combined with magnetic beads. *Int. J. Clin. Oncol.* **2012**, *17*, 89–95. [CrossRef]
31. Camaggi, C.M.; Zavatto, E.; Gramantieri, L.; Camaggi, V.; Strocchi, E.; Righini, R.; Merina, L.; Chieco, P.; Bolondi, L. Serum albumin-bound proteomic signature for early detection and staging of hepatocarcinoma: Sample variability and data classification. *Clin. Chem. Lab. Med.* **2010**, *48*, 1319–1326. [CrossRef] [PubMed]
32. Kaur, H.; Dhall, A.; Kumar, R.; Raghava, G.P.S. Identification of Platform-Independent Diagnostic Biomarker Panel for Hepatocellular Carcinoma Using Large-Scale Transcriptomics Data. *Front. Genet.* **2020**, *10*, 1306. [CrossRef] [PubMed]
33. Lee, N.P.; Chen, L.; Lin, M.C.; Tsang, F.H.; Yeung, C.; Poon, R.T.; Peng, J.; Leng, X.; Beretta, L.; Sun, S.; et al. Proteomic expression signature distinguishes cancerous and nonmalignant tissues in hepatocellular carcinoma. *J. Proteome Res.* **2009**, *8*, 1293–1303. [CrossRef] [PubMed]
34. Chen, X.L.; Zhou, L.; Yang, J.; Shen, F.K.; Zhao, S.P.; Wang, Y.L. Hepatocellular carcinoma-associated protein markers investigated by MALDI-TOF MS. *Mol. Med. Rep.* **2010**, *3*, 589–596. [CrossRef]
35. Bruix, J.; Sherman, M. Management of hepatocellular carcinoma. *Hepatology* **2005**, *42*, 1208–1236. [CrossRef]
36. Morgan, T.A.; Maturen, K.E.; Dahiya, N.; Sun, M.R.M.; Kamaya, A. US LI-RADS: Ultrasound liver imaging reporting and data system for screening and surveillance of hepatocellular carcinoma. *Abdom. Radiol.* **2018**, *43*, 41–55. [CrossRef]

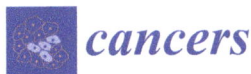

Article

Multitarget Stool mRNA Test for Detecting Colorectal Cancer Lesions Including Advanced Adenomas

Elizabeth Herring [1,2], Éric Tremblay [1,2], Nathalie McFadden [2,3], Shigeru Kanaoka [4] and Jean-François Beaulieu [1,2,*]

1. Laboratory of Intestinal Physiopathology, Faculty of Medicine and Health Sciences, Université de Sherbrooke, Sherbrooke, QC J1H 5N4, Canada; elizabeth.herring@usherbrooke.ca (E.H.); eric.tremblay@usherbrooke.ca (É.T.)
2. Centre de Recherche du Centre Hospitalier, Universitaire de Sherbrooke, Sherbrooke, QC J1H 5N4, Canada; nathalie.mc.fadden@usherbrooke.ca
3. Department of Surgery, Faculty of Medicine and Health Sciences, Université de Sherbrooke, Sherbrooke, QC J1H 5N4, Canada
4. Department of Gastroenterology, Hamamatsu Medical Center, Naka-ku, Hamamatsu 432-8580, Japan; kanaoka@hmedc.or.jp
* Correspondence: jean-francois.beaulieu@usherbrooke.ca; Tel.: +1-819-821-8000

Simple Summary: Colorectal cancer is still one of the deadliest cancers, even though its detection at early stages has been shown to be a key factor for reducing mortality. Screening methods are available, but their efficacy for detecting early-stage lesions is limited. In the present discovery stage study, we used a targeted mRNA assay in the stools to optimize the identification of patients bearing precancerous lesions as well as colorectal cancers at curable stages with only five targets, thus compatible with standard multiplex PCR. Although further validation is required, this assay has high potential for improving colorectal cancer screening efficacy.

Abstract: Current approved non-invasive screening methods for colorectal cancer (CRC) include FIT and DNA-FIT testing, but their efficacy for detecting precancerous lesions that are susceptible to progressing to CRC such as advanced adenomas (AA) remains limited, thus requiring further options to improve the detection of CRC lesions at earlier stages. One of these is host mRNA stool testing. The aims of the present study were to identify specific stool mRNA targets that can predict AA and to investigate their stability under a clinical-like setting. A panel of mRNA targets was tested on stool samples obtained from 102 patients including 78 CRC stage I-III and 24 AA as well as 32 healthy controls. Area under the receiver operating characteristic (ROC) curves were calculated to establish sensitivities and specificities for individual and combined targets. Stability experiments were performed on freshly obtained specimens. Six of the tested targets were found to be specifically increased in the stools of patients with CRC and three in the stools of both AA and CRC patients. After optimization for the choice of the 5 best markers for AA and CRC, ROC curve analysis revealed overall sensitivities of 75% and 89% for AA and CRC, respectively, for a $\geq$95% specificity, and up to 75% and 95% for AA and CRC, respectively, when combined with the FIT score. Targets were found to be stable in the stools up to 3 days at room temperature. In conclusion, these studies show that the detection of host mRNA in the stools is a valid approach for the screening of colorectal cancerous lesions at all stages and is applicable to a clinical-like setup.

Keywords: colorectal cancer; advanced adenoma; screening; stool; mRNA

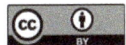

1. Introduction

Colorectal cancer (CRC) is one of the few cancer types for which screening has been proven to reduce cancer mortality in average-risk individuals [1]. Indeed, the spread of the disease in terms of local invasion as well as to lymph nodes and distant organs at the time of diagnosis is an important prognostic factor, with five-year survival rates of more than 90% for individuals with localized lesions but only ~10% for those having their CRC metastasized to distal organs [2]. Early detection is thus a key factor in reducing mortality from CRC [3,4]. Advanced adenomas (AA) are also important to detect since they are considered to be the precursors of CRC [5,6], while non-advanced adenomas (<1 cm without advanced histology) may not be associated with increased colorectal cancer risk [6]. Several screening regiments for CRC and AA are recommended such as fecal occult blood testing and colonoscopy. While colonoscopy remains the gold standard for the detection of colorectal lesions, compliance is not optimal owing to discomfort and unpleasant preparation procedures [7]. The risk of complications, cost and access are other limitations of this procedure [8]. On the other hand, the improved immunological version of fecal occult blood testing also referred to as the fecal immunochemical test (FIT), which detects human hemoglobin, has been used for some time with some success [1] but poor precursor lesion detection rates (66–80% sensitivity for CRC but only 10–28% for AA) albeit an excellent specificity (93–95%) limits its effectiveness [3,9–12]. It is therefore imperative to explore alternate or complementary strategies with the potential to improve CRC screening performance, especially for the detection of cancers at their early stages and AA.

In this context, a number of initiatives have been undertaken over the last ten years, from stool testing as a noninvasive approach [1] to the implementation of personalized CRC screening [13] trying to meet with desirable features for a CRC screening test [3]. Interestingly, many of the stool-based testing strategies are based on the high rate of tumor cell exfoliation into the colon-rectal lumen, a parameter that appears to be independent of blood release [14–17]. One of the best documented strategies is the FDA-approved multi-target stool DNA test, an approach based on the detection of specific DNA aberrations from the CRC cells shed into the stools in combination with FIT, which results in an improvement of sensitivity for both CRC (92.3%) and AA (42.4%) detection compared to FIT alone, although achieved through a reduction in specificity to 87% thus generating almost three times more false positives [18]. At first sight, the cost–benefit of such new methods for the medical system may temper screening recommendations [19] but the high cost of CRC treatment, particularly for more advanced disease, is considered to improve the cost-effectiveness of CRC screening [20,21]. Furthermore, higher threshold costs for a biomarker test that could significantly increase the sensitivity of AA detection while maintaining reasonable specificity, would likely be cost-effective relative to currently available noninvasive tests [22,23].

Still based on the significant exfoliation of dysplastic cells from colorectal lesions into the lumen, host mRNA has also been investigated in the stools as a potential biomarker. While isolated from purified exfoliated colonocytes [24] or directly extracted from the stools [25,26], host mRNA has been found to be a reliable source of biomarkers for detecting colorectal cancers. Further analysis confirmed the target mRNAs originated from the tumor or surrounding mucosa and that expression was affected by the number of exfoliated tumor cells, exfoliation of inflammatory cells, tumor size and transcript expression level in the tumor but not primary vs. distal location [27]. More recently, based on the analysis of a series of transcripts previously reported to be upregulated in CRC cells [27–29] or linked to CRC recurrence [30], it has been demonstrated that the inclusion of a multitarget mRNA assay significantly strengthens both sensitivity and specificity for CRC detection [31,32]. Droplet digital PCR was also evaluated as a potential alternative to qPCR for stool mRNA multiplex analysis [33]. However, one important question that remains to be tested for the validation of a multitarget stool mRNA test pertains to AA detection since, up to now, *ITGA6* is the only target found to be overrepresented in stool samples of patients bearing AA [32]. Another aspect that needs to be evaluated before considering a potential clinical implementation is the robustness of the test under realistic preservation conditions, as mRNA are considered to be relatively susceptible to degradation in the stools [34,35].

2. Materials and Methods

2.1. Patients and Samples

Two sets of patient samples were used in the study. Both sets were analyzed retrospectively. The first set of samples was collected from patients and healthy controls from the Hamamatsu University School of Medicine with written informed consent. The study was approved by the Institutional Research Ethics Committee of the Hamamatsu University School of Medicine. Complete information about this set has been provided in previous studies [31–33] which was further investigated to find the new data reported in this paper. Briefly, the study cohort used herein included 24 patients with AA defined as being 10 mm or larger at their greatest dimension and 78 patients with CRC (24 stage I, 32 stage II and 22 stage III) diagnosed by colonoscopy and histopathology as well as 32 healthy controls. For controls and AA, stool samples were collected before colonoscopy. The FIT was performed on all patients and controls as described [32].

The second set of samples was collected from 3 healthy controls and 3 patients diagnosed with CRC stage II or III by colonoscopy and histopathology from the Centre Hospitalier Universitaire de Sherbrooke (CHUS) with written informed consent. The study was approved by the Institutional Research Ethics Committee of the CHUS. This set of samples was used for mRNA target stability experiments. Each sample was split into 13 aliquots stored under various conditions for up to 5 days as follows: #1, 5 days at $-80\ °C$ used as control; #2, 5 days at $-20\ °C$; #3, 5 days at $-20\ °C$ with a thaw/freeze cycle; #4–8, 1–5 days at $4\ °C$ and #9–13, 1–5 days at $23\ °C$.

2.2. RNA Isolation, Reverse Transcription, Preamplification, and PCR Amplification

RNA was isolated from fecal samples and reverse transcribed as described previously [27,36]. For preamplification, the TaqMan PreAmp Master Kit (Applied Biosystems, Thermo Fisher Scientific, Mississauga, ON, Canada) was used to provide unbiased, multiplex preamplification of specific amplicons for analysis with TaqMan gene expression assays [33]. Commercially available TaqMan primer and probe mixtures were used for the preamplification of the 27 preselected targets as described before [33] and detailed in Table 1. Quantitative polymerase chain reaction (qPCR) was performed using the TaqMan Gene Expression Assay with conditions described previously [31].

2.3. Data Presentation and Statistical Analysis

Stool mRNA data were calculated as copy number per µL of reaction. For each transcript, a standard reference curve was generated using a serial fivefold dilution of a cDNA stock solution of the target sequence quantified on a NanoDrop 1000 Spectrophotometer (NanoDrop, Wilmington, DE, USA). Prism 8 was used for calculating statistics. Comparison mRNA expression (in copy number) in stool controls and patients with AA and CRC stage I-III lesions were expressed as median with interquartile range and analyzed by the Kruskal–Wallis test followed by Dunn's multiple comparison test. Area under the receiver operating characteristic (ROC) curves were calculated to establish sensitivities and specificities for each marker expressed in % with a 95% confidence interval. Scores were calculated for each marker on a scale of 0 to 3 on the basis of three cut-off values established from the ROC curve: (the lower cut-off corresponding to a sensitivity of 80%, medium cut-off corresponding to a specificity of 90% and higher cut-off corresponding to a specificity of 99%) as established previously [32]. Statistical significance was defined as $p < 0.05$.

Table 1. List of specific targets tested.

Gene Name	TaqMan Assay I.D.	Consistently Detected in Stools	Over-Represented CRC Only	Over-Represented AA and CRC
BGN	Hs00156076_m1			
CEACAM5	Hs00944025_m1	Y		Y
CTNNB1	Hs00355049_m1			
DYNC2H1	Hs00941787_m1			
FAP	Hs00990806_m1			
GADD45B	Hs00169587_m1	Y	Y	
GLI1	Hs00171790_m1			
HMAN1B1	Hs01032463_m1			
HNRNPA2B1	Hs00955384_m1			
INHBA	Hs04187260_m1			
ITGA1	Hs00235006_m1	Y		
ITGA2	Hs01673848_m1	Y		
ITGA6A	Hs01041013_m1	Y	Y	
ITGA6	Hs01041011_m1	Y		Y
KI67	Hs01032434_m1			
KIF3A	Hs01126351_m1			
KIF7	Hs00419527_m1			
MACC1	Hs00766186_m1	Y		Y
MLH1	Hs00179866_m1	Y		
MSH1	Hs00954125_m1	Y		
MTR	Hs01090031_m1			
MYBL2	Hs00942543_m1	Y	Y	
MYC	Hs00153408_m1	Y	Y	
PTGS2	Hs00153133_m1	Y	Y	
S100A4	Hs00243202_m1	Y	Y	
VDAC2	Hs01075603_m1			

All primer and probe mixtures were first tested on a subset of stool samples including controls, AA and CRC to select those that were consistently detectable in the stools. Further analysis on the whole set of samples allowed the selection of those specifically enriched in CRC and AA or only CRC.

3. Results

In this study, we first screened 27 specific targets chosen on the basis of their reported over expression in colorectal cancerous lesions. Preliminary evaluation of these using a subset of 30 samples (10 controls, 10 AA and 10 CRC) revealed that 14 were consistently detected in the stools of patients bearing colorectal lesions (Table 1). Further testing with other primer and probe mixtures for poorly detected targets was tried but not further studied herein, since 14 appeared to be enough to run the validation assay considering that for a clinical assay, the multiplex PCR capacity is limited to four to five targets depending on the equipment provided by the manufacturer.

Further investigation of the 14 targets was performed on the set of 132 samples obtained from healthy controls ($n = 32$) and patients bearing colorectal lesions ($n = 24$ AA and 78 CRC). As detailed in Table 1, six of the targets were found to be significantly over-represented in samples from patients with CRC while three identified patients bearing AA or CRC. As shown in Figure 1, the median copy numbers for the transcripts of the first group which included *GADD45B*, *ITGA2*, *MYBL2*, *MYC*, *PTGS2* and *S100A4* were found to be significantly increased in the stools of patients with CRC as compared with the controls, while only three, including *CEACAM5*, *ITGA6* and *MACC1*, were found to be over-represented also in patients with AA.

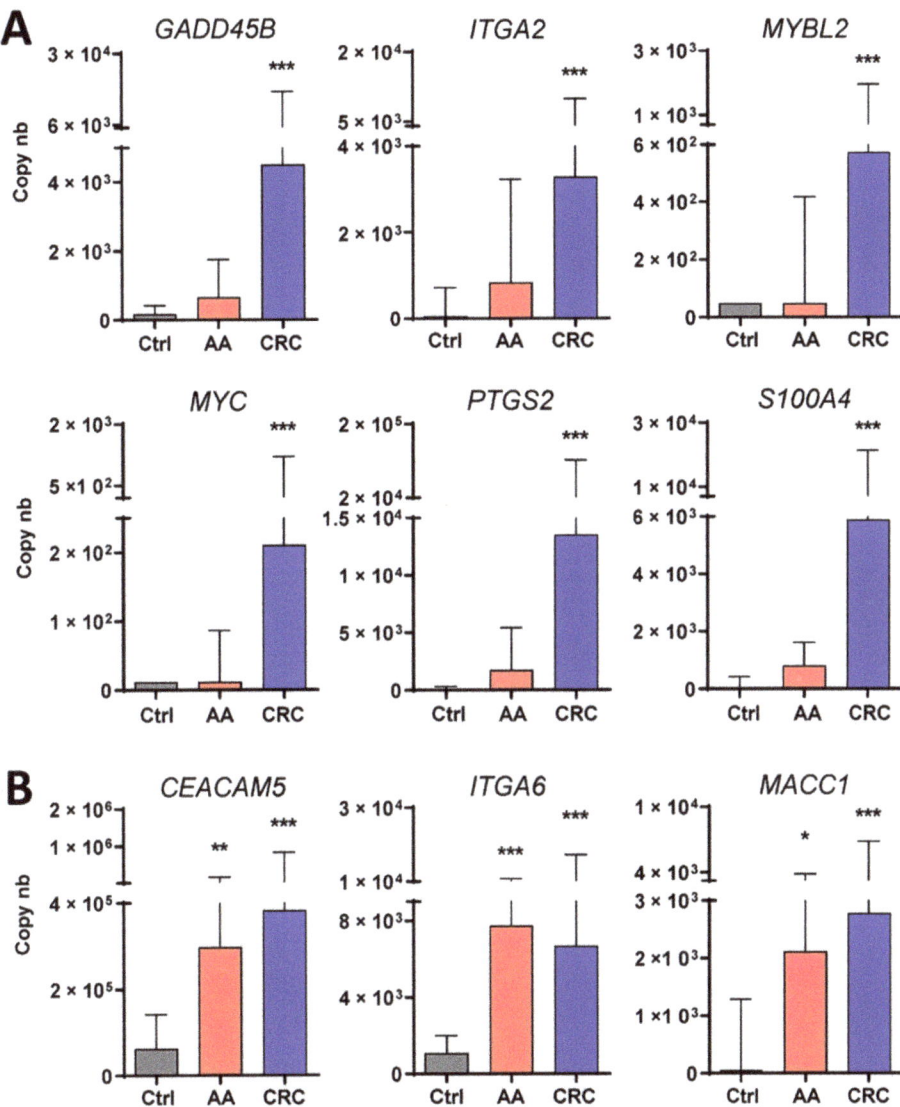

Figure 1. Detection and analysis of selected mRNA targets found to be overrepresented in stool samples of patients with colorectal cancer (CRC) stages I-III (**A**) or advanced adenomas (AA) (**B**). A significant increase was observed for the targets *GADD45B*, *ITGA2*, *MYBL2*, *MYC*, *PTGS2* and *S100A4* in CRC stages I-III as compared to controls (Ctrl) while for three of the targets, *CEACAM5*, *ITGA6* and *MACC1*, a significant increase was observed in samples from patients with CRC stages I-III or AA as compared to controls (Ctrl). Results are expressed as median (interquartile range) of copy number relative to control patients. * $p < 0.05$, ** $p < 0.001$ and *** $p < 0.0005$ using the Kruskal–Wallis test.

ROC curves were calculated for each marker. As expected from the expression levels between control, AA and CRC, the area under the curve (AUC) values were ≥0.8 for all markers for identifying CRC and three markers for identifying AA (Figure 2). The regrouping of the targets was then calculated for the two groups of markers, which can identify CRC only or AA and CRC. As copy numbers varied considerably between the targets, from ~200 for MYC to 40,000 for CEACAM5, individual scores were determined for all targets by attributing a value of 0 to 3 for each patient sample based on the ROC curve cut-off values of the targets, as described in Materials and Methods. Then, an overall score for the each of the two groups of markers was determined for controls and patients with AA or CRC. The overall score for the six markers of the first group significantly recognized the samples from CRC patients vs. those of the controls while the overall scores of the three markers of the second group distinguished the samples from patients bearing CRC or AA from those of the controls (Figure 3).

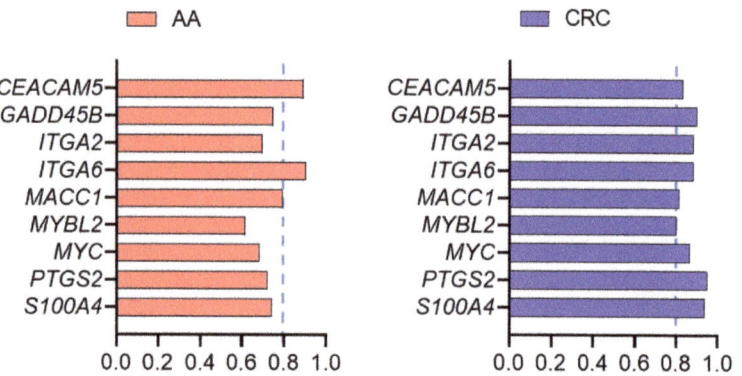

Figure 2. ROC curves were determined for the nine targets characterized in Figure 1 and areas under the curve were calculated to identify those equal or above 0.8 (dotted lines) for AA and CRC.

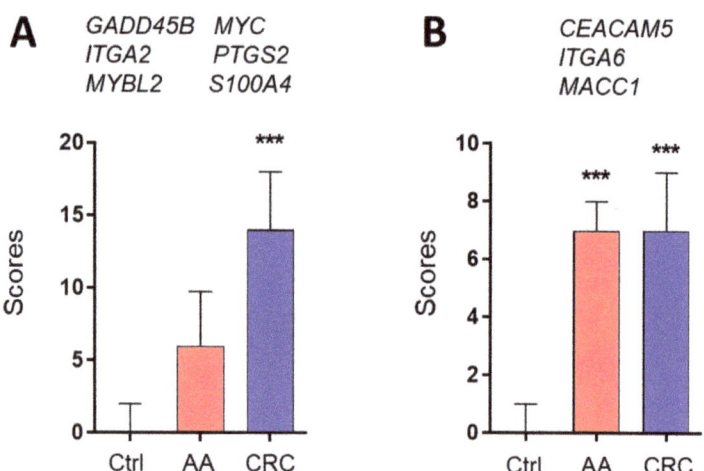

Figure 3. Based on the data from Figures 1 and 2, scores were calculated for the two groups of markers using an algorithm for combining the six targets significant for CRC (**A**) and the three targets significant for AA and CRC (**B**) lesions relative to controls. Results are expressed as median (interquartile range) of scores relative to control patients. *** $p < 0.0005$ using the Kruskal–Wallis test.

ROC curves were then produced for the two groups of targets significant for CRC (Figure 3A, Group A) and for AA and CRC (Figure 3B, Group B). As shown in Table 2 (upper two rows) for >95% specificity, group A (Gr. A) displayed 85.2% sensitivity for CRC but only 45% for AA while group B (Gr. B) showed 79% and 75% sensitivity (for 95% specificity) for CRC and AA, respectively.

Table 2. Selection of the best combinations of targets.

		AA						CRC					
		AUC	Sen [1]	Spe [1]	YI [2]	Sen [3] Spe ≥95%	Spe [4] Sen ≥80%	AUC	Sen [1]	Spe [1]	YI [2]	Sen [3] Spe ≥95%	Spe [4] Sen ≥80%
Gr. A		0.819	79.1	87.10	0.66	45.30	51.61	0.969	85.19	96.97	0.86	85.19	100.0
Gr. B		0.917	91.67	83.87	0.76	75.00	83.87	0.914	79.01	96.97	0.76	79.01	83.87
Gr. B	+ GADD45B	0.900	75.00	87.88	0.63	70.83	72.73	0.923	79.01	96.97	0.76	79.01	87.88
Gr. B	+ ITGA2	0.900	79.17	90.91	0.70	70.83	66.67	0.929	83.95	96.97	0.81	83.95	96.97
Gr. B	+ MYBL2	0.915	79.17	93.94	0.73	75.00	78.79	0.924	85.19	93.94	0.79	80.25	96.97
Gr. B	+ MYC	0.918	83.33	93.94	0.77	66.67	93.94	0.939	85.19	94.94	0.79	80.25	96.97
Gr. B	+ PTGS2	0.905	79.17	90.32	0.70	66.67	70.97	0.944	86.42	93.55	0.80	81.48	96.97
Gr. B	+ S100A4	0.910	79.17	93.94	0.73	75.00	87.88	0.952	86.42	93.94	0.80	81.48	96.97
Gr. B	+ ITGA2 + S100A4	0.897	79.17	90.91	0.69	70.83	84.85	0.958	86.42	93.94	0.80	82.72	96.97
Gr. B	+ ITGA2 + S100A4	0.890	75.00	93.55	0.69	66.67	80.65	0.952	87.65	93.55	0.81	83.95	100.0
Gr. B	**+ PTGS2 + S100A4**	**0.910**	**83.33**	**87.10**	**0.70**	**75.00**	**87.10**	**0.961**	**88.89**	**96.77**	**0.86**	**88.89**	**96.97**

Gr A: GADD45B + ITGA2 + MYBL2 + MYC + PTGS2 + S100A4. Gr B: CEACAM5 + ITGA6 + MACC1. [1] Sensitivities (Sen) and Specificities (Spe) were determined based on optimal cut-off values. [2] YI: Youden Index. [3] Sensitivity for specificity ≥95%. [4] Specificity for sensitivity ≥80%. Bold (last row): Best combination.

Considering that the detection 75% of the AA could be achieved using the three markers of the group B (i.e., *CEACAM5*, *ITGA6* and *MACC1*), we then assayed various combinations of markers belonging to the group A in order to improve CRC detection using a maximum of 5 targets while keeping AA detection at 75% (Table 2). The results show that adding the two markers *S100A4* and *PTGS2* significantly improved the rate of CRC detection up to 89% (for 95% specificity) (Table 2, lower row). Corresponding ROC curves are provided in Figure 4A. FIT positivity was 29 % in AA (7/24) and 72% in CRC stage I-III (56/72). Interestingly, considering the result of the FIT in combination with the multi-target score further increased CRC detection up to 95% (for a 97% specificity), but had no significant effect on AA detection (Figure 4B).

As the ultimate goal of the study was to evaluate the feasibility of using the multi-target mRNA stool test in a clinical set-up, we evaluated the stability of the mRNA targets in stool samples subjected to various conditions of preservation that mimic the clinical reality. Stool samples were obtained from three controls and three patients diagnosed with CRC. Four of the identified targets in stools were selected for testing, including two for each group identified above: *CEACAM5*, *ITGA6*, *ITGA2*, and *PTGS2*. Conditions to be tested included conventional freezing at −20 °C with and without a thaw cycle, conservation at 4 °C and conservation at room temperature (23 °C), for a 5-day period. As shown in Figure S1, the mRNA targets were found to be relatively stable under all frozen and cooled conditions over the 5-day period while some individual variations were observed in samples maintained at room temperature. Score compilation of the data confirmed the relative stability of the targets for all conditions including ambient temperature for at least 3 days (Figure 5).

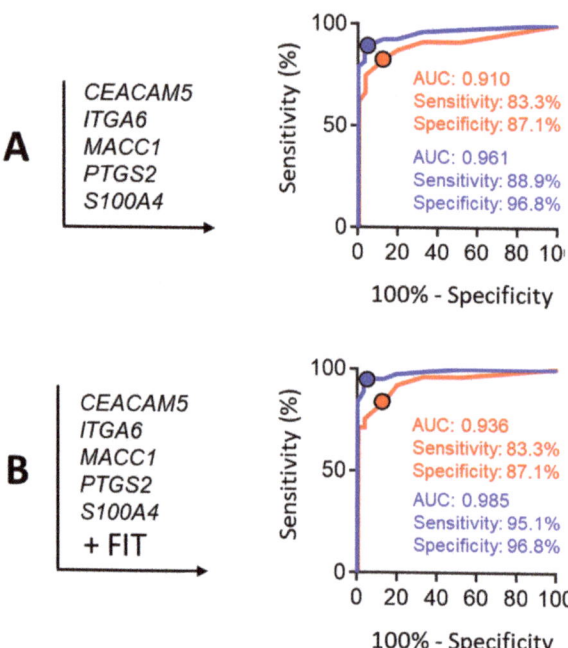

Figure 4. ROC curve analysis of an optimized combination of five of the targets for the detection of patients with AA or CRC as selected from data presented in Table 2. (**A**) ROC curve analysis of the combination of the three targets identified for detecting AA and CRC, CEACAM5, ITGA6 and MACC1 with the two stronger targets for detecting CRC, PTGS2 and S100A4, for AA and CRC. (**B**) Same combination as in A but including the FIT component. AUC is indicated and sensitivity and specificity are provided in % (95% CI).

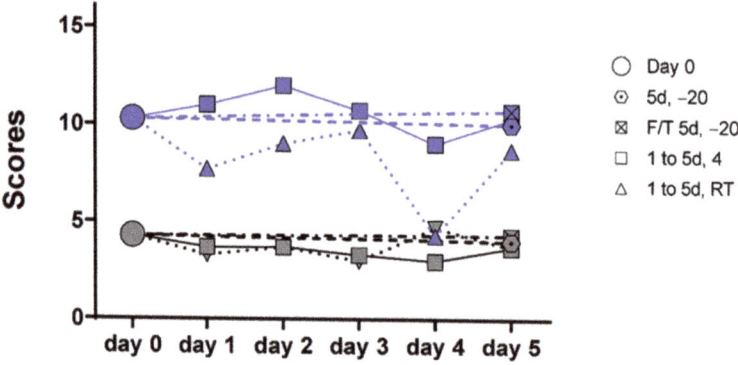

Figure 5. Target stability analyses in stool samples over a 5-day period. Target stability was tested under various conditions of conservation and target detection was monitored throughout the 5 days in samples maintained at −20 °C with (F/T 5d, −20) and without (5d −20) a thaw cycle, at 4 °C (1 to 5d, 4) and at room temperature (1 to 5d, RT). Data for individual targets in copy number are provided in Figure S1. Cumulative scores including the 4 tested targets PTGS2, CEACAM5, ITGA2 and ITGA6 showed that overall, the targets were relatively stable for the five days under all cooled conditions and for three days at room temperature for both controls (Gray symbols) and CRC (Blue symbols).

4. Discussion

In this study, we confirm that a multitarget stool mRNA test represents a powerful assay for detecting patients with colorectal cancers and demonstrate its usefulness to also detect high risk adenomas. One interest of the procedure relies on its relative simplicity considering that high sensitivities and specificities can be obtained with a selection of only five targets, thus compatible with multiplex PCR in stool samples, an approach already in place in the clinic to investigate gastrointestinal infections [37,38].

One strength of the multitarget stool mRNA test presented herein is that transcripts are directly isolated from the stools by conventional extraction methods [25,32] thus being compatible with automation rather than procedures that require enrichment protocols for exfoliated colorectal cells prior to RNA extraction and processing [25,39]. Another strength is the relatively low number of targets required to optimize the assay. It is worth mentioning that an important part of this proof-of-concept study was finding specific targets to identify samples from patients with AA among others that appear to be overrepresented in CRC and then selecting the strongest combination to allow the detection of both AA and CRC. Indeed, some of the targets have been previously assessed for CRC detection [25,32] but it is noteworthy that one of the best markers identified herein for CRC detection, *S100A4*, is reported for the first time. In the same direction, *ITGA6* has been previously reported to be a good candidate for the improvement of AA detection [32] while the current study show that sensitivity and specificity for AA detection can be further improved by combining *ITGA6* with *CEACAM5* and *MACC1*, two targets not yet tested before for this purpose. Further study in this direction would be assisted by the development of specific algorithms where a specific weight is assigned to each marker.

While we agree that our study is preliminary, based on a retrospective analysis of a cohort of patients, as addressed below, it is nevertheless interesting to contextualize the findings that this study, relying on the use of only five mRNA targets, allowed the detection of 75% of the samples obtained from patients with AA and 89% of the samples obtained from patients with CRC, using a specificity of $\geq$95%. We chose to express the data using this optimal specificity which generates less than 5% of false positives in order to allow a fair comparison to other tests such as FIT as detailed above. Incidentally, integration of the FIT component to the mRNA data increased CRC sensitivity up to 95%, consistent with the fact that the origins of exfoliated cells and blood in the stools are likely to be different [14–17]. Overall, a multitarget stool mRNA-FIT test allows the detection of 75% of the AA and 95% of the CRC with less than 4% of false positives. These numbers, although from a preliminary study, compared advantageously to any other screening test for colorectal cancerous lesions. As shown with the inclusion of the FIT component, diversification of target types improves sensitivity. In this context, it would be interesting to investigate the potential complementarity of the multitarget stool mRNA test with others approaches also involving stool-derived nucleic acids [18,40,41] or proteins [15,42]. Incidentally, although the extra costs and specific organizational requirements of the multitarget stool mRNA test relative to the FIT are difficult to evaluate at this time, they should be substantially reduced if performed in conjunction with another nucleic acid-based stool test such as the already implemented multi-target stool DNA test [18].

Another finding from this study is the possibility of including a factor for predicting AA vs. CRC, which could provide pertinent information ahead of colonoscopy. Indeed, considered separately, the combination of the three targets *CEACAM5*, *ITGA6* and *MACC1* selected to predict AA provided 75% and 79% sensitivity (for 95% specificity) for AA and CRC, respectively and the two targets *S100A4* and *PTGS2* selected to improve CRC detection provided 29% and 80% sensitivity (for 95% specificity) for AA and CRC prediction, respectively, suggesting that using distinct repertoires of targets for AA and CRC could be used to improve patient stratification for colonoscopy. Specific analysis of *S100A4* and *PTGS2* scores for patients identified as positive in the multi-target stool mRNA test could contribute to discriminating between patients carrying AA vs. those with CRC considering that, for instance, a patient with a score >4.5 for *S100A4* and *PTGS2* displays a 17% probability of having an AA vs. 73% odds of having a CRC.

Finally, the assessment of target stability revealed that stool sample collection to perform the multitarget stool mRNA test does not require specific conditions, being relatively stable for at least 3 days, even at room temperature. Part of this relatively surprising observation may result from the possibility that mRNA degradation is prevented in exfoliated cells, which are the main source of host mRNA in the stools [25,39]. Another part results from the procedure used for selecting the mRNA targets. Incidentally, it was not surprising that only half of the 27 selected targets were amplified in stool samples. The efficient amplification of these targets was also dependent on the use of the TaqMan Gene Expression Assay which was found to be more sensitive and specific than conventional qPCR for stool samples [31] while requiring relatively short intact mRNA sequences.

The limitations of this study, as mentioned above, include the relatively small size of the cohort of patients providing the two sets of samples from only two sites and the fact that the samples were obtained retrospectively. Future investigations should include a larger and multicentric prospective study. However, the relatively low incidence of CRC in the asymptomatic population to be screened complicates this kind of study. Low scale prospective analyses on higher risk cohorts such as FIT positive patients could then be considered.

5. Conclusions

In conclusion, this study demonstrates the usefulness of host mRNAs as biomarkers to identify patients carrying curable colorectal cancers as well as precancerous lesions. In the context where various stool-based screening approaches are already implemented or in progress, with their strengths and weaknesses, we suggest that the inclusion of a multitarget stool mRNA component could contribute to getting closer to the "desirable features of a screening test" [3].

Supplementary Materials: The following are available online at https://www.mdpi.com/2072-6694/13/6/1228/s1, Figure S1: Target stability analyses in stool samples over a 5-day period.

Author Contributions: J.-F.B. designed the study and wrote the manuscript. E.H. and É.T. conducted the experiments and performed the statistical analyses. N.M. and S.K. contributed samples and analyzed the clinical data. All authors have read and agreed to the published version of the manuscript.

Funding: The work was supported by the Canadian Institutes of Health Research, grants number PPP133373, MOP97836 and PJT1773403 and by the Canada Chair Program, an internal grant from the Centre de recherche du Centre Hospitalier Universitaire de Sherbrooke and a research grant from ALIGO Innovation, a Quebec-based valorization society. None of these funding bodies had any role in the design of the study or the collection, analysis, and interpretation of data nor in the writing of the manuscript.

Institutional Review Board Statement: Two sets of patient samples were used in this study. The first set of samples was collected from patients and healthy controls from the Hamamatsu University School of Medicine with written informed consent. The study was approved by the Institutional Research Ethics Committee of the Hamamatsu University School of Medicine for sample collection and use as well as the Institutional Research Ethics Committee of the Centre Hospitalier Universitaire de Sherbrooke (CHUS) for the handling and analyses of the samples. The second set of samples was collected from healthy controls and patients diagnosed with CRC at the CHUS with written informed consent. The study was approved by the Institutional Research Ethics Committee of the CHUS on 9 December 2016 (ethic protocol # 90–18) and then renewed yearly.

Informed Consent Statement: Informed consent was obtained from all subjects involved in the study.

Data Availability Statement: The data presented in this study are available on request from the corresponding author.

Acknowledgments: The authors thank Maude Gerard for her help in the recruitment of patients for the Sherbrooke arm and Yvan Côté and Jorge Ganopolsky for suggestions in the design of the experiments to evaluate mRNA stability in stools.

Conflicts of Interest: The authors Elizabeth Herring, Éric Tremblay and Jean-François Beaulieu are inventors of the intellectual property owned by the Université de Sherbrooke. The other authors have no conflict of interest to declare.

References

1. Ladabaum, U.; Dominitz, J.A.; Kahi, C.; Schoen, R.E. Strategies for colorectal cancer screening. *Gastroenterology* **2020**, *158*, 418–432. [CrossRef]
2. Manfredi, S.; Bouvier, A.M.; Lepage, C.; Hatem, C.; Dancourt, V.; Faivre, J. Incidence and patterns of recurrence after resection for cure of colonic cancer in a well defined population. *Br. J. Surg.* **2006**, *93*, 1115–1122. [CrossRef]
3. Robertson, D.J.; Imperiale, T.F. Stool testing for colorectal cancer screening. *Gastroenterology* **2015**, *149*, 1286–1293. [CrossRef] [PubMed]
4. Willyard, C. Screening: Early alert. *Nature* **2015**, *521*, S4–S5. [CrossRef]
5. Brenner, H.; Hoffmeister, M.; Stegmaier, C.; Brenner, G.; Altenhofen, L.; Haug, U. Risk of progression of advanced adenomas to colorectal cancer by age and sex: Estimates based on 840,149 screening colonoscopies. *Gut* **2007**, *56*, 1585–1589. [CrossRef] [PubMed]
6. Click, B.; Pinsky, P.F.; Hickey, T.; Doroudi, M.; Schoen, R.E. Association of colonoscopy adenoma findings with long-term colorectal cancer incidence. *JAMA* **2018**, *319*, 2021–2031. [CrossRef]
7. Schroy, P.C., 3rd; Lal, S.; Glick, J.T.; Robinson, P.A.; Zamor, P.; Heeren, T.C. Patient preferences for colorectal cancer screening: How does stool DNA testing fare? *Am. J. Manag. Care* **2007**, *13*, 393–400.
8. Lin, J.S.; Piper, M.A.; Perdue, L.A.; Rutter, C.M.; Webber, E.M.; O'Connor, E.; Smith, N.; Whitlock, E.P. Screening for colorectal cancer: Updated evidence report and systematic review for the US preventive services task force. *JAMA* **2016**, *315*, 2576–2594. [CrossRef]
9. Allison, J.E.; Fraser, C.G.; Halloran, S.P.; Young, G.P. Population screening for colorectal cancer means getting FIT: The past, present, and future of colorectal cancer screening using the fecal immunochemical test for hemoglobin (FIT). *Gut Liver* **2014**, *8*, 117–130. [CrossRef]
10. Hundt, S.; Haug, U.; Brenner, H. Comparative evaluation of immunochemical fecal occult blood tests for colorectal adenoma detection. *Ann. Intern. Med.* **2009**, *150*, 162–169. [CrossRef]
11. Lee, J.K.; Liles, E.G.; Bent, S.; Levin, T.R.; Corley, D.A. Accuracy of fecal immunochemical tests for colorectal cancer: Systematic review and meta-analysis. *Ann. Intern. Med.* **2014**, *160*, 171–181. [CrossRef]
12. Laanani, M.; Coste, J.; Blotiere, P.O.; Carbonnel, F.; Weill, A. Patient, procedure, and endoscopist risk factors for perforation, bleeding, and splenic injury after colonoscopies. *Clin. Gastroenterol. Hepatol.* **2019**, *17*, 719–727.e13. [CrossRef]
13. Robertson, D.J.; Ladabaum, U. Opportunities and challenges in moving from current guidelines to personalized colorectal cancer screening. *Gastroenterology* **2019**, *156*, 904–917. [CrossRef]
14. Yu, Y.J.; Majumdar, A.P.; Nechvatal, J.M.; Ram, J.L.; Basson, M.D.; Heilbrun, L.K.; Kato, I. Exfoliated cells in stool: A source for reverse transcription-PCR-based analysis of biomarkers of gastrointestinal cancer. *Cancer Epidemiol. Biomark. Prev.* **2008**, *17*, 455–458. [CrossRef]
15. Ang, C.S.; Baker, M.S.; Nice, E.C. Mass spectrometry-based analysis for the discovery and validation of potential colorectal cancer stool biomarkers. *Methods Enzymol.* **2017**, *586*, 247–274. [CrossRef]
16. Berger, B.M.; Ahlquist, D.A. Stool DNA screening for colorectal neoplasia: Biological and technical basis for high detection rates. *Pathology* **2012**, *44*, 80–88. [CrossRef]
17. Koga, Y.; Yasunaga, M.; Katayose, S.; Moriya, Y.; Akasu, T.; Fujita, S.; Yamamoto, S.; Baba, H.; Matsumura, Y. Improved recovery of exfoliated colonocytes from feces using newly developed immunomagnetic beads. *Gastroenterol. Res. Pract.* **2008**, *2008*, 605273. [CrossRef] [PubMed]
18. Imperiale, T.F.; Ransohoff, D.F.; Itzkowitz, S.H.; Levin, T.R.; Lavin, P.; Lidgard, G.P.; Ahlquist, D.A.; Berger, B.M. Multitarget stool DNA testing for colorectal-cancer screening. *N. Engl. J. Med.* **2014**, *370*, 1287–1297. [CrossRef]
19. Ransohoff, D.F.; Sox, H.C. Clinical practice guidelines for colorectal cancer screening: New recommendations and new challenges. *JAMA* **2016**, *315*, 2529–2531. [CrossRef] [PubMed]
20. Lansdorp-Vogelaar, I.; van Ballegooijen, M.; Zauber, A.G.; Habbema, J.D.; Kuipers, E.J. Effect of rising chemotherapy costs on the cost savings of colorectal cancer screening. *J. Natl. Cancer Inst.* **2009**, *101*, 1412–1422. [CrossRef]
21. Neumann, P.J.; Cohen, J.T.; Weinstein, M.C. Updating cost-effectiveness—The curious resilience of the $50,000-per-QALY threshold. *N. Engl. J. Med.* **2014**, *371*, 796–797. [CrossRef]
22. Imperiale, T.F.; Kahi, C.J. Cost-effectiveness of future biomarkers for colorectal cancer screening: Quantified futility or call for innovation? *Clin. Gastroenterol. Hepatol.* **2018**, *16*, 483–485. [CrossRef]
23. Haug, U.; Knudsen, A.B.; Lansdorp-Vogelaar, I.; Kuntz, K.M. Development of new non-invasive tests for colorectal cancer screening: The relevance of information on adenoma detection. *Int. J. Cancer* **2015**, *136*, 2864–2874. [CrossRef]

24. Koga, Y.; Yasunaga, M.; Moriya, Y.; Akasu, T.; Fujita, S.; Yamamoto, S.; Kozu, T.; Baba, H.; Matsumura, Y. Detection of colorectal cancer cells from feces using quantitative real-time RT-PCR for colorectal cancer diagnosis. *Cancer Sci.* **2008**, *99*, 1977–1983. [CrossRef]
25. Kanaoka, S.; Yoshida, K.; Miura, N.; Sugimura, H.; Kajimura, M. Potential usefulness of detecting cyclooxygenase 2 messenger RNA in feces for colorectal cancer screening. *Gastroenterology* **2004**, *127*, 422–427. [CrossRef]
26. Takai, T.; Kanaoka, S.; Yoshida, K.; Hamaya, Y.; Ikuma, M.; Miura, N.; Sugimura, H.; Kajimura, M.; Hishida, A. Fecal cyclooxygenase 2 plus matrix metalloproteinase 7 mRNA assays as a marker for colorectal cancer screening. *Cancer Epidemiol. Biomark. Prev.* **2009**, *18*, 1888–1893. [CrossRef]
27. Hamaya, Y.; Yoshida, K.; Takai, T.; Ikuma, M.; Hishida, A.; Kanaoka, S. Factors that contribute to faecal cyclooxygenase-2 mRNA expression in subjects with colorectal cancer. *Br. J. Cancer* **2010**, *102*, 916–921. [CrossRef]
28. Dydensborg, A.B.; Teller, I.C.; Groulx, J.F.; Basora, N.; Pare, F.; Herring, E.; Gauthier, R.; Jean, D.; Beaulieu, J.F. Integrin alpha6Bbeta4 inhibits colon cancer cell proliferation and c-Myc activity. *BMC Cancer* **2009**, *9*, 223. [CrossRef]
29. Groulx, J.F.; Giroux, V.; Beausejour, M.; Boudjadi, S.; Basora, N.; Carrier, J.C.; Beaulieu, J.F. Integrin alpha6A splice variant regulates proliferation and the Wnt/beta-catenin pathway in human colorectal cancer cells. *Carcinogenesis* **2014**, *35*, 1217–1227. [CrossRef]
30. You, Y.N.; Rustin, R.B.; Sullivan, J.D. Oncotype DX((R)) colon cancer assay for prediction of recurrence risk in patients with stage II and III colon cancer: A review of the evidence. *Surg. Oncol.* **2015**, *24*, 61–66. [CrossRef] [PubMed]
31. Herring, E.; Kanaoka, S.; Tremblay, E.; Beaulieu, J.F. A stool multitarget mRNA assay for the detection of colorectal neoplasms. *Methods Mol. Biol.* **2018**, *1765*, 217–227. [CrossRef]
32. Beaulieu, J.F.; Herring, E.; Kanaoka, S.; Tremblay, E. Use of integrin alpha 6 transcripts in a stool mRNA assay for the detection of colorectal cancers at curable stages. *Oncotarget* **2016**, *7*, 14684–14692. [CrossRef]
33. Herring, E.; Kanaoka, S.; Tremblay, E.; Beaulieu, J.F. Droplet digital PCR for quantification of ITGA6 in a stool mRNA assay for the detection of colorectal cancers. *World J. Gastroenterol.* **2017**, *23*, 2891–2898. [CrossRef] [PubMed]
34. Reck, M.; Tomasch, J.; Deng, Z.; Jarek, M.; Husemann, P.; Wagner-Dobler, I.; Consortium, C. Stool metatranscriptomics: A technical guideline for mRNA stabilisation and isolation. *BMC Genomics* **2015**, *16*, 494. [CrossRef]
35. Stauber, J.; Shaikh, N.; Ordiz, M.I.; Tarr, P.I.; Manary, M.J. Droplet digital PCR quantifies host inflammatory transcripts in feces reliably and reproducibly. *Cell. Immunol.* **2016**, *303*, 43–49. [CrossRef] [PubMed]
36. Dydensborg, A.B.; Herring, E.; Auclair, J.; Tremblay, E.; Beaulieu, J.-F. Normalizing genes for quantitative RT-PCR in differentiating human intestinal epithelial cells and adenocarcinomas of the colon. *Am. J. Physiol. Gastrointest. Liver Physiol.* **2006**, *290*, G1067–G1074. [CrossRef] [PubMed]
37. Maas, J.; Dorigo-Zetsma, J.W.; de Groot, C.J.; Bouter, S.; Plotz, F.B.; van Ewijk, B.E. Detection of intestinal protozoa in paediatric patients with gastrointestinal symptoms by multiplex real-time PCR. *Clin. Microbiol. Infect.* **2014**, *20*, 545–550. [CrossRef]
38. Becker, S.L.; Chatigre, J.K.; Gohou, J.P.; Coulibaly, J.T.; Leuppi, R.; Polman, K.; Chappuis, F.; Mertens, P.; Herrmann, M.; N'Goran, E.K.; et al. Combined stool-based multiplex PCR and microscopy for enhanced pathogen detection in patients with persistent diarrhoea and asymptomatic controls from Cote d'Ivoire. *Clin. Microbiol. Infect.* **2015**, *21*, 591.e1–591.e10. [CrossRef] [PubMed]
39. Barnell, E.K.; Kang, Y.; Wurtzler, E.M.; Griffith, M.; Chaudhuri, A.A.; Griffith, O.L.; Geneoscopy, S. Noninvasive detection of high-risk adenomas using stool-derived eukaryotic RNA sequences as biomarkers. *Gastroenterology* **2019**, *157*, 884–887.e3. [CrossRef]
40. Rengucci, C.; De Maio, G.; Menghi, M.; Benzi, F.; Calistri, D. Evaluation of colorectal cancer risk and prevalence by stool DNA integrity detection. *J. Vis. Exp.* **2020**. [CrossRef]
41. Ahmed, F.E.; Ahmed, N.C.; Gouda, M.M.; Vos, P.W.; Bonnerup, C. RT-qPCR for fecal mature MicroRNA quantification and validation. *Methods Mol. Biol.* **2018**, *1765*, 203–215. [CrossRef] [PubMed]
42. Alvarez-Chaver, P.; Otero-Estevez, O.; Paez de la Cadena, M.; Rodriguez-Berrocal, F.J.; Martinez-Zorzano, V.S. Proteomics for discovery of candidate colorectal cancer biomarkers. *World J. Gastroenterol.* **2014**, *20*, 3804–3824. [CrossRef] [PubMed]

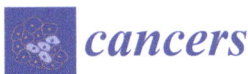

Review

Novel Biomarkers of Gastric Adenocarcinoma: Current Research and Future Perspectives

Nadja Niclauss [1,*,†], Ines Gütgemann [2,†], Jonas Dohmen [1], Jörg C. Kalff [1] and Philipp Lingohr [1]

[1] Department of General, Visceral, Vascular and Thoracic Surgery, University Hospital Bonn, 53127 Bonn, Germany; jonas.dohmen@ukbonn.de (J.D.); kalff@uni-bonn.de (J.C.K.); philipp.lingohr@ukbonn.de (P.L.)
[2] Department of Pathology, University Hospital Bonn, 53127 Bonn, Germany; ines.guetgemann@ukb.uni-bonn.de
* Correspondence: nadja.niclauss@ukbonn.de; Tel.: +49-228-28715857
† These authors contributed equally to this work.

Simple Summary: Gastric cancer is characterized by poor survival rates despite surgery and chemotherapy. Current research focuses on biomarkers to improve diagnosis and prognosis, and to enable targeted treatment strategies. The aim of our review was to give an overview over the wide range of novel biomarkers in gastric cancer. These biomarkers are targets of a specific treatment, such as antibodies against human epidermal growth factor receptor 2. Other promising biomarkers for targeted therapies that have shown relevance in clinical trials are vascular endothelial growth factor, programmed cell death protein 1, and Claudin 18.2. There is a vast number of biomarkers based on DNA, RNA, and protein expression, as well as detection of circulating tumor cells and the immune tumor microenvironment.

Abstract: Overall survival of gastric cancer remains low, as patients are often diagnosed with advanced stage disease. In this review, we give an overview of current research on biomarkers in gastric cancer and their implementation in treatment strategies. The HER2-targeting trastuzumab is the first molecular targeted agent approved for gastric cancer treatment. Other promising biomarkers for targeted therapies that have shown relevance in clinical trials are VEGF and Claudin 18.2. Expression of MET has been shown to be a negative prognostic factor in gastric cancer. Targeting the PD-1/PD-L1 pathway with immune checkpoint inhibitors has proven efficacy in advanced gastric cancer. Recent technology advances allow the detection of circulating tumor cells that may be used as diagnostic and prognostic indicators and for therapy monitoring in gastric cancer patients. Prognostic molecular subtypes of gastric cancer have been identified using genomic data. In addition, transcriptome profiling has allowed a comprehensive characterization of the immune and stromal microenvironment in gastric cancer and development of novel risk scores. These prognostic and predictive markers highlight the rapidly evolving field of research in gastric cancer, promising improved treatment stratification and identification of molecular targets for individualized treatment in gastric cancer.

Keywords: gastric cancer; advanced gastric cancer; biomarker; targeted therapy

1. Introduction

Gastric cancer (GC), based on GLOBOCAN 2020 data [1], is the fifth most common cancer and the fourth most common cause of cancer-related death in the world. Gastric adenocarcinomas account for 5.6% of all new cancer cases and 7.7% of all cancer deaths worldwide [1]. H. pylori infection is the strongest known risk factor for gastric cancer [2]; another pathogen associated with gastric cancer is the Epstein–Barr virus [3]. The incidence of gastric cancer has steadily declined worldwide over the past 50 years, due to prevention and treatment of H. pylori infection and changing of food preservation and diet [4]. Surgery associated with chemotherapy still offers the best chance for curative therapy. Due to earlier detection of GC and achievements in chemotherapy and targeted therapy, mortality has decreased in recent decades. Still, the overall survival of gastric cancer remains low, with a reported 5-year survival rate of 32% in all stages combined, and of only 6% in metastatic disease [5]. This is mostly due to the fact that gastric cancer is usually diagnosed in an advanced and unresectable stage. If the cancer is diagnosed and treated before it has spread outside the stomach, the 5-year survival rate is 70% [5]. Therefore, most current new strategies aim to detect gastric cancer at an early stage, or to treat gastric cancer at an advanced stage. Biomarkers are playing a crucial role in these strategies. Cancer biomarkers can be soluble molecules derived from tumor cells, or can be soluble or cell-bound molecules that are expressed by nontumorous cells. Genetic, epigenetic, proteomic, glycomic, and imaging biomarkers can be used for cancer diagnosis, prognosis, and epidemiology [6]. In recent decades, multiple novel biomarkers have been identified in GC, and biomedical sciences and technology have developed at a rapid pace. The Cancer Genome Atlas (TCGA) project has identified four major genomic subtypes of GC: Epstein–Barr Virus (EBV)-infected tumors, tumors with microsatellite instability (MSI), genomically stable tumors, and chromosomally unstable tumors, which might provide a guide to targeted agents [7].

This review intends to give an overview of the literature on current and newly identified biomarkers and their roles in targeted therapies in gastric cancer (i.e., their function as predictive markers). PubMed was searched for articles using the terms 'biomarker' and 'gastric cancer' on 28 March 2021. We analyzed English articles from the last 10 years including clinical trials and randomized controlled trials. We obtained 295 articles. We excluded 150 articles that did not mention biomarkers in gastric or esophagogastric cancer or did not differentiate results between either gastric or esophagogastric and other carcinomas. The resulting 145 articles were analyzed. Another 49 articles were cited that were found relevant to this article. Articles treating gastro-esophageal junction (GEJ) adenocarcinoma were included in this review. Furthermore, clinical implementation of these biomarkers for early diagnosis, prognosis, and prediction of drug efficacy is discussed.

2. Treatment-Related Biomarkers—Molecular Targeted Therapy
2.1. Human Epidermal Growth Factor Receptor 2

Human epidermal growth factor receptor 2 (HER2), also called ERBB2, is a receptor tyrosine-protein kinase. It is an important biomarker and key driver of tumorigenesis in GC [8]. HER2-positive tumors show *HER2* gene amplification that is generally, although not always, associated with protein overexpression, leading to tumorigenesis [9]. *HER2* acts as an oncogene, mainly because high-level amplification of the gene induces protein overexpression in the cellular membrane and subsequent acquisition of advantageous properties for a malignant cell [10]. *HER2* gene amplification can be detected by fluorescence in situ hybridization (ISH), whereas overexpression of HER2 protein is commonly assessed by immunohistochemistry (IHC). Concordance between positive gene amplification and protein overexpression has been observed in 96% of GC, whereby positive *HER2* amplification was defined as a *HER2*/chromosome 17 centromere (CEP17) ratio ≥ 2.0 [11].

HER2-positivity rates by IHC in GC range between 10.9 and 27% [11–16]. HER2-positivity rates are higher in papillary and tubular adenocarcinoma compared to poorly differentiated adenocarcinoma or signet-ring cell carcinoma [13]. For clinical use, it has been proposed to test the HER2 status in all adenocarcinoma of the stomach and carcinomas of the GEJ by IHC first. In inconclusive cases, *HER2* amplification status needs to be assessed with ISH [17].

HER2-targeted therapy has dramatically improved outcomes for HER2-positive gastric cancer. Trastuzumab is a monoclonal antibody targeting the HER2-receptor, causing downregulation of HER2. The Trastuzumab for Gastric Cancer (ToGA) trial showed improved overall survival (OS) of patients treated with trastuzumab in combination with cisplatin and a fluoropyrimidine compared to chemotherapy alone in patients with HER2-overexpressing advanced gastric or GEJ cancer (13.8 vs. 11.1 months, $p = 0.005$) [8]. A subgroup analysis of Japanese patients confirmed the benefit of adding trastuzumab to chemotherapy [18]. Trastuzumab in combination with chemotherapy is the standard of care when treating HER2-positive metastatic gastric and GEJ cancers. Furthermore, it is the first molecular targeted agent approved as standard treatment in gastric cancer.

A retrospective analysis compared OS in advanced GC patients according to HER2 status and exposure to trastuzumab. It showed longer OS of HER2-positive patients treated with trastuzumab than HER2-negative patients (24.7 vs. 13.9 months, $p = 0.03$), with trastuzumab having a significant impact on OS. Interestingly, HER2-positive patients not treated with trastuzumab showed similar OS as HER-negative patients (13.5 vs. 13.9 months, $p = 0.91$). The authors concluded that trastuzumab improved prognosis of HER2-positive beyond that of HER2-negative AGC patients, but HER2 status itself without targeted therapy might have a small impact on survival in advanced GC [19].

Li et al. analyzed whether clinicopathological factors were predictive for progression-free survival (PFS) of patients with trastuzumab-based first-line therapy. They found only liver metastasis and poor performance status to be independently associated with worse PFS [20].

Antibody–drug conjugates with trastuzumab that have been developed and tested are listed in Table 1 [21–24].

Table 1. Targeted therapies and treatment outcomes.

Target	Study	Design	Patient Number	Treatment Aim	Outcome
HER2	Bang, Y.J. et al. [8]	RCT (phase 3)	594	Trastuzumab + CT vs. CT alone in HER2(+) AGC (ToGA trial)	OS: 13.8 vs. 11.1 months ($p = 0.005$) PFS: 6.7 vs. 5.5 months ($p = 0.0002$) ORR: 47 vs. 35% ($p = 0.002$)
	Sawaki, A. et al. [18]	RCT (phase 3)	101	Trastuzumab + CT vs. CT alone in HER2(+) AGC (subgroup analysis of ToGA trial)	OS: 15.9 vs. 17.7 months PFS: 6.2 vs. 5.6 months ORR: 64.4 vs. 58.5%
	Shitara, K. et al. [19]	Retrospective case series	364	Trastuzumab + CT in HER2(+) vs. CT in HER2(−) AGC (1), CT in HER2(+) vs. HER2(−) AGC (2)	OS: 24.7 vs. 13.9 months ($p = 0.03$) (1) OS: 13.5 vs. 13.9 months ($p = 0.91$) (2)
	Li, Q. et al. [20]	Prospective observational study	107	Trastuzumab as first-line treatment in HER2(+) AGC	OS: 16 months PFS: 7.7 months ORR: 58.9%
	Shitara, K. et al. [21]	RCT (phase 2)	187	Trastuzumab deruxtecan vs. CT in previously treated HER2(+) AGC	OS: 12.5 vs. 8.4 months ($p = 0.01$) ORR: 51 vs. 14% ($p < 0.001$)
	Thuss-Patience, P.C. et al. [22]	RCT (phase 2/3)	182	Trastuzumab emtansine vs. Taxane as second-line therapy in HER2(+) AGC (GATSBY study)	OS: 7.9 vs. 8.6 months ($p = 0.86$)
	Shah, M.A. et al. [23]	RCT (phase 2/3)	182	Biomarker analysis of the GATSBY study: Trastuzumab emtansine vs. Taxane as second-line therapy in HER2(+) AGC	Subgroup with high HER2 expression in IHC: OS: 9.5 vs. 8.3 months

Table 1. Cont.

Target	Study	Design	Patient Number	Treatment Aim	Outcome
HER2	Shitara, K. et al. [24]	RCT (phase 2/3)	82	Trastuzumab emtansine vs. taxane as second-line therapy in HER2(+) AGC (subgroup analysis of GATSBY study)	OS: 11.8 vs. 10 months
	Horita, Y. et al. [25]	Phase 2	28	Paclitaxel + trastuzumab in previously treated HER2(+) AGC	OS: 9.6 months PFS: 4.6 months ORR: 21.4%
	Makiyama, A. et al. [26]	RCT (phase 2)	91	Paclitaxel + trastuzumab vs. Paclitaxel as first-line therapy of HER2(+) AGC	OS: 10 months ($p = 0.20$) PFS: 3.7 vs. 3.2 months ($p = 0.33$) ORR: 33 vs. 32% ($p = 1.00$)
	Ryu, M.H. et al. [27]	Phase 2	55	Trastuzumab + capecitabine + oxaliplatin in HER2(+) AGC	OS: 21 months PFS: 9.8 months ORR: 67%
	Gong, J. et al. [28]	Phase 2	51	Trastuzumab + oxaliplatin + capecitabine as first-line therapy in HER2(+) AGC	OS: 19.5 months PFS: 9.2 months ORR: 66.7%
	Rivera, F. et la [29]	Phase 2	41	Xelox + trastuzumab as first-line therapy of HER2(+) AGC	OS: 13.8 months PFS: 7.1 months ORR: 46.7%
	Roviello, G. et al. [30]	Phase 2	15	DOF (docetaxel, oxaliplatin, 5-FU) + trastuzumab in HER2(+) AGC	OS: 19.4 months PFS: 9.2 months ORR: 60%
	Mondaca, S. et al. [31]	Phase 2	26	mDCF (docetaxel, cisplatin and 5-FU) + trastuzumab as first-line therapy in HER2(+) metastatic GC	OS: 24.9 months PFS: 13 months ORR: 65%
	Kagawa, S. et al. [32]	Phase 2	23	Trastuzumab + docetaxel as first-line therapy in HER2(+) AGC	OS: 17.5 months PFS: 6.7 months ORR: 39.1%
	Takahari, D. et al. [33]	Phase 2	75	Trastuzumab + S-1 + oxaliplatin in HER2(+) AGC	OS: 18.1 months PFS: 8.8 months ORR: 70.7%
	Yuki, S. et al. [34]	Phase 2	42	Trastuzumab + S-1 + oxaliplatin as treatment of HER2(+) advanced or recurrent GC	OS: 27.6 months PFS: 7.0 months ORR: 82.1%
	Kataoka, H. et al. [35]	Phase 2	22	Trastuzumab + S-1 + cisplatin in HER2(+) AGC	OS: 15.3 months PFS: 7.5 months ORR: 41.2%
	Miura, Y. et al. [36]	Phase 2	44	Trastuzumab + S-1 + cisplatin in HER2(+) AGC	OS: 16.5 months PFS: 5.9 months ORR: 61%
	Endo, S. et al. [37]	Prospective observational study	15	Trastuzumab + cisplatin + S-1 in HER2(+) AGC	OS: 14.4 months
	Kimura, Y. et al. [38]	Phase 2	51	Trastuzumab + S-1 in patients 65 years or older with HER2(+) AGC	OS: 15.8 months PFS: 5.1 months ORR: 40.8%

Table 1. Cont.

Target	Study	Design	Patient Number	Treatment Aim	Outcome
HER2	Shah, M.A. et al. [39]	RCT (Phase 3b)	248	Standard-of-care vs. higher-dose trastuzumab + CT as first-line therapy in HER2(+) metastatic GC (HELOISE trial)	OS: 12.5 vs. 10.6 months ($p = 0.2401$)
	Tabernero, J. et al. [40]	RCT (phase 3)	780	Pertuzumab + trastuzumab + CT vs. placebo + trastuzumab + CT as first-line therapy of HER2(+) AGC (JACOB trial)	OS: 17.5 vs. 14.2 months ($p = 0.057$)
	Liu, T. et al. [41]	RCT (phase 3)	163	Pertuzumab + trastuzumab + CT vs. placebo + trastuzumab + CT as first-line therapy of HER2(+) metastatic GC (subgroup analysis of JACOB trial)	OS: 18.7 vs. 16.1 months PFS: 10.5 vs. 8.6 months ORR: 68.9 vs. 55.7%
	Oh, D.Y. et al. [42]	Phase 2	27	Dacomitinib in previously treated HER2(+) AGC	OS: 7.1 months PFS: 2.1 months ORR: 7.4%
	Kim, T.Y. et al. [43]	Phase 2	32	Poziotinib + trastuzumab + paclitaxel as second-line therapy in HER2(+) AGC	OS: 29.5 weeks PFS: 13 weeks ORR: 21.9%
EGFR HER2	Iqbal, S. et al. [44]	Phase 2	47	Lapatinib as first-line therapy in advanced or metastatic GC	OS: 4.8 months PFS: 1.9 months ORR: 9%
	Satoh, T. et al. [45]	RCT (phase 3)	261	Lapatinib + paclitaxel vs. paclitaxel alone as second-line therapy in HER2(+) AGC	OS: 11 vs. 8.9 months ($p = 0.10$) PFS: 5.4 vs. 4.4 months ($p = 0.24$) ORR: 27 vs. 9% ($p < 0.001$)
	Lorenzen, S. et al. [46]	RCT (phase 2)	37	Lapatinib + capecitabine vs. lapatinib alone in HER2(+) AGC	ORR: 11.1% (LAP + CAP) (study closed for futility)
	Hecht, J.R. et al. [47]	RCT (phase 3)	545	Lapatinib + capecitabine/oxaliplatin vs. placebo + capecitabine/oxaliplatin in HER2(+) AGC	OS: 12.2 vs. 10.5 months (NS) PFS: 6.0 vs. 5.4 months ($p = 0.038$) ORR: 53 vs. 39% ($p = 0.003$)
	Moehler, M. et al. [48]	RCT (phase 2)	29	Lapatinib + ECF/ECX vs. placebo + ECF/ECX as first-line therapy in metastatic GC patients EGFR(+) and/or HER2(+)	OS: 13.8 vs. 10.1 months (NS) PFS: 8 vs. 5.9 months (NS) ORR: 42.9 vs. 21.4%
	LaBonte, M.J. et al. [49]	Phase 2	68	Lapatinib as first-line therapy in AGC independent of HER2 status	OS: 6.3 months PFS: 3.3 months ORR: 17.9%
	Sanchez-Vega, F. et al. [50]	Prospective observational study	20	Afatinib in trastuzumab-resistant HER2(+) metastatic GC	OS: 7 months PFS: 2 months ORR: 25%

Table 1. *Cont.*

Target	Study	Design	Patient Number	Treatment Aim	Outcome
EGFR	Waddell, T. et al. [51]	RCT (phase 3)	553	Panitumumab + CT vs. CT alone in advanced EG cancer (REAL3 trial)	OS: 8.8 vs. 11.3 months ($p = 0.013$) PFS: 6.0 vs. 7.4 months ($p = 0.068$) ORR: 46 vs. 42% ($p = 0.42$)
	Stahl, M. et al. [52]	RCT (phase 2)	160	Panitumumab + CT vs. placebo + CT in untreated locally advanced esophagogastric cancer	Similar histological response and R0 resection rate.
	Satoh, T. et al. [53]	RCT (phase 2)	82	Nimotuzumab + irinotecan vs. irinotecan alone as second-line therapy in AGC	OS: 251 vs. 232 days ($p = 0.978$) PFS: 73 vs. 85 days ($p = 0.567$) ORR: 18.4 vs. 10.3%
	Lordick, F. et al. [54]	Phase 2	52	Cetuximab + CT as first-line therapy in metastatic GC	OS: 9.5 months PFS: 7.6 months ORR: 65%
	Moehler, M. et al. [55]	Phase 2	49	Cetuximab + irinotecan/folinic acid/5-FU as first-line therapy of HER2(+) AGC	OS: 16.5 months PFS: 9 months ORR: 46% (higher response in EGFR-expressing tumors, PTEN expression associated with longer PFS and OS)
	Lordick, F. et al. [56]	RCT (phase 3)	904	Cetuximab + capecitabine-cisplatin vs. capecitabine-cisplatin in unresectable or metastatic GC or EGJ cancer (EXPAND trial)	PFS: 4.4 vs. 5.6 months ($p = 0.32$)
	Zhang, X. et al. [57]	Phase 2	47	Cetuximab + cisplatin/capecitabine in untreated unresectable or metastatic GC	OS: 10.8 months PFS: 5.2 months ORR: 53.2%
	Liu X et al. [58]	Phase 2	61	Cetuximab + modified FOLFIRI as second-line therapy in metastatic GC	OS: 8.6 months ORR: 33.3%
VEGF	Wilke, H. et al. [59]	RCT (phase 3)	665	Ramucirumab + paclitaxel vs. placebo + paclitaxel as second-line therapy in AGC	OS: 9.6 vs. 7.4 months ($p = 0.017$) PFS: 4.4 vs. 2.9 months ($p < 0.0001$) ORR: 28 vs. 16% ($p = 0.0001$)
	Ohtsu, A. et al. [60]	RCT (phase 3)	774	Bevacizumab + CT vs. placebo + CT as first-line therapy in AGC (AVAGAST trial)	OS: 12.1 vs. 10.1 months ($p = 0.1002$) PFS: 6.7 vs. 5.3 months ($p = 0.0037$) ORR: 46 vs. 37.4% ($p = 0.0315$)

Table 1. Cont.

Target	Study	Design	Patient Number	Treatment Aim	Outcome
VEGF	Meulendijks, D. et al. [61]	Phase 2	60	Bevacizumab + CT as first-line therapy in HER2(−) GC	OS: 12 months PFS: 8.3 months ORR: 70%
	Meulendijks, D. et al. [62]	Phase 2	25	Bevacizumab + trastuzumab + CT as first-line therapy in HER2(+) AGC	OS: 17.9 months PFS: 10.8 months ORR: 74%
VEGF PDGF	Moehler, M. et al. [63]	Phase 2	51	Sunitinib monotherapy in pretreated AGC	OS: 5.8 months PFS: 1.3 months ORR: 4%
	Moehler, M. et al. [64]	RCT (phase 2)	91	Sunitinib + FOLFIRI vs. placebo + FOLFIRI as second- or third-line therapy in AGC	OS: 10.4 vs. 8.9 months ($p = 0.21$) PFS: 3.5 vs. 3.3 months ($p = 0.66$)
FGFR VEGF PDGF	Won, E. et al. [65]	Phase 2	32	Nintedanip as second-line therapy in metastatic EG cancer	OS: 14.2 months PFS: 1.9 months ORR: 0%
FGFR	Van Cutsem, E. et al. [66]	RCT	71	AZD4547 vs. paclitaxel as second-line therapy in AGC with FGFR2 polysomy or gene amplification (SHINE study)	OS: 5.5 vs. 6.6 months ($p = 0.8156$) PFS: 1.8 vs. 3.5 months ($p = 0.9581$) ORR: 2.6 vs. 23.3% ($p = 0.9970$)
HGFR/MET	Iveson, T. et al. [67]	RCT (phase 2)	121	Rilotumumab (2 different concentrations) vs. placebo in advanced or metastatic GC	PFS: 5.7 vs. 4.2 months ($p = 0.016$)
	Zhu, M. et al. [68]	RCT (phase 2)	121	Rilotumumab + ECX vs. placebo + ECX in MET-positive patients	High rilotumumab vs. placebo vs. low rilotumumab: OS: 13.4 vs. 5.7 and 8.1 months ($p = 0.017$) PFS: 7.0 vs. 4.4 and 5.5 months ($p = 0.017$)
	Catenacci, D.V. et al. [69]	RCT (phase 3)	609	Rilotumumab + epirubicin/cisplatin/capecitabine vs. placebo + epirubicin/cisplatin/capecitabine as first-line therapy in MET(+) AGC	OS: 8.8 vs. 10.7 months ($p = 0.003$) (study stopped early)
	Shah, M.A. et al. [70]	RCT (phase 3)	499	Onartuzumab + mFOLFOX6 vs. placebo + mFOLFOX6 in HER2-negative, MET-positive gastroesophageal adenocarcinoma	OS: 11.0 vs. 11.3 months ($p = 0.24$) PFS: 6.7 vs. 6.8 months ($p = 0.43$) ORR: 46.1 vs. 40.6% ($p = 0.25$)

Table 1. Cont.

Target	Study	Design	Patient Number	Treatment Aim	Outcome
Claudin 18.2	Sahin, U. et al. [71]	RCT (phase 2)	161	Zolbetuximab + CT + vs. CT alone in Claudin 18.2(+) advanced or recurrent GC (FAST trial)	Overall: PFS: 7.5 vs. 5.3 months ($p < 0.0005$) OS: 13.0 vs. 8.3 months ($p < 0.0005$) ≥70% Claudin 18.2(+): PFS: 9.0 vs. 5.7 months ($p < 0.0005$) OS: 16.5 vs. 8.9 months ($p < 0.0005$)
ATM	Bang, Y.J. et al. [72]	RCT (phase 2)	124	Olaparib + paclitaxel vs. placebo + paclitaxel in recurrent or metastatic GC	OS—overall: 13.1 vs. 8.3 months ($p = 0.005$) OS—ATM low: not reached vs. 8.2 months ($p = 0.002$) PFS: 3.91 vs. 3.55 months ($p = 0.131$) ORR: 26.4 vs. 19.1% ($p = 0.162$)
AKT	Bang, Y.J. et al. [73]	RCT (phase 2)	153	Ipatasertib + mFOLFOX6 vs. placebo + mFOLFOX6 in advanced or metastatic GC	PFS: 6.6 vs. 7.5 months ($p = 0.56$)
HDAC	Yoo, C. et al. [74]	Phase 2	45	Vorinostat + capecitabine + cisplatin as first-line therapy in AGC	OS: 12.7 months PFS: 5.9 months ORR: 42%
MMP9	Shah, M.A. et al. [75]	Phase 2	40	Andecaliximab + mFOLFOX6 in advanced GC	PFS: 7.8 months ORR: 48%
MMP9	Shah, M.A. et al. [76]	RCT (phase 3)	432	Andecaliximab + mFOLFOX vs. placebo + mFOLFOX	OS: 12.5 vs. 11.8 months ($p = 0.56$) PFS: 7.5 vs. 7.1 months ($p = 0.10$) ORR: 51 vs. 41%
PD-1/PD-L1	Muro, K. et al. [77]	Phase 1b	36	Pembrolizumab in PD-L1(+) AGC	ORR: 22%
PD-1/PD-L1	Fuchs, C.S. et al. [78]	Phase 2	259	Pembrolizumab in previously treated AGC (KEYNOTE-059 trial)	OS: 5.6 months (PD-L1(+)/(−): 5.8/4.9 months) PFS: 2.0 months ORR: 11.6% (PD-L1(+)/(−): 15.5/6.4%, $p = 0.02$)
PD-1/PD-L1	Kim, S.T. et al. [79]	Phase 2	61	Pembrolizumab in metastatic GC	ORR: 85.7% in MSI-H, 100% in EBV+
PD-1/PD-L1	Kawazoe, A. et al. [80]	Phase 2b	54	Pembrolizumab + S-1 + oxaliplatin in PD-L1(+) HER2-negative AGC	PFS: 9.4 months ORR: 72.2%
PD-1/PD-L1	Wang, F. et al. [81]	Phase 1b/2	76	1: Toripalimab (chemo-refractory) 2: Toripalimab + CT (CT-naïve) in AGC	1: OS: 4.8 months, PFS: 1.9 months, ORR: 12.1% 2. OS: not reached; PFS: 5.8 months; ORR: 66.7%;

Table 1. Cont.

Target	Study	Design	Patient Number	Treatment Aim	Outcome
PD-1/PD-L1	Kang, Y.K. et al. [82]	RCT (phase 3)	493	Nivolumab or placebo in CT-refractory AGC (ATTRACTION-2 trial)	OS: 5.26 vs. 4.14 months ($p < 0.0001$) PFS: 1.61 vs. 1.45 months ($p < 0.0001$) ORR: 11.2 vs. 0%
	Huang, J. et al. [83]	Phase 1	30	SHR-1210 in recurrent or metastatic GC refractory or intolerant to previous CT	ORR: 23.3%
	Moehler, M. et al. [84]	Phase 3	499	Avelumab vs. chemotherapy after first-line induction chemotherapy in patients with gastric or GEJ cancer	OS: 10.4 vs. 10.9 months ($p = 0.18$) OS in PD-L1(+): 16.2 vs. 17.7 months ($p = 0.64$)
PD-1/PD-L1 HER2	Janjigian, Y.Y. et al. [85]	Phase 2	37	Pembrolizumab + trastuzumab as first-line therapy in HER2(+) metastatic GC	PFS: 70% at 6 months
	Catenacci, D.V. et al. [86]	Phase 1b-2 trial	95	Pembrolizumab + margetuximab in locally advanced or metastatic HER2(+), PD-L1-unselected GE cancer	ORR: 18.48%
PD-1/PD-L1 CTLA-4	Kelly, R.J. et al. [87]	RCT (phase 2)	63	Durvalumab + tremelimumab vs. durvalumab alone vs. tremelimumab alone as scond-line therapy in CT-refractory AGC	OS: 9.2 vs. 3.4 vs. 7.7 months PFS: 1.8 vs. 1.6 vs. 1.7 months ORR: 7.4 vs. 0 vs. 8.3%
CIK-cells	Shi, L. et al. [88]	Non-randomized controlled trial	151	3 cycles of CIK-cell therapy vs. no CIK-cell therapy after curative gastrectomy and adjuvant chemotherapy for gastric adenocarcinoma	Intestinal type— 5-year OS: 46.8 vs. 31.4%, $p = 0.045$ 5-year DFS: 42.4 vs. 15.7%, $p = 0.023$ Diffuse or mixed-type— 5-year OS: 7.4 vs. 7.7%, $p = 0.97$ 5-year DFS: 3.7 vs. 0%, $p = 0.96$

Studies with biomarkers and relevance as to molecular targeted therapies are listed and grouped depending on the targeted biomarker. Study design, patient number, treatment aim, and treatment outcomes including overall survival, progression-free survival and overall response rate, if available, are shown. Abbreviations: AGC—advanced gastric cancer; CIK-cells—cytokine-induced killer cells; CPS—combined positivity score; CT—chemotherapy; DFS—disease-free survival; EGFR—epidermal growth factor receptor; EGJC—esophagogastric junction cancer; FGFR—fibroblast growth factor receptor; GC—gastric cancer; HDAC—histone deacetylase; HER2—human epidermal growth factor receptor 2; HGFR—hepatocyte growth factor receptor; MMP9—matrix metalloproteinase-9; ORR—overall response rate; OS—overall survival; PARP—poly ADP ribose polymerase; PD-1—programmed cell death protein 1; PD-L1—programmed cell death ligand 1; PDGF—platelet-derived growth factor; PFS—progression-free survival; RCT—randomized controlled trial; VEGF—vascular endothelial growth factor.

The use of trastuzumab in combination with paclitaxel in patients with tumor progression after first-line chemotherapy with or without trastuzumab did not show benefit on OS, PFS, and overall response rate (ORR) compared to chemotherapy alone in patients with HER2-positive advanced gastric or GEJ cancer [25,26].

Several phase 2 trials have tested different chemotherapies in combination with trastuzumab as first line therapy in advanced or metastatic gastric or GEJ cancer. Studies that combined trastuzumab and different chemotherapies and treatment outcomes are summarized in Table 1 [27–39].

Pertuzumab, another monoclonal antibody against HER2, was added to first-line trastuzumab and chemotherapy in the JACOB trial, and did not show a significant survival benefit [40,41].

While the irreversible pan-HER inhibitor dacomitinib showed only a limited response [42], poziotinib, another irreversible pan-HER inhibitor targeting EGFR, HER2, and HER4, showed an objective response rate of about 20% [43] (Table 1). The dual blockade with a pan-HER inhibitor and trastuzumab might therefore be a promising strategy in trastuzumab resistance.

Several studies that analyzed the impact of HER2 status on survival and treatment response are listed in Table 2.

Table 2. Biomarkers and their impacts on outcomes.

Biomarker	Study	Design	Patient Number	Aim	Outcome
HER2	Iqbal, S. et al. [44]	Phase 2	47	Lapatinib as first-line therapy in advanced or metastatic GC	HER2(+) vs. HER(−): OS 6.8 vs. 3.0 months ($p = 0.0031$) IL-8 high vs. IL-8 low expression: OS 3.0 vs. 5.6 months ($p = 0.016$)
	Shitara, K. et al. [19]	Prospective observational study	364	Impact of HER2 status and trastuzumab treatment on prognosis of AGC	HER2(+) + trastuzumab vs. HER(−): OS 24.7 vs. 13.9 months ($p = 0.03$) HER2(+) w/o trastuzumab vs. HER2(−): OS 13.5 vs. 13.9 months ($p = 0.091$)
	Okines, A.F. et al. [11]	RCT	415	Prognostic and predictive impact of HER2 status (tissue samples from MAGIC trial)	HER2 status not prognostic and not predictive for response to CT
	Matsumoto, T. et al. [13]	Phase 2	89	HER2 expression in AGC with extensive LNM, correlation between HER2 status and survival	HER2(+) vs. HER2(−): 3-year OS 66.7 vs. 38.7% ($p = 0.022$) Multivariate analysis: HER2 status not prognostic
	Press, M.F. et al. [14]	RCT	487	Screening of adenocarcinoma for HER2-amplification, lapatinib in HER2(+) EG cancer	16.1% HER2 amplification, HER2 amplification levels correlated with PFS ($p = 0.035$), but not with OS
	Feizy, A. et al. [16]	Prospective observational study	210	Association of HER2 expression and survival	No association between HER2 expression and survival ($p = 0.88$)
	Kim, S.T. et al. [89]	Phase 2	32	Capecitabine + oxaliplatin + lapatinib in HER2(+) AGC	High vs. low level HER2 amplification: predictive for treatment response ($p = 0.02$)
	Shah, M.A. et al. [23]	RCT (phase 2/3)	182	Biomarker analysis of the GATSBY study: Trastuzumab emtansine vs. taxane as second-line therapy in HER2-positive AGC	High vs. low HER2 expression associated with longer OS; high HER2 expression predictor of OS

Table 2. Cont.

Biomarker	Study	Design	Patient Number	Aim	Outcome
EGFR HER2	Sanchez-Vega, F. et al. [50]	Phase 2	20	Afatinib in trastuzumab-resistant HER2(+) EG cancer	Treatment response associated with EGFR + HER2 coamplification
EGFR	Luber, B. et al. [90]	Phase 2	39	Cetuximab + oxaliplatin/leucovorin/5-fluorouracil in 1st line metastatic EGJC or GC	Increased EGFR gene copy numbers associated with better OS ($p = 0.011$)
	Moehler, M. et al. [55]	Phase 2	49	Cetuximab + irinotecan/folinic acid/5-FU as first-line therapy of HER2(+) AGC	EGFR-expressing vs. nonexpressing tumors: ORR 84 vs. 23% ($p = 0.041$)
	Zhang, X. et al. [57]	Phase 2	47	Cetuximab + cisplatin/capecitabine in untreated AGC	High vs. low EGFR expression: OS: 16.6 vs. 9.5 months ($p = 0.12$), PFS: 7.1 vs. 4.0 months ($p = 0.078$)
	Liu, X. et al. [58]	Phase 2	61	Cetuximab + modified FOLFIRI in metastatic GC	EGFR(+) vs. EGFR(−): similar ORR and OS
	Stahl, M. et al. [52]	RCT (phase 2)	160	Panitumumab + CT vs. placebo + CT in untreated locally advanced EG cancer	Shorter PFS and OS with EGFR expression
VEGF	Moehler, M. et al. [63]	Phase 2	51	Sunitinib monotherapy in pretreated AGC	VEGF-C expression vs. no expression: PFS: 1.2 vs. 2.9 months ($p = 0.012$)
	Van Cutsem, E. et al. [91]	RCT	774	Bevacizumab + CT vs. placebo + CT (AVAGAST study), correlations between BM and clinical outcomes	Placebo group: baseline low vs. high VEGF-A: OS: 12.9 vs. 8.3 months. Bevacizumab group: baseline high vs. low VEGF-A: higher OS ($p = 0.07$)
	Moehler, M. et al. [64]	RCT (phase 2)	91	Sunitinib + FOLFIRI vs. placebo + FOLFIRI as second- or third-line therapy in AGC	Baseline low vs. high VEGF-A: PFS: 166 vs. 91 days ($p = 0.017$) Baseline low vs. high VEGFR2: PFS: 107 vs. 167 days ($p = 0.044$)
	Liu, X. et al. [58]	Phase 2	61	Cetuximab + modified FOLFIRI in metastatic GC	Low vs. high baseline plasma VEGF: ORR: 55 vs. 5.3% ($p = 0.001$), OS: 12 vs. 5 months ($p < 0.0001$), PFS: 14.0 vs. 6.8 months ($p = 0.035$)
	Van Cutsem, E. et al. [92]	RCT	637	Biomarker analysis from RAINBOW trial (2nd line ramucirumab + CT vs. placebo + CT in AGC)	VEGF not predictive for ramucirumab efficacy.

Table 2. Cont.

Biomarker	Study	Design	Patient Number	Aim	Outcome
FGFR	Kim, S.T. et al. [93]	Phase 2	66	Pazopanib + CT in metastatic or recurrent GC	FGFR2(+) vs. FGFR2(−): PFS: 8.5 vs. 5.6 months ($p = 0.05$) OS: 13.2 vs. 11.4 months ($p = 0.055$) ORR: 85.7 vs. 59.6%
	Won, E. et al. [65]	Phase 2	32	Nintedanib as second-line therapy in metastatic EG cancer	FGFR2(+) vs. FGFR2(−): PFS: 3.5 vs. 1.9 months ($p = 0.92$)
HGFR/MET	Stahl, M. et al. [52]	RCT (phase 2)	160	Panitumumab + CT vs. placebo + CT in untreated locally advanced EG cancer	Shorter PFS and OS with MET expression.
	Sanchez-Vega, F. et al. [50]	Phase 2	20	Afatinib in trastuzumab-resistant HER2(+) EG cancer	Resistance associated with MET amplification.
PD-1/PD-L1	Fuchs, C.S. et al. [78]	Phase 2	259	Pembrolizumab in previously treated unselected AGC (KEYNOTE-059 trial)	PFS: 2.1 vs. 2.0 months in PD-L1(+) vs. PD-L1(−) ORR: 15.5 vs. 6.4% in PD-L1(+) vs. PD-L1(−)
	Kim, S.T. et al. [79]	Phase 2	61	Pembrolizumab in metastatic GC	ORR: 50 vs. 0% in PD-L1(+) vs. PD-L1(−) ($p < 0.001$)
	Wang, F. et al. [81]	Phase 1b/2	76	Toripalimab (chemo-refractory) or Toripalimab + CT (CT-naïve) in AGC	PD-L1 overexpression not associated with survival
	Huang, J. et al. [83]	Phase 1	30	SHR-1210 in recurrent or metastatic GC refractory to CT	ORR: 23.1% in PD-L1(+) and 26.7% in PD-L1(−) ($p = 1.0$)
	Choi, Y.Y. et al. [94]	RCT	592	PD-L1 expression as prognostic and predictive BM (BM study of CLASSIC trial)	Multivariate analysis of DFS: stromal PD-L1 independent prognostic factors ($p = 0.044$)

Studies with biomarkers and their impacts on outcomes are shown. Studies are grouped depending on the biomarker. Study design, patient number, treatment or study aim, and outcomes including overall survival, progression-free survival, and overall response rate, if available, are shown. Only biomarkers that have already been addressed by targeted therapies (Table 1) are shown. Abbreviations: AGC—advanced gastric cancer; CT—chemotherapy; DFS—disease-free survival; EGFR—epidermal growth factor receptor; EG—esophagogastric; EGJC—esophagogastric junction cancer; FGFR—fibroblast growth factor receptor; GC—gastric cancer; HDAC—histone deacetylase; HER2—human epidermal growth factor receptor 2; HGFR—hepatocyte growth factor receptor; LNM—lymph node metastasis; MMP9—matrix metalloproteinase-9; ORR—overall response rate; OS—overall survival; PARP—poly ADP ribose polymerase; PD-1—programmed cell death protein 1; PD-L1—programmed cell death ligand 1; PDGF—platelet-derived growth factor; PFS—progression-free survival; RCT—randomized controlled trial; TGF-a—transforming growth factor-alpha; VEGF—vascular endothelial growth factor.

Taken together, the HER2 status itself without associated treatment has no direct impact on survival in patients with advanced GC, and is therefore not a prognostic factor [11,13,16]. Nevertheless, HER2 has shown to be a predictive biomarker, as high HER2 expression is associated with better treatment response [23,89]. Furthermore, HER2 expression is associated with longer survival in patients with advanced GC following HER2-directed treatment [19,44].

Treatment response to the tyrosine kinase inhibitor afatinib is associated with EGFR and HER2 coamplification [50].

2.2. Epidermal Growth Factor Receptor

Epidermal growth factor receptor (EGFR) overexpression is reported in 27–55% of GC, and it is associated with shortened overall survival by multivariate analysis [51].

Lapatinib is a dual tyrosine kinase inhibitor that blocks both the HER2 and epidermal growth factor receptor (EGFR) pathways. In a phase 2 trial, lapatinib was tested as first-line single therapy in metastatic GC and showed only modest activity, with a PFS of 1.9 months and an ORR of 9% (Table 1) [44]. Addition of lapatinib has not proven to be superior to conventional chemotherapy in terms of OS and PFS, neither in first- nor in second-line treatment of advanced GC [45–48]. In a phase 2 trial with lapatinib and capecitabine as first-line treatment, lapatinib induced no changes in gene expression, and no associations between single nucleotide polymorphisms and treatment outcome were found [49].

Panitumumab, a monoclonal antibody to EGFR, has shown no advantage in terms of histological response, OS, and PFS in patients with untreated advanced esophageal, gastric, or GEJ cancer when added to conventional first-line chemotherapy, compared to chemotherapy alone (Table 1) [51,52].

Similarly, nimotuzumab, also a monoclonal antibody to EGFR, in combination with irinotecan has shown no superiority in PFS compared to irinotecan alone as second-line therapy in advanced GC (Table 1). Interestingly, there was a trend toward better response rate, OS, and PFS with nimotuzumab in the subgroup with high EGFR expression levels [53].

Cetuximab, another monoclonal antibody directed against EGFR, is primarily known as a treatment in metastatic colorectal cancer. Several nonrandomized phase 2 trials without a control group have investigated cetuximab in combination with conventional chemotherapy. As a first-line treatment, overall response rates (ORR) between 45 and 65%, PFS between 5 and 9 months, and OS between 9 and 17 months have been reported (Table 1) [54,55,57]. In the randomized EXPAND trial, cetuximab was tested in combination with capecitabine and cisplatin compared to chemotherapy alone in previously untreated advanced GC without any survival benefit [56]. As a second-line therapy, addition of cetuximab to conventional chemotherapy has shown more limited treatment response (Table 1) [58].

Studies analyzing the impact of EGFR expression on survival and treatment response showed inconsistent results (Table 2). EGFR expression was associated with better OS and a higher response rate in advanced GC under EGFR-directed therapy [55,90], while other studies showed no impact of EGFR expression on survival and treatment response [57,58]. Taken together, it remains unclear if EGFR is a prognostic or predictive biomarker.

2.3. Vascular Endothelial Growth Factor

Vascular endothelial growth factor (VEGF) plays a role in pathogenesis and progression of GC.

Ramucirumab, a monoclonal antibody that binds to VEGF receptor-2, was tested in the RAINBOW trial in combination with paclitaxel. This was a randomized placebo-controlled and double-blind study of 665 patients with advanced gastric or GEJ cancer with disease progression on or after first-line chemotherapy. Compared to paclitaxel alone, overall survival was significantly longer with ramucirumab (Table 1) [59].

Bevacizumab, a monoclonal antibody to VEGF, was tested in the AVAGAST study in untreated patients with advanced GC. Adding bevacizumab to chemotherapy did not improve OS, but led to a longer PFS and higher ORR compared to chemotherapy alone [60]. Meulendijks et al. investigated the efficacy of bevacizumab in combination with chemotherapy in untreated advanced gastric and GEJ cancer in two phase 2 trials without a control group. In HER2-negative patients PFS was 8.3 months and OS was 12 months, while in HER2-positive patients, a combination of trastuzumab and bevacizumab led to a PFS of 10.8 months and an OS of 17.9 months (see Table 1) [61,62].

Sunitinib, a tyrosine kinase inhibitor targeting platelet-derived growth factor (PDGF) receptor and VEGFR, was tested as monotherapy in pretreated patients with advanced

GC. It was associated with very limited tumor response (Table 1) [63]. Sunitinib did not improve PFS or response as an adjunct to FOLFIRI compared to FOLFIRI alone in chemotherapy-resistant GC [64].

Foretinib, another multikinase inhibitor targeting MET and VEGFR-2, lacked efficacy in metastatic GC [95].

Several studies have analyzed the impact of VEGF on survival in advanced GC (Table 2). They consistently showed a negative association between VEGF levels and survival, indicating that VEGF is a negative prognostic biomarker [58,63,64,91]. In a biomarker study from the RAINBOW trial, all analyzed biomarkers including VEGF were not predictive for ramucirumab efficacy [92].

2.4. Fibroblast Growth Factor Receptor

Won et al. tested the efficacy of a combined inhibition of VEGF receptors 1–3, PDGF receptor, and fibroblast growth factor receptor (FGFR) 1–3 with the tyrosine-kinase inhibitor nintedanip. In patients with metastatic esophageal or GEJ adenocarcinoma and disease progression on first-line chemotherapy, treatment with nintedanip showed no partial or complete response (Table 1) [65].

The selective FGFR 1–3 tyrosine kinase inhibitor AZD4547 was tested as a second-line therapy in patients with advanced GC in the randomized controlled SHINE study, and did not improve PFS compared to paclitaxel (Table 1) [66].

The prognostic value of FGFR was analyzed in advanced GC treated with multikinase inhibitors (Table 2). FGFR2 expression was a significant prognostic factor for PFS with pazopanib, while there was only a trend to better PFS with nintedanip [65,93].

2.5. Hepatocyte Growth Factor Receptor

Hepatocyte growth factor receptor (HGFR), also called c-Mesenchymal-Epithelial Transition (MET), is a tyrosine kinase receptor. MET overexpression is highly heterogenous and uncommon in GC by immunohistochemistry [96].

The MET signaling pathway plays an integral role in GC. An aberrant, overactivated MET pathway promotes disease progression, and serves as a common mechanism of resistance to HER-targeted therapy. Beyond anti-HER2 therapy, the MET pathway seems to be a culprit of cancer invasiveness, with MET-overexpressing tumors having poorer prognosis [97].

Rilotumumab, a monoclonal antibody to MET, was tested against placebo in combination with chemotherapy in advanced or metastatic gastric or GEJ adenocarcinoma without testing MET status. PFS was longer with rilotumumab (Table 1) [67]. Zhu and colleagues found that high rilotumumab exposure was associated with better PFS compared to low exposure and placebo among patients with MET-positive tumors (Table 1) [68]. A randomized phase 3 trial testing rilotumumab against placebo in combination with chemotherapy was stopped early due to higher mortality in the rilotumumab group (Table 1) [69]. MET positivity was defined in both trials as 25% or more of membranous staining of tumor cells in IHC.

Several other tyrosine kinase inhibitors targeting the HGF/MET pathway were studied in MET-positive gastric cancer, but no substantial benefit was proven [98]. Thus, onartuzumab was tested in a phase 3 trial against placebo in combination with chemotherapy in HER2-negative, MET-positive gastroesophageal cancer and showed no improvement in survival or response rates (Table 1) [70].

MET expression has been shown to be a prognostic factor in locally advanced gastric and GEJ cancer treated with chemotherapy and panitumumab, as it was associated with shorter PFS and OS (Table 2) [52]. Resistance to the kinase inhibitor afatinib was associated with MET amplification in advanced GC (Table 2) [50]. Hence, MET might be predictive for decreased treatment response.

2.6. Claudin 18.2

In normal tissue, the tight junction molecule Claudin 18.2 is only expressed on the membrane of differentiated epithelial cells of the gastric mucosa. Its expression is activated in primary and GC and GC metastases, but also in malignancies of the pancreas, esophagus, ovaries, and the lung [98]. Claudin 18.2 expression is found in 77–87% of primary GC, and in 51–80% of lymph node metastasis [98,99]. The exclusive expression of Claudin 18.2 in differentiated gastric cells, in combination with the fact that transient gastrointestinal toxicity is a frequent and manageable adverse event, makes this molecule highly attractive as a target for the development of safe and potent drugs [98].

The monoclonal antibody zolbetuximab targets Claudin 18.2. In the FAST trial, patients with advanced gastric, GEJ, or esophageal adenocarcinoma and with moderate-to-strong Claudin 18.2 expression in ≥40% of tumor cells received chemotherapy with or without zolbetuximab. Patients treated with zolbetuximab had significantly higher PFS and OS, with an even more pronounced difference in the subpopulation with very high Claudin 18.2 expression (Table 1) [71]. The ongoing SPOTLIGHT study compares the effect of zolbetuximab against placebo in combination with chemotherapy as a first-line therapy in Claudin-18.2-positive and HER-2-negative advanced gastric or GEJ cancer [100].

2.7. Ataxia Teleangiectasia Mutated

Ataxia telangiectasia mutated (ATM) is a key activator of DNA damage response. GC cell lines with low levels of ATM are sensitive to the poly ADP ribose polymerase (PARP) inhibitor olaparib, which prevents tumor cells from repairing DNA damage from chemotherapy. Olaparib was tested against placebo in combination with paclitaxel in patients with metastatic GC and showed improved OS in both the overall population and the population with low ATM levels, but no difference in PFS or response rates (Table 1) [72].

2.8. AKT

Ipatasertib is a small molecule inhibitor of AKT, a key component of the PI3K/AKT pathway. When tested in a randomized controlled trial in combination with FOLFOX6 against placebo, it did not improve PFS. No benefit was observed in biomarker-selected patients (PTEN-low, PI3K/AKT-activated tumors) [73].

2.9. Histone Deacetylase

Vorinostat, an inhibitor of histone deacetylase (HDAC), was investigated in combination with capecitabine and cisplatin as a first-line chemotherapy in advanced GC, and showed an ORR of 42% and a 6-month PFS rate of 44%. As in a previous phase 3 study with capecitabine and cisplatin with a 6-month PFS rate of 40%, the addition of vorinostat was not likely to enhance efficacy. A biomarker analysis using Western blotting included plasma levels of atecyl-H3, HDAC2, and p21. None of these three biomarkers correlated with PFS, but high baseline acetyl-H3 and p21 were significantly associated with worse OS [74].

2.10. Matrix Metalloproteinase-9

Matrix metalloproteinases are proteases involved in degradation and remodeling of the extracellular matrix and basement membranes. Matrix metalloproteinase-9 (MMP9), which is expressed heterogeneously by tumor epithelia and infiltrating inflammatory cells, has been associated with loss-of-tumor suppression activity, as well as oncogenic activity [75].

Andecaliximab, a monoclonal antibody targeting MMP9, showed encouraging results in a phase 2 trial, but failed to show improved OS in the ensuing randomized GAMMA-1 trial (Table 1) [76].

2.11. Immunotherapy

Programmed cell death protein 1 (PD-1) is located at the surface of immune cells, and functions as an immune checkpoint by regulating the immune response. Programmed cell death ligand 1 (PD-L1) binds to PD-1 and inhibits the immune response through inhibition of T-cell receptor-mediated lymphocyte proliferation and cytokine secretion, among other mechanisms [101]. PD-L1 expression is measured with IHC, and PD-L1 positivity is defined as a combined positivity score (CPS) ≥ 1, where CPS is the number of PD-L1-positive cells (tumor cells, lymphocytes, and macrophages) divided by the total number of viable tumor cells, multiplied by 100 [102].

In the molecular evaluation of gastric adenocarcinoma as part of the TCGA project, PD-L1/2 expression was elevated in EBV-positive tumors, suggesting that PD-L1/2 antagonists should be tested in this subgroup [7]. This was confirmed by Liu and colleagues, who found PD-L1 expression significantly associated with MSI, EBV-positive, and H. pylori status. There was a greater proportion of PD-L1 CPS ≥ 1 tumors among MSI-H versus microsatellite stable (MSS), EBV-positive versus EBV-negative, and H. pylori-positive as compared to H. pylori-negative tumors. PD-L1 CPS ≥ 1 was observed in 49.7% of EBV-negative and MSS tumors [102].

Pembrolizumab, a monoclonal antibody to PD-1, was tested in the phase 1b KEYNOTE-012 trial in patients with PD-L1-positive recurrent or metastatic gastric or GEJ adenocarcinoma, and showed an objective response rate of 22% and a rate of grade 3–4 treatment-related adverse events of 13% [77]. In the following phase 2 KEYNOTE-059 trial, pembrolizumab was tested in 259 patients with disease progression after two or more lines of chemotherapy. PD-L1 expression was assessed in tumor biopsy samples by immunohistochemistry. Tumors were considered PD-L1 positive if the combined positive score (number of PD-L1-positive cells including tumor cells, macrophages, and lymphocytes divided by the total number of tumor cells, multiplied by 100) was 1 or greater. Response to pembrolizumab treatment was observed in both PD-L1-positive and -negative tumors, but was higher in patients with PD-L1-positive compared to PD-L1-negative tumors (15.5 vs. 6.4%, $p = 0.02$). There was no difference in OS between patients with PD-L1-positive and PD-L1-negative tumors (5.8 vs. 4.9 months) (Table 1) [78].

Kim et al. observed very high ORR with pembrolizumab in patients with MSI-high (85.7%) and EBV-positive (100%) metastatic GC [79]. These results were in line with higher immunogenicity of MSI or virally induced tumors in other localizations, such as gynecologic malignancies [103].

More recently Kawazoe et al. tested pembrolizumab in combination with the oral fluorouracil derivate S-1 plus oxaliplatin as a first-line treatment in patients with PD-L1-positive and HER2-negative advanced gastric or GEJ cancer, and observed high ORR (Table 1) [80].

A recent single-arm phase 2 trial investigated the combination of pembrolizumab with a HER2-targeting antibody as a proof of concept of synergistic antitumor activity. Janjigian et al. tested trastuzumab and pembrolizumab plus conventional chemotherapy as a first-line therapy in HER2-positive metastatic gastric or GEJ cancer. The PFS at 6 months was 70% [85]. The combination of pembrolizumab and trastuzumab is currently being further tested in the ongoing KEYNOTE-811 randomized controlled trial [104].

Margetuximab, a novel anti-HER2 monoclonal antibody, was evaluated in a single-arm phase 1b-2 trial in combination with pembrolizumab in HER2-positive, PD-L1-unselected gastric or GEJ cancer on progression after chemotherapy with trastuzumab. This phase 1b/2 trial showed a considerable ORR of 18.5%. This study confirmed that combined targeting of HER2 and PD-1/PD-L1 could yield antitumor activity greater than that with either approach alone [86].

The anti-PD-L1 antibody durvalumab and the anti-CTLA-4 antibody tremelimumab were tested alone or in combination in patients with chemotherapy-refractory gastric or GEJ cancer. ORR and PFS were low and did not differ between treatment arms (Table 1) [87].

Toripalimab, a monoclonal antibody to PD-1, was given as monotherapy in a group of patients with chemo-refractory GC, and in combination with chemotherapy in a group of chemotherapy-naïve patients. With toripalimab, monotherapy ORR was 12.1%, while in combination with chemotherapy, the ORR was 66.7% (Table 1) [81].

In the ATTRACTION-2 trial, the PD-1 antibody nivolumab was tested against placebo in patients with advanced gastric or GEJ cancer refractory to two or more regimens of chemotherapy. OS was significantly longer with nivolumab compared to placebo at 2-year follow-up. The authors concluded that nivolumab might be a new treatment option for heavily pretreated patients with advanced gastric or GEJ cancer (Table 1) [82].

The CheckMate 577 trial showed that Nivolumab was efficient as an adjuvant treatment in patients with resected esophageal or GEJ cancer who had received neoadjuvant chemoradiotherapy and had residual pathological disease. Disease-free survival was 22.4 months with nivolumab compared to 11 months with placebo ($p < 0.001$) [105].

The JAVELIN Gastric 100 trial, which tested the PD-L1 antibody avelumab against chemotherapy maintenance after first-line induction chemotherapy in locally advanced or metastatic gastric or GEJ cancer, showed no superior OS with avelumab, both in an overall and PD-L1-positive population [84].

The anti-PD-1 antibody SHR-1210 was tested as a second-line treatment in advanced GC, and showed an ORR of 26.7% [83].

Studies analyzing treatment outcome dependent on PD-L1 status are shown in Table 2. ORR was higher in patients with PD-L1-positive (defined as a combined positive score of 1 or greater) compared to PD-L1-negative tumors treated with pembrolizumab [78,79]. Furthermore, PD-L1 positivity was independently associated with longer disease-free survival, regardless of PD-L1-directed treatment [94].

There was no association of PD-L1 expression with treatment outcome in advanced GC treated with toripalimab and SHR-1210 [81,83].

In conclusion, PD-L1 is a prognostic biomarker and predictive for response to pembrolizumab therapy. Based on the results of the KEYNOTE-059 trial, pembrolizumab was approved by the U.S. Food and Drug Administration (FDA) for the treatment of patients with recurrent, locally advanced, or metastatic gastric or GEJ adenocarcinoma with disease progression on or after two or more systemic therapies, and whose tumors express PD-L1 [78,106]. As mentioned above, there might be a role of combined targeting of HER2 and PD-1/PD-L1. The recently published CheckMate 577 trial showed that nivolumab is also highly efficient as an adjuvant treatment in patients at risk for recurrence, regardless of PD-L1 expression [105]. Therefore, the main role of immunotherapy may be to prevent recurrence, rather than to treat metastatic or advanced disease in the future.

Adjuvant immunotherapy with autologous cytokine-induced killer cells has been assessed in a nonrandomized study for patients after gastrectomy and subsequent chemotherapy for locally advanced GC. Compared to a control group without immunotherapy, patients treated with cytokine-induced killer cells had longer 5-year disease-free survival. For patients with intestinal-type tumors, OS and disease-free survival were significantly higher for patients with immunotherapy. Subgroup analysis of patients with diffuse or mixed-type tumors showed no survival benefit from adjuvant immunotherapy (Table 1) [88].

3. Diagnostic and Potential Target Biomarkers

3.1. DNA Methylation and Gene Expression

DNA methylation is an epigenetic mechanism leading to carcinogenesis in GC through silencing of tumor-suppressor genes and activation of oncogenes [107].

Pirini et al. found lower global DNA methylation levels in endoscopic biopsies with gastric cancer than in those with gastritis [108].

DNA methylation in the long interspersed nucleotide element-1 (*LINE-1*) is a good indicator of global DNA methylation. *LINE-1* methylation has been shown to be lower in GC tissue than in matched noncancerous gastric mucosa. In addition, analysis of *LINE-1* methylation in GC specimens of 203 patients revealed that *LINE-1* hypomethylation was significantly associated with lower OS [109].

Reprimo-like (*RPRML*) is a member of the reprimo gene family that is a group of poorly understood single-exon intronless genes, and whose loss of expression is related to increased cell proliferation and growth in gastric cancer [110]. Alarcon and colleagues observed that circulating methylated *RPRML* DNA in plasma samples significantly distinguished patients with GC from cancer-free controls, and that downregulation of *RPRML* expression was associated with poor survival in advanced GC [111].

Bcl-2 homologous antagonist killer (BAK) is a protein belonging to the BCL2 family and encoded by the *BAK1* gene. BAK promotes cell death by apoptosis. Kubo et al. showed that higher BAK protein expression in gastric cancer is associated with better chemotherapeutic histopathological response to docetaxel, and with longer survival [112].

The tumor-suppressor characteristics of cyclin-dependent kinase 10 (CDK10) have been demonstrated in nasopharyngeal carcinoma and breast cancer. You et al. investigated the expression status of CDK10 and its prognostic significance in GC. They found that CDK10 protein expression was decreased in GC, and loss of CDK10 expression correlated with advanced tumor stage and unfavorable OS. CDK10 protein expression was an independent predictor for survival [113].

The role of breast cancer 1 (*BRCA1*) gene expression by IHC in sporadic gastric cancer was investigated by Kim et al. They found reduced expression of the *BRCA1* gene associated with more advanced-stage disease, perineural invasion, and decreased disease-free survival. *BRCA1* nuclear expression < 5% was predictive for the benefit of adjuvant chemotherapy [114].

Li et al. investigated genotypic distribution of toll-like receptor 4 (*TLR4*) gene polymorphisms in Chinese patients with GC and patients with atrophic gastritis. The *TLR4-2081G/A* gene polymorphism was negatively associated with occurrence of GC, indicating an influence on GC risk [115].

Alterations of deubiquitinating enzymes have been discussed in the pathogenesis of various tumors [116]. Expression of ubiquitin-specific protease 42 (USP42) mRNA was demonstrated to be higher in GC than in nontumorous tissues, and correlated with tumor size, TNM stage, lymph node metastasis, and OS of patients with GC [116]. The expression of proteasome-associated deubiquitinating enzyme UCHL5 was analyzed in a large cohort study of 650 patients with GC undergoing surgery. Positive UCHL5 protein expression was associated with better survival in the subgroup of patients with tumors <5 cm, disease stages I-II, and age 66 years or older [117].

Two studies investigated the role of biomarkers in treatment of patients with advanced GC refractory to chemotherapy with the mechanistic target of rapamycin (mTOR) inhibitor everolimus, which inhibits the ability of mTOR to phosphorylate the ribosomal protein S6, and thereby inhibits cell-cycle progression. Both studies found high expression of phospho-S6 ribosomal protein (Ser240/4) associated with better clinical response or stable disease, and prolonged PFS [118,119].

The excision repair cross-complementing gene 1 (ERCC1) is a key enzyme in the nucleotide excision repair pathway that serves as a DNA repair mechanism. High expression of ERCC1 mRNA in endoscopic biopsies of primary GC was shown to be associated with poor prognosis, and was an independent prognostic factor for OS [120]. Several potential predictive factors of the response to 5-fluorouracil (5-FU) or prognostic factors have been reported in the metabolic pathway of 5-FU and folic acid. These include thymidylate synthase (TS) and the cytosolic enzyme dihydropyrimidine dehydrogenase (DPD). High mRNA expression of TS and DPD has been shown to predict a poor clinical outcome of treatment with 5-FU [120].

Tsuburaya et al. analyzed mRNA expression of TS, DPD, topoisomerase I, ERCC1, and thymidine phosphorylase (TP) in tumor specimens of 126 patients with advanced GC. In patients treated with S-1 plus irinotecan compared to S-1 alone, low TS, low ERCC1, and high TP mRNA levels were associated with a better prognosis [121].

Sasako et al. analyzed expression of genes involved in pyrimidine metabolism, TS, DPD, TP, and orotate phosphoribosyltransferase (OPRT). Expression of these genes was determined in patients enrolled in a trial testing S-1 as an adjuvant chemotherapy for gastric cancer. Results showed that high TS and DPD expression were associated with a better OS, whereas TP and OPRT expression were not associated with survival [122].

Hirakawa et al. analyzed protein expression of damage DNA binding protein complex subunit 2 (DDB2), which serves as an initial damage recognition factor during nucleotide excision repair, and ERCC1 by IHC in tumor tissues pretreated with the combination chemotherapy of docetaxel, cisplatin, and the oral fluorouracil derivate S-1. High expression of DDB2 and ERCC1 was more frequent in tissues of nonresponders compared to responders (p = 0.0065 and p = 0.029, respectively). The authors showed that a combination of DDB2 and ERCC1 expression could predict response or nonresponse to chemotherapy in 82.5% [123].

3.2. Multiple Gene Expression Signatures

With next-generation sequencing (NGS), valuable tools to study GC at the molecular level have been developed. With multiomics data from genome, transcriptome, proteome, and epigenome levels, GC can be stratified to subtypes and correlated to therapeutic outcomes [124].

Roh et al. performed a biomarker analysis on tumor samples collected from the CLASSIC trial that compared capecitabine plus oxaliplatin-based adjuvant chemotherapy to surgery alone after D2 gastrectomy [125]. The authors developed a single patient classifier (SPC) assay using a combination of gene expression of nine genes, MSI status, and EBV association to predict prognosis and responsiveness of adjuvant chemotherapy [126]. In this study, the SPC-assay score and MSI status were independent prognostic factors for disease-free survival (DFS), while EBV status was not a prognostic factor [127].

Smyth et al. analyzed 200 genes by mRNA expression from tissue samples from the MAGIC trial, in which patients had been pretreated with chemotherapy [128]. They developed a seven-gene signature assay allowing stratification of patients into two risk groups according to survival. Median OS in the high- and low-risk groups were 10.2 and 80.9 months, respectively. Risk groups and lymph node metastases (LNMs) were independent prognostic factors for OS. In patients treated with surgery only from the MAGIC trial, none of the seven genes were associated with OS. Therefore, the seven-gene signature assay might help to predict prognosis in pretreated gastric, lower esophageal, or GEJ cancer patients [129].

Sundar et al. analyzed tissue samples from patients with metastatic GC that were treated with a PD-1 inhibitor. They measured alternate promoter utilization, an epigenetic phenomenon that might be associated with immune evasion in early GC. High alternate promoter utilization was found in 33% of GC, and was associated with a lower response rate and survival. They concluded that alternate promoter utilization is a potential mechanism of resistance to immune checkpoint inhibition and a novel predictive biomarker for immunotherapy [130].

Li and colleagues performed a multiomics characterization of molecular features of GC. They performed whole-genome, whole-exome, and RNA sequencing on tumor samples from 35 GC patients before and after undergoing neoadjuvant chemotherapy. Increased MSI and mutational burden were observed in nonresponse tumors, indicating that MSI-H status may serve as a predictive marker for nonresponse to neoadjuvant chemotherapy [131]. These results were in line with previous studies indicating that MSI-H status and mismatch repair (MMR) deficiency were associated with less benefit from chemotherapy. Furthermore, a significant positive prognostic effect of MSI-H status for patients with resected gastric cancer without chemotherapy has been shown [132]. On the other hand, strong immunogenicity and widespread expression of immune-checkpoint ligands make the MSI subtype more vulnerable to the immunotherapeutic approach [133]. After analysis of individual mutated genes, only mutations of the *C10orf71* gene were associated with treatment resistance. Analysis of somatic copy number alterations revealed that amplification of the *MYC* gene, a proto-oncogene, was associated with better response to chemotherapy, while amplification of another proto-oncogene, MDM2, was associated with nonresponse [131].

Biopsies from untreated advanced gastric, GEJ, or esophageal adenocarcinoma from the REAL3 trial were assessed for *KRAS*, *BRAF*, and *PIK3CA* mutations, and *PTEN* expression. In the REAL3 trial, the therapeutic efficacy of the EGFR-antibody panitumumab was assessed in combination with chemotherapy, and showed no increase in OS [52]. Furthermore, these biomarkers were assessed in patients from the MAGIC trial. Here, peri-operative epirubicin, cisplatin, and 5-fluorouracil improved survival in patients with resectable lower esophageal, gastric, or GEJ adenocarcinoma [128]. None of the tested biomarkers predicted resistance to treatment combined with panitumumab from the REAL3 trial, or were associated with survival in patients from the MAGIC trial [134].

The NanoString gene expression system captures and counts individual mRNA transcripts by direct measurement of mRNA expression levels without enzymatic reactions or bias [135]. Das et al. used the NanoString gene expression platform to analyze 105 gastric tumors from a randomized cohort that was treated with irinotecan plus S-1 (IRI-S) versus S-1 alone [121]. Increased expression level of CD14 was significantly associated with a younger age of patients. Expression levels of the chemokines CCL5 and CXCL12 were high in the diffuse type of GC. Increased mRNA expression of *ADAMTS1*, *CCL19*, and *CXCL12* was associated with peritoneal metastasis, suggesting that these genes related to the tumor microenvironment may play a significant role in tumor progression. Elevated expression levels of the *DPYD* gene, encoding the pyrimidine catabolic enzyme in the 5-FU pathway, was associated with a younger patient age and the diffuse type of GC. Higher expression of *Wnt5A* and lower expression of *PTRF* were associated with unresectable GC and measurable lesions, respectively. *Wnt5A* downregulation was identified as a predictor of improved PFS in S-1 but not in IRI-S treatment [136].

Microarrays of biopsies from advanced GC patients before chemotherapy were used to identify biomarkers for predicting efficacy of S-1, cisplatin, and docetaxel combinatory chemotherapy. A four-gene signature was identified, including platelet-derived growth factor subunit B (*PDGFB*), polycomb group ring finger 3 (*PCGF3*), cytokine-inducible SH2-containing protein (*CISH*), and annexin A5 (*ANXA5*). *PDGFB* plays an essential role in the regulation of cell proliferation. *PCGF3* is related to the signaling pathways regulating pluripotency of stem cells. *CISH* acts as regulator of cytokine signal transduction. *ANXA5* encodes an anticoagulant protein acting as indirect inhibitor of the thromboplastin-specific complex. These four genes identified early- and nonresponders to chemotherapy with an accuracy of 100%, and hence may serve as markers for efficacy of chemotherapy [137].

3.3. Noncoding RNA

Different noncoding RNAs, such as long noncoding RNA (lncRNA), circular RNA (circRNA), and microRNA (miRNA), are involved in GC development [138].

The HOX transcript antisense intergenic RNA (HOTAIR), an lncRNA, has shown to play an important role during GC tumorigenesis [139]. Du and colleagues investigated genetic variations of HOTAIR and association with GC risk. They found the single nucleotide polymorphism rs4759314 to be significantly associated with increased GC risk [140].

lncRNA and miRNA have been shown to be involved in GC progression: MiRNAs function through regulation of gene expression, and their dysregulated expression has been linked to tumor development and progression [141].

MiR-34 is downregulated in GC, and has been identified as a tumor suppressor in GC [142]. Pan et al. analyzed the role of miR-34 polymorphisms in GC risk. They found that the genotype miR-34b/c rs 44938723 might have a protective effect on GC risk [143]. Mu and colleagues identified miR-193b and miR-196a as promising prognostic markers in GC [144].

MiR-26a was found to be downregulated in GC, and decreased miR-26a expression correlated with poor clinical prognosis. It was suggested that miR-26a functions as a tumor suppressor in GC development and progression, and might be a prognostic biomarker and potential therapeutic target [145].

Malhotra et al. examined 1032 microRNAs expressed in 29 cases of previously untreated advanced esophagogastric cancer. They could not identify an association between tumor epithelial microRNA expression and disease progression [146].

Ahn et al. found specific miRNA single-nucleotide polymorphisms associated with GC susceptibility and prognosis in the Korean population depending on diffuse- or intestinal-type GC [147].

A systematic review identified eight consistently upregulated miRNAs (miR-21, miR-223, miR-18a, miR-214, miR-93, miR-25, miR-106b, and miR-191) and five miRNAs that were consistently downregulated (miR-375, miR-564, miR-155, miR-148a, and miR-92) in GC. Furthermore, miR-940 and the combination of miR-21, miR-93, miR-106a, and miR-106b were identified as a diagnostic biomarker for GC, while miR-204 and miR-15a were associated with poor survival in GC [148].

Another study investigated whether circRNA is involved in pathological processes of GC. The authors found circRNA Has_circ_0000745 was downregulated in GC tissues and in plasma from patients with GC. Therefore, its expression level in plasma in combination with the CEA level might be a promising diagnostic marker for GC [149].

3.4. Protein Expression

The adhesion molecule cadherin-17 (CDH17) is a potential marker for GC. It has been shown to be upregulated in GC, and higher expression by IHC was associated with poorer OS [150].

Human leucocyte antigen (HLA)-G expression, which is primarily seen in the placenta and induces immune tolerance in pregnancy, has been reported in several human cancers, including GC. HLA-G may represent one of the ways tumor cells escape immunosurveillance. Immunohistochemistry in 52 GC patients showed that HLA-G-positive tumors were associated with poorer OS than HLA-G-negative tumors, and HLA-G expression was an independent predictor of OS [151].

Di Bartolomeo et al. found osteopontin overexpression by IHC to be associated with a higher risk of tumor recurrence and metastases in radically resected GC. Osteopontin overexpression was an independent prognostic factor for PFS and OS [152].

Similarly, caveolin-1 expression was associated with progression and poor prognosis in GC patients after radical gastrectomy [153].

The prognostic value of 2,3-dioxygenase in GC was analyzed by Liu and colleagues: 2,3-dioxygenase expression in GC tissue after gastrectomy was an independent prognostic factor, and high expression was associated with poor OS [154].

Expression of stromal monocarboxylate transporter 4 (MCT4), a plasma membrane transporter, and the enzyme carbonic anhydrase IX have been investigated in GC specimens of 143 patients. High stromal MCT4 expression was found in 50.3% and high carbonic anhydrase IX in 51.7% of patients. High stromal MCT and carbonic anhydrase IX expression were correlated with advanced TNM stage. High stromal MCT expression was an independent predictor of poor OS and DFS. Contrarily, carbonic anhydrase IX expression was not predictive for survival [155].

Somatostatin receptor subtype 2A (SSTR2A) and human epidermal growth factor receptor 2 (HER2) expression in GC tissues of 51 patients were analyzed by Romiti et al. They observed SSTR2A expression in 74.5% of patients with a predominance in well and moderately differentiated GC. HER2 expression, which was positive in 35% of patients, was associated with SSTR2 expression in 95% of all HER2+ cases [156].

Autocrine motility factor receptor (AMFR) is a cell-surface cytokine receptor that is involved in numerous physiological and pathological processes, including cell motility, signal transduction, and protein ubiquitination [157]. Huang et al. investigated the expression of AMFR in GC and its clinical significance. AMFR expression, which was positive in 59.8% of GC, was associated with invasion depth and LNM, and reduced OS. AMFR expression was also an independent predictor for OS and DFS. Therefore, expression of AMFR was a risk factor for poor prognosis in GC patients after resection [157].

The proteins C-X-C chemokine receptor type 4 (CXCR-4) and VEGF receptor-3 have been identified as potential new biomarkers for advanced esophagogastric carcinoma associated with lymphangiogenesis, invasion, and metastasis [158]. Thomaidis et al. analyzed the expression levels of CXCR-4 and VEGF receptor-3 in 72 patients with advanced gastric or GEJ cancer treated with fluorouracil, leucovorin, and either oxaliplatin (FLO) or cisplatin (FLP). Patients with strong expression of CXCR-4 end VEGF receptor-3 showed a trend toward better OS when treated with FPL. In contrast, patients with weak CXCR-4 and VEGF receptor-3 expression had significantly better OS when treated with FLO [158].

The protein trefoil factor 3 (TFF3) is normally not expressed in gastric mucosa, while it may be detected in cases of GC [159]. TFF3 expression in GC correlates with the occurrences of lymph node metastasis, muscularis propria invasion ($\geq$T2), worse TNM stage, and histological type, which indicates that TFF3 may be an adverse factor in GC progression and metastasis [159].

The cytokine macrophage migration inhibitory factor (MIF) is highly expressed in various tumors, including GC, and stimulates proliferation and inhibits apoptosis in cancer cells [160]. He and colleagues observed higher MIF expression in GC compared to adjacent normal tissue, and showed that MIF expression was an independent prognostic factor for poor patient survival, as well as advanced clinical stage [160].

3.5. Serum Biomarkers

Serum biomarkers are usually analyzed by enzyme-linked immunosorbent assay (ELISA). However, ELISA tests have limited detection sensitivity ($\geq$1 pM), which is insufficiently sensitive for the detection of small amounts of biomarkers in the early stages of disease or infection [161].

Angiopoietin-2 is a key driver of tumor angiogenesis. Its prognostic and predictive role was assessed retrospectively in a biomarker study of the AVAGAST trial, which had shown improved PFS but not OS with addition of bevacizumab to conventional chemotherapy in patients with advanced GC [60]. Low baseline plasma levels of angiopoietin-2 were associated with longer OS (13.7 vs. 10 months, p = 0.0055). While baseline angiopoietin-2 was an independent prognostic marker for OS, angiopoietin-2 levels did not predict efficacy of bevacizumab [162].

Serum pepsinogen is an established marker of chronic atrophic gastritis. Its predictive value for the development of GC was studied in the Hisayama study, which followed 2446 community-dwelling Japanese aged 40 or older for 10 years who underwent a screening examination regardless of previous history of gastritis. The authors found a serum pepsinogen I level of 59 ng/mL or less and a pepsinogen I/II ratio of 3.9 or less as most predictive for GC development, independently from H. pylori infection status and history of peptic ulcer [163]. Although various cut-off values have been suggested, pepsinogen I $\leq$70 ng/mL and pepsinogen I/II ratio $\leq$ 3 have been proposed for the prediction of chronic atrophic gastritis and GC, and have been confirmed in several meta-analyses [164].

Nagel et al. analyzed serum levels of cytokeratin-18 fragments in patients enrolled in the SUN-CASE study by comparing sunitinib or placebo as adjunct to standard chemotherapy. They found that baseline full-length cytokeratin-18 correlated with treatment failure and PFS. The cytokeratin-18 fragment M30 at day 14 was identified as an independent predictor of treatment response [165].

Serum levels of vascular adhesion protein-1 (VAP-1) were measured before treatment of operable and metastatic GC. Decreased VAP-1 levels were associated with shortened OS [166].

Chemerin is a chemokine linked to adipogenesis and chemotaxis of the innate immune system. Plasma chemerin levels analyzed in 196 GC patients before surgery were found to be higher than in 196 matched healthy controls. Plasma chemerin level was an independent predictor for OS and DFS in GC patients, with a high chemerin level associated with poor OS [167].

C-C motif chemokine ligand 22 (CCL22) is a protein secreted by dendritic cells and macrophages that interacts with cell-surface chemokine receptors. CCL22 serum levels and CCL22 expression in tumor beds were shown to be higher in GC patients than in healthy controls. Furthermore, a high CCL22 serum level before surgery was an independent risk factor for early recurrence [168].

Xu et al. found a preoperative C-reactive protein/albumin ratio of 0.131 or greater to be a predictor of early recurrence (<12 months) and of response to postoperative adjuvant chemotherapy [169]. Another study found the preoperative C-reactive protein/prealbumin ratio to be predictive of recurrence, with a higher predictive value than the C-reactive protein/albumin ratio [170].

Visfatin, also called pre-B-cell colony-enhancing factor (PBEF), is a proinflammatory cytokine secreted by adipocytes, macrophages, and inflamed endothelial tissue. High expression levels of visfatin have been found in tissues of several cancers, including GC, and were shown to be associated with poor OS [171]. Lu et al. showed higher visfatin levels in plasma of GC patients compared to healthy individuals, and found preoperative visfatin levels in GC patients to serve as an independent predictor of OS [172].

3.6. Peritoneal Biomarkers

Measurement of carcinoembryonic antigen (CEA) in peritoneal fluid can be used to detect cancer cells in the fluid. Fujiwara et al. determined CEA mRNA using the technique of transcriptase-reverse transcriptase concerted reaction (TRC). They observed CEA mRNA in 54% of peritoneal fluids obtained during resection of GC in 137 patients. Presence of CEA mRNA was associated with poorer OS, and it was an independent prognostic factor for survival [173].

Peritoneal lavage fluids of 140 patients with advanced GC undergoing surgery were analyzed by RT-PCR targeting the markers CEA and CK-20 mRNA. In patients with negative lavage cytology, those with both CEA and CK-20 positivity showed a poorer OS. By multivariate analysis CEA alone correlated with peritoneal recurrence, CK-20 alone correlated with OS and combination of CEA and CK-20 correlated with peritoneal recurrence and OS after surgery [174].

Xie et al. compared CEA expression levels in samples of peritoneal washing fluids during D2 resection of GC with or without complete mesogastric excision. CEA expression level after gastrectomy was lower in the group with complete mesogastric excision. In patients with low CEA expression before gastrectomy, D2 gastrectomy with complete mesogastric excision was associated with better disease-free survival [175].

3.7. Cell Biomarkers

Circulating tumor cells (CTCs) are metastatic cells that are released from the primary tumor into the blood stream, and are easily accessible in a liquid biopsy from peripheral blood. Several studies have shown that peripheral blood CTCs are useful to predict prognosis and monitor therapy in GC patients [176].

Pernot et al. used immunomagnetic and fluorescence imaging technology for the isolation and enumeration of CTCs in peripheral blood from patients with advanced gastric and GEJ cancer. The authors found CTC counts were significantly associated with worse survival at baseline and during treatment, with the optimal threshold at 2 CTCs [177]. This was confirmed by Sclafani and colleagues, who assessed the prevalence of CTCs in metastatic esophagogastric cancer. They found an increased response rate to chemotherapy and increased PFS and OS in patients with less than 2 CTCs compared to more than 2 CTCs detected at baseline [178].

CD44 has been identified as a GC stem cell marker. Li et al. analyzed CD44 expression on CTCs by fluorescence microscopy in peripheral blood samples from 45 GC patients before treatment. They found the presence of CD44-positive CTCs and TNM stage were independent predictors for recurrence of GC [179].

3.8. Tumor Microenvironment

The tumor microenvironment (TME) corresponds to the aggregation of tumor cells and neighboring nontumor cells, such as stromal and immune cells, extracellular matrix, and soluble factors. The TME has been shown to play a crucial role in tumorigenesis by activating immune cells to favor tumor growth and progression. Thus, tumor-associated macrophages and tumor-associated neutrophils can exert protumoral functions by enhancing tumor cell invasion and metastasis, angiogenesis, and extracellular matrix remodeling while inhibiting antitumoral immune surveillance [180].

Immunohistochemical analysis of 52 primary GC tissues revealed that high numbers of tumor-infiltrating Tregs and low numbers of tumor infiltrating CD8+ T cells were associated with shortened OS [151].

Tada et al. analyzed peripheral blood mononuclear cells (PBMCs) and tumor-infiltrating lymphocytes (TILs) in primary advanced GC before and after VEGFR2-targeting therapy with ramucirumab. They observed reduced effector regulatory T cells (Treg cells) and reduced PD-1 expression by CD8+ T cells in TILs compared to PBMCs after therapy. Before therapy, effector Treg cells in TILs were more frequent in patients with partial response or stable disease than those with progressive disease. Thus, effector Treg cell frequency in TILs could represent a novel biomarker for stratifying clinical responders [181].

Analysis of circulating and selected intratumoral immune cells was correlated with the Lauren classification subtype and prognosis in patients with untreated advanced GC [182]. Diffuse or mixed-type advanced GC showed lower rates of CD8+ TILs, circulating natural killer (NK) cells, and Treg cells than the intestinal type of GC. While Treg cells were not a prognostic factor, higher CD8+ TIL and NK cell numbers were associated with better OS [182].

Zeng and colleagues analyzed the TME infiltration patterns of 1524 GC patients and developed the TME score as an independent prognostic biomarker and a predictive factor for response to immune-checkpoint inhibitors. The high-TME-score GC subtype was characterized by immune activation, while the low-TME-score subtype was considered T-cell suppressive and associated with worse prognosis [183].

Li and colleagues [184] evaluated the prognostic significance of major stromal and immune cells within the TME. They identified NK cells, fibroblasts, and endothelial cells as the most robust prognostic markers, and developed a TME risk score by combining these cell types. Higher TME risk scores were consistently associated with worse survival.

Zhang and colleagues used transcriptome profiling to predict peritoneal recurrence of advanced GC. They developed an immune cell infiltration score that was an independent predictor for peritoneal recurrence [185].

Furthermore, Li et al. investigated the relationship between regulatory B (Breg) cells in peripheral blood and clinical outcome in XELOX-treated patients with advanced GC. Patients with decreased Breg frequencies after XELOX treatment had a longer PFS than those with increased Breg frequencies (7 vs. 5 months, $p = 0.01$) [186].

Platelet-to-lymphocyte ratio (PLR) has been reported to be a prognostic biomarker of GC [187]. Chen and colleagues analyzed the prognostic value of PLR in patients before neoadjuvant therapy and gastric resection. They observed better DFS and OS in patients with low PLR compared to high PLR, with a cutoff PLR value of 162 [188].

Finally, high preoperative neutrophil/lymphocyte ratio (NLR) (4 or more) in primary gastric cancer has been identified as independent risk factor for reduced survival ($p = 0.003$) [189].

4. Discussion

Our review gives an overview of the wide range of novel biomarkers in GC. As shown, multiple targeted therapies beyond HER2-antibodies have already been developed, and show promising results in GC.

An attempt to compare therapies targeting different biomarkers remains difficult. HER2 remains, to date, the most relevant biomarker in the targeted therapy of GC. Other promising biomarkers for targeted therapies that have shown relevance in clinical trials are VEGF, PD-1, and Claudin 18.2. Expression of MET has been shown to be a negative prognostic factor in GC.

There is a vast number of biomarkers based on DNA, RNA, and protein expression analyses, as well as detection of CTCs and more recently, the immune TME that has been proven to be prognostic factors and may be used for therapeutic stratification in the future.

Up to now, it has been difficult to predict which of these numerous biomarkers will be useful in which clinical scenario. One of the problems is the multitude of molecular markers to be assessed in a single tumor.

An efficient way to assess multiple markers is molecular profiling: Kim and colleagues performed molecular profiling on a cohort of 93 patients with advanced or metastatic GC using next-generation sequencing (NGS) and IHC. IHC comprised analysis of expression of 10 proteins, including the mismatch repair (MMR) proteins MLH1, PMS2, MSH2, and MSH6; the receptor tyrosine kinases HER2, EGFR, and MET; as well as PTEN and p53. NGS was performed with a commercially available assay that enabled detection of variants in 52 genes relevant to solid tumors. In this prospective study, one group of patients was treated with matched therapy based on NGS or IHC results. Matched therapy based on NGS included trastuzumab for *ERBB2* amplification, Akt inhibitor for *PIK3CA* mutation, and FGFR inhibitor for *FGFR2* amplification. Matched therapy based on IHC consisted of trastuzumab for ERBB2 amplification, pembrolizumab for MMR deficiency, pan-ERBB inhibitor for EGFR+, and PI3Kbeta inhibitor for PTEN loss. The nonmatched group received either ramucirumab or standard chemotherapy. The overall response rate was higher with matched compared to nonmatched therapy (55.6 vs. 13.1%, $p = 0.001$) with a trend to higher PFS with matched therapy (7.1 vs. 5.2 months, $p = 0.7$). The authors concluded that, as the matched group experienced significantly better responses and survival, their pilot study justified the need for further umbrella trials in GC [190]. Umbrella trials are prospective clinical trials that test multiple targeted interventions for a single disease based on predictive biomarkers or other predictive patient risk factors [191].

Future studies should include gene panels and not only gene classifiers to cover a large number of genes and potential targets for future therapy.

Genomic profiling often presents practical challenges due to tissue availability [190]. There is certainly great potential for circulating biomarkers from liquid biopsies due to their availability. Beyond CTC and circulating tumor DNA, other circulating biomarkers such as RNA, proteins, and metabolites are still in early phases of development, and need to be explored further before broad clinical use as screening or monitoring markers [192].

From an economical point of view, molecular profiling might at this point be reserved for patients with GC resistant to chemotherapy or with metastatic disease. As techniques of molecular profiling are further improved, however, they will become more readily available and less expensive in the future.

5. Conclusions

In conclusion and from a clinical point of view, biopsies from patients with locally advanced or metastatic GC should be tested for HER2 overexpression, as trastuzumab is indicated in HER2-positive tumors in combination with palliative chemotherapy. Before instauration of palliative chemotherapy, tumors should also be tested for Claudin 18.2 overexpression, as targeted therapy to Claudin 18.2 has proven efficacy. In case of resistance to first-line chemotherapy, VEGF is a promising target. Tumors refractory to two or more regimens of chemotherapy should be tested for PD-L1 expression, as immune checkpoint inhibitors have proven efficacy. MSI-high tumors have shown to be especially responsive to immunotherapy. Testing tumors for MET expression might be predictive for decreased treatment response.

Author Contributions: Conceptualization, N.N., I.G. and P.L.; methodology, N.N. and I.G.; writing—original draft preparation, N.N., I.G. and P.L.; writing—review and editing, N.N., I.G., J.D., J.C.K. and P.L. All authors have read and agreed to the published version of the manuscript.

Funding: This research received no external funding.

Conflicts of Interest: The authors declare no conflict of interest.

References

1. Sung, H.; Ferlay, J.; Siegel, R.L.; Laversanne, M.; Soerjomataram, I.; Jemal, A.; Bray, F. Global Cancer Statistics 2020: GLOBOCA Estimates of Incidence and Mortality Worldwide for 36 Cancers in 185 Countries. *CA Cancer J. Clin.* **2021**, *71*, 209–249. [CrossRef]
2. Wroblewski, L.E.; Peek, R.M.; Wilson, K.T. Helicobacter pylori and gastric cancer: Factors that modulate disease risk. *Clin. Microbiol. Rev.* **2010**, *23*, 713–739. [CrossRef] [PubMed]
3. Van Cutsem, E.; Sagaert, X.; Topal, B.; Haustermans, K.; Prenen, H. Gastric cancer. *Lancet* **2016**, *388*, 2654–2664. [CrossRef]
4. Rawla, P.; Barsouk, A. Epidemiology of gastric cancer: Global trends, risk factors and prevention. *Gastroenterol. Rev.* **2019**, *14*, 26–38. [CrossRef] [PubMed]
5. Stomach Cancer Survival Rates. Available online: https://www.cancer.org/cancer/stomach-cancer/detection-diagnosis-staging/survival-rates (accessed on 2 March 2021).
6. Mishra, A.; Verma, M. Cancer biomarkers: Are we ready for the prime time? *Cancers* **2010**, *2*, 190–208. [CrossRef] [PubMed]
7. Cancer Genome Atlas Research Network. Comprehensive molecular characterization of gastric adenocarcinoma. *Nature* **2014**, *513*, 202–209. [CrossRef]
8. Bang, Y.J.; Van Cutsem, E.; Feyereislova, A.; Chung, H.C.; Shen, L.; Sawaki, A.; Lordick, F.; Ohtsu, A.; Omura, Y.; Satoh, T.; et al. Trastuzumab in combination with chemotherapy versus chemotherapy alone for treatment of HER2-positive advanced gastric or gastro-oesophageal junction cancer (ToGA): A phase 3, open-label, randomized controlled trial. *Lancet* **2010**, *376*, 687–697. [CrossRef]
9. Meric-Bernstam, F.; Johnson, A.M.; Dumbrava, E.E.; Raghav, K.; Balaji, K.; Bhatt, M.; Murthy, R.K.; Rodon, J.; Piha-Paul, S.A. Advances in HER2-Targeted Therapy: Novel Agents and Opportunities Beyond Breast and Gastric Cancer. *Clin. Cancer Res.* **2019**, *25*, 2033–2041. [CrossRef]
10. Gravalos, C.; Jimeno, A. HER2 in gastric cancer: A new prognostic factor and a novel therapeutic target. *Ann. Oncol.* **2008**, *19*, 1523–1529. [CrossRef]
11. Okines, A.F.; Thompson, L.C.; Cunningham, D.; Wotherspoon, A.; Reis-Filho, J.S.; Langley, R.E.; Waddell, T.S.; Noor, D.; Eltahir, Z.; Wong, R.; et al. Effect of HER2 on prognosis and benefit from perioperative chemotherapy in early oesophago-gastric adenocarcinoma in the MAGIC trial. *Ann. Oncol.* **2013**, *24*, 1253–1261. [CrossRef] [PubMed]
12. Van Cutsem, E.; Bang, Y.J.; Feng-Yi, F.; Xu, J.M.; Lee, K.W.; Jiao, S.C.; Chong, J.L.; Lopez-Sanchez, R.I.; Price, T.; Gladkov, O.; et al. HER2 screening data from ToGA: Targeting HER2 in gastric and gastroesophageal junction cancer. *Gastric Cancer* **2015**, *18*, 476–484. [CrossRef]
13. Matsumoto, T.; Sasako, M.; Mizusawa, J.; Hirota, S.; Ochiai, A.; Kushima, R.; Katai, H.; Tanaka, Y.; Fukushima, N.; Nashimoto, A.; et al. HER2 expression in locally advanced gastric cancer with extensive lymph node (bulky N2 or paraaortic) metastasis (JCOG1005-A trial). *Gastric Cancer* **2015**, *18*, 467–475. [CrossRef] [PubMed]
14. Press, M.F.; Ellis, C.E.; Gagnon, R.C.; Grob, T.J.; Buyse, M.; Villalobos, I.; Liang, Z.; Wu, S.; Bang, Y.J.; Qin, S.K.; et al. HER2 Status in Advanced or Metastatic Gastric, Esophageal, or Gastroesophageal Adenocarcinoma for Entry to the TRIO-013/LOGIC Trial of Lapatinib. *Mol. Cancer Ther.* **2017**, *16*, 228–238. [CrossRef] [PubMed]
15. Kim, W.H.; Gomes-Izquierdo, L.; Vilardell, F.; Chu, K.M.; Soucy, G.; Dos Santos, L.V.; Monges, G.; Viale, G.; Brito, M.J.; Osborne, S.; et al. HER2 status in Gastric and Gastroesophageal Junction Cancer: Results of the Large, Multinational HER-EAGLE Study. *Appl. Immunohistochem. Mol. Morph* **2018**, *26*, 239–245. [CrossRef] [PubMed]
16. Feizy, A.; Karami, A.; Eghdamzamiri, R.; Moghimi, M.; Taheri, H.; Mousavinasab, N. HER2 Expression Status and Prognostic, Diagnostic, and Demographic Properties of Patients with Gastric Cancer: A Single Center Cohort Study from Iran. *Asian Pac. J. Cancer Prev.* **2018**, *19*, 1721–1725.
17. Lordick, F.; Al-Batran, S.E.; Dietel, M.; Gaiser, T.; Hofheinz, R.D.; Kirchner, T.; Kreipe, H.H.; Lorenzen, S.; Möhler, M.; Qaas, A.; et al. HER2 testing in gastric cancer: Results of a German expert meeting. *J. Cancer Res. Clin. Oncol.* **2017**, *143*, 835–841. [CrossRef]
18. Sawaki, A.; Ohashi, Y.; Omuro, Y.; Satoh, T.; Hamamoto, Y.; Boku, N.; Miyata, Y.; Takiuchi, H.; Yamaguchi, K.; Sasaki, Y.; et al. Efficacy of trastuzumab in Japanese patients with HER2-positive advanced gastric or gastroesophageal junction cancer: A subgroup analysis of the Trastuzumab for Gastric Cancer (ToGA) study. *Gastric Cancer* **2012**, *15*, 313–322. [CrossRef]
19. Shitara, K.; Yatabe, Y.; Matsuo, K.; Sugano, M.; Kondo, C.; Takahiri, D.; Ura, T.; Tajika, M.; Ito, S.; Muro, K. Prognosis of patients with advanced gastric cancer by HER2 status and trastuzumab treatment. *Gastric Cancer* **2013**, *16*, 261–267. [CrossRef]

20. Li, Q.; Li, H.; Jiang, H.; Feng, Y.; Cui, Y.; Wang, Y.; Ji, Y.; Yu, Y.; Li, W.; Xu, C.; et al. Predictive factors of trastuzumab-based chemotherapy in HER2 positive advanced gastric cancer: A single-center prospective observational study. *Clin. Transl. Oncol.* **2018**, *20*, 695–702. [CrossRef]
21. Shitara, K.; Bang, Y.J.; Iwasa, S.; Sugimoto, N.; Ryu, M.-H.; Sakai, D.; Chung, H.-C.; Kawakami, H.; Yabusaki, H.; Lee, J.; et al. Trastuzumab Deruxtecan in Previously Treated HER2-Positive Gastric Cancer. *N. Engl. J. Med.* **2020**, *382*, 2419–2430. [CrossRef]
22. Thuss-Patience, P.C.; Shah, M.A.; Ohtsu, A.; Van Cutsem, E.; Ajani, J.A.; Castro, H.; Mansoor, W.; Chung, H.C.; Bodoky, G.; Shitara, K.; et al. Trastuzumab emtansine versus taxane use for previously treated HER2-positive locally advanced or metastatic gastric or gastro-oesophageal junction adenocarcinoma (GATSBY): An international randomised, open-label, adaptive, phase 2/3 study. *Lancet Oncol.* **2017**, *18*, 640–653. [CrossRef]
23. Shah, M.A.; Kang, Y.K.; Thuss-Patience, P.C.; Ohtsu, A.; Ajani, J.A.; Van Cutsem, E.; Hoersch, S.; Harle-Yge, M.L.; de Haas, S.L. Biomarker analysis of the GATSBY study of trastuzumab emtansine versus a taxane in previously treated HER2-positive advanced gastric/gastroesophageal junction cancer. *Gastric Cancer* **2019**, *22*, 803–816. [CrossRef]
24. Shitara, K.; Honma, Y.; Omuro, Y.; Yamaguchi, K.; Chin, K.; Muro, K.; Nakagawa, S.; Kawakami, S.; Hironaka, S.; Nishina, T. Efficacy of trastuzumab emtansine in Japanese patients with previously treated HER2-positive locally advanced or metastatic gastric or gastroesophageal junction adenocarcinoma: A subgroup analysis of the GATSBY study. *Asia Pac. J. Clin. Oncol.* **2020**, *16*, 5–13. [CrossRef]
25. Horita, Y.; Nishino, M.; Sugimoto, S.; Kida, A.; Mizukami, A.; Yano, M.; Arihara, F.; Matsuda, K.; Matsuda, M.; Sakai, A. Phase II clinical trial of second-line weekly paclitaxel plus trastuzumab for patients with HER2-positive metastatic gastric cancer. *Anticancer Drugs* **2019**, *30*, 98–104. [CrossRef]
26. Makiyama, A.; Sukawa, Y.; Kashiwada, T.; Kawada, J.; Hosokawa, A.; Horie, Y.; Tsuji, A.; Moriwaki, T.; Tanioka, H.; Shinozaki, K.; et al. Randomized, Phase II Study of Trastuzumab Beyond Progression in Patients with HER2-Positive Advanced Gastric or Gastroesophageal Junction Cancer: WJOG7112G (T-ACT Study). *J. Clin. Oncol.* **2020**, *38*, 1919–1927. [CrossRef]
27. Ryu, M.H.; Yoo, C.; Kim, J.G.; Ryoo, B.Y.; Park, Y.S.; Park, S.R.; Han, H.S.; Chung, I.J.; Song, E.K.; Lee, K.H.; et al. Multicenter phase II study of trastuzumab in combination with capecitabine and oxaliplatin for advanced gastric cancer. *Eur. J. Cancer* **2015**, *51*, 482–488. [CrossRef] [PubMed]
28. Gong, J.; Liu, T.; Fan, Q.; Bai, L.; Feng, B.; Qin, Y.; Wang, J.; Xu, N.; Cheng, Y.; Bai, Y.; et al. Optimal regimen of trastuzumab in combination with oxaliplatin/ capecitabine in first-line treatment of HER2-positive advanced gastric cancer (CGOG1001): A multicenter, phase II trial. *BMC Cancer* **2016**, *16*, 68. [CrossRef] [PubMed]
29. Rivera, F.; Romero, C.; Jimenez-Fonseca, P.; Izquierdo-Manuel, M.; Salud, A.; Martinez, E.; Jorge, M.; Arrazubi, V.; Mendez, J.C.; Garcia-Alfonso, P.; et al. Phase II study to evaluate the efficacy of Trastuzumab in combination with Capecitabine and Oxaliplatin in first-line treatment of HER2-positive advanced gastric cancer: HERXO trial. *Cancer Chemother. Pharm.* **2019**, *83*, 1175–1181. [CrossRef]
30. Roviello, G.; Petrioli, R.; Petrioli, R.; Nardone, V.; Rosellini, P.; Multari, A.G.; Conca, R.; Aieta, M. Docetaxel, oxaliplatin, 5FU, and trastuzumab as first-line therapy in patients with human epidermal receptor 2-positive advanced gastric or gastroesophageal junction cancer: Preliminary results of a phase II study. *Medicine* **2018**, *97*, e10745. [CrossRef] [PubMed]
31. Mondaca, S.; Margolis, M.; Sanchez-Vega, F.; Jonsson, P.; Riches, J.C.; Ku, G.Y.; Hechtman, J.F.; Tuvy, Y.; Berger, M.F.; Shah, M.A.; et al. Phase II study of trastuzumab with modified docetaxel, cisplatin, and 5 fluorouracil in metastatic HER2-positive gastric cancer. *Gastric Cancer* **2019**, *22*, 355–362. [CrossRef]
32. Kagawa, S.; Muraoka, A.; Kambara, T.; Nakayama, H.; Hamano, R.; Tanaka, N.; Noma, K.; Tanakaya, K.; Kishimoto, H.; Shigeyasu, K.; et al. A multi-institution phase II study of docetaxel and S-1 in combination with trastuzumab for HER2-positive advanced gastric cancer (DASH study). *Cancer Chemother. Pharm.* **2018**, *81*, 387–392. [CrossRef] [PubMed]
33. Takahari, D.; Chin, K.; Ishizuka, N.; Takashima, A.; Minashi, K.; Kadowaki, S.; Nishina, T.; Nakajima, T.E.; Amagai, K.; Machida, N.; et al. Multicenter phase II study of trastuzumab with S-1 plus oxaliplatin for chemotherapy-naïve, HER2-positive advanced gastric cancer. *Gastric Cancer* **2019**, *22*, 1238–1246. [CrossRef]
34. Yuki, S.; Shinozaki, K.; Kashiwada, T.; Kusumoto, T.; Iwatsuki, M.; Satake, H.; Kobayashi, K.; Esaki, T.; Nakashima, Y.; Kawanaka, H.; et al. Multicenter phase II study of SOX plus trastuzumab for patients with HER2(+) metastatic or recurrent gastric cancer: KSCC/HGCSG/CCOG/PerSeUS 1501B. *Cancer Chemother. Pharm.* **2020**, *85*, 217–223. [CrossRef] [PubMed]
35. Kataoka, H.; Mori, Y.; Shimura, H.; Nishie, H.; Natsume, M.; Mochizuki, Y.; Hirata, Y.; Sobue, S.; Mizushima, T.; Sano, H.; et al. A phase II prospective study of the trastuzumab combined with 5-weekly S-1 and CDDP therapy for HER2-positive advanced gastric cancer. *Cancer Chemother. Pharm.* **2016**, *77*, 957–962. [CrossRef] [PubMed]
36. Miura, Y.; Sukawa, Y.; Hironaka, S.; Mori, M.; Nishikawa, K.; Tokunaga, S.; Okuda, H.; Sakamoto, T.; Taku, K.; Nishikawa, T.; et al. Five-weekly S-1 plus cisplatin therapy combined with trastuzumab therapy in HER2-positive gastric cancer: A phase II trial and biomarker study (WJOG7212G). *Gastric Cancer* **2018**, *21*, 84–95. [CrossRef]
37. Endo, S.; Kurokawa, M.; Gamoh, M.; Kimura, Y.; Matsuyama, J.; Taniguchi, H.; Takeno, A.L.; Kawabata, R.; Kawada, J.; Masuzawa, T.; et al. Trastuzumab with S-1 Plus Cisplatin in HER2-positive Advanced Gastric Cancer Without Measurable Lesions: OGSG 1202. *Anticancer Res.* **2019**, *39*, 1059–1065. [CrossRef] [PubMed]
38. Kimura, Y.; Fujii, M.; Masuishi, T.; Nishikawa, K.; Kunisaki, C.; Matsusaka, T.; Segawa, Y.; Nakamura, M.; Sasaki, K.; Nagao, N.; et al. Multicenter phase II study of trastuzumab plus S-1 alone in elderly patients with HER2-positive advanced gastric cancer (JACCRO GC-06). *Gastric Cancer* **2018**, *21*, 421–427. [CrossRef] [PubMed]

39. Shah, M.A.; Xu, R.H.; Bang, Y.J.; Hoff, P.M.; Liu, T.; Herraez-Baranda, L.A.; Xia, F.; Garg, A.; Shing, M.; Tabernero, J. HELOISE: Phase IIIb Randomized Multicenter Study Comparing Standard-of-Care and Higher-Dose Trastuzumab Regimens Combined with Chemotherapy as First-Line Therapy in Patients with Human Epidermal Growth Factor Receptor 2-Positive Metastatic Gastric or Gastroesophageal Junction Adenocarcinoma. *J. Clin. Oncol.* **2017**, *35*, 2558–2567.
40. Tabernero, J.; Hoff, P.M.; Shen, L.; Ohtsu, A.; Shah, M.A.; Cheng, K.; Song, C.; Wu, H.; Eng-Wong, J.; Kim, K.; et al. Pertuzumab plus trastuzumab and chemotherapy for HER2-positive metastatic gastric or gastro-oesophageal junction cancer (JACOB): Final analysis of a double-blind, randomised, placebo-controlled phase 3 study. *Lancet Oncol.* **2018**, *19*, 1372–1384. [CrossRef]
41. Liu, T.; Qin, Y.; Li, J.; Xu, R.; Xu, J.; Yang, S.; Qin, S.; Bai, Y.; Wu, C.; Mao, Y.; et al. Pertuzumab in combination with trastuzumab and chemotherapy for Chinese patients with HER2-positive metastatic gastric or gastroesophageal junction cancer: A subpopulation analysis of the JACOB trial. *Cancer Commun.* **2019**, *39*, 38. [CrossRef]
42. Oh, D.Y.; Lee, K.W.; Cho, J.Y.; Kang, W.K.; Im, S.A.; Kim, J.W.; Bang, Y.J. Phase II trial of dacomitinib in patients with HER2-positive gastric cancer. *Gastric Cancer* **2016**, *19*, 1095–1103. [CrossRef]
43. Kim, T.Y.; Han, H.S.; Lee, K.W.; Zang, D.Y.; Rha, S.Y.; Park, Y.I.; Kim, J.-S.; Lee, K.H.; Park, S.H.; Song, E.K.; et al. A phase I/II study of poziotinib combined with paclitaxel and trastuzumab in patients with HER2-positive advanced gastric cancer. *Gastric Cancer* **2019**, *22*, 1206–1214. [CrossRef]
44. Iqbal, S.; Goldman, B.; Fenoglio-Preiser, C.; Lenz, H.J.; Zhang, W.; Danenberg, K.D.; Shibata, S.I.; Blanke, C.D. Southwest Oncology Group study S0413: A phase II trial of lapatinib (GW572016) as first-line therapy in patients with advanced or metastatic gastric cancer. *Ann. Oncol.* **2011**, *22*, 2610–2615. [CrossRef] [PubMed]
45. Satoh, T.; Xu, R.H.; Chung, H.C.; Sun, G.P.; Doi, T.; Xu, J.M.; Tsuji, A.; Omuro, Y.; Li, J.; Wang, J.W.; et al. Lapatinib plus paclitaxel versus paclitaxel alone in the second-line treatment of HER2-amplified advanced gastric cancer in Asian populations: TyTAN—A randomized, phase III study. *J. Clin. Oncol.* **2014**, *32*, 2039–2049. [CrossRef] [PubMed]
46. Lorenzen, S.; Riera Knorrenschild, J.; Haag, G.M.; Pohl, M.; Thuss-Patience, P.; Bassermann, F.; Helbig, U.; Weißinger, F.; Schnoy, E.; Becker, K.; et al. Lapatinib versus lapatinib plus capecitabine as second-line treatment in human epidermal growth factor receptor 2-amplified metastatic gastro-oesophageal cancer: A randomised phase II trial of the Arbeitsgemeinschaft Internistische Onkologie. *Eur. J. Cancer* **2015**, *51*, 569–576. [CrossRef]
47. Hecht, J.R.; Bang, Y.J.; Qin, S.K.; Chung, H.C.; Xu, J.M.; Park, J.O.; Jeziorski, K.; Shparyk, Y.; Hoff, P.M.; Sobrero, A.; et al. Lapatinib in Combination with Capecitabine Plus Oxaliplatin in Human Epidermal Growth Factor Receptor 2-Positive Advanced or Metastatic Gastric, Esophageal, or Gastroesophageal Adenocarcinoma: TRIO-013/LOGiC—A Randomized Phase III Trial. *J. Clin. Oncol.* **2016**, *34*, 443–451. [CrossRef]
48. Moehler, M.; Schad, A.; Maderer, A.; Atasoy, A.; Mauer, M.E.; Caballero, C.; Thomaidis, T.; Mahachie John, J.M.; Lang, I.; Van Cutsem, E.; et al. Lapatinib with ECF/X in the first-line treatment of metastatic gastric cancer according to HER2neu and EGFR status: A randomized placebo-controlled phase II study (EORTC 40071). *Cancer Chemother. Pharm.* **2018**, *82*, 733–739. [CrossRef] [PubMed]
49. LaBonte, M.J.; Yang, D.; Zhang, W.; Wilson, P.M.; Nagarwala, Y.M.; Koch, K.M.; Briner, C.; Kaneko, T.; Rha, S.Y.; Gladkov, O.; et al. A Phase II Biomarker-Embedded Study of Lapatinib plus Capecitabine as First-line Therapy in Patients with Advanced or Metastatic Gastric Cancer. *Mol. Cancer Ther.* **2016**, *15*, 2251–2258. [CrossRef]
50. Sanchez-Vega, F.; Hechtman, J.F.; Castel, P.; Ku, G.Y.; Tuvy, Y.; Won, H.; Fong, C.J.; Bouvier, N.; Nanjangud, G.J.; Soong, J.; et al. EGFR and MET Amplifications Determine Response to HER2 Inhibition in ERBB2-Amplified Esophagogastric Cancer. *Cancer Discov.* **2019**, *9*, 199–209. [CrossRef] [PubMed]
51. Waddell, T.; Chau, I.; Cunningham, D.; Gonzalez, D.; Okines, A.F.; Wotherspoon, A.; Saffery, C.; Middleton, G.; Wadsley, J.; Ferry, D.; et al. Epirubicin, oxaliplatin, and capecitabine with or without panitumumab for patients with previously untreated advanced oesophagogastric cancer (REAL3): A randomised, open-label phase 3 trial. *Lancet Oncol.* **2013**, *14*, 481–489. [CrossRef]
52. Stahl, M.; Maderer, A.; Lordick, F.; Mihaljevic, A.L.; Kanzler, S.; Hoehler, T.; Thuss-Patience, P.; Mönig, S.; Kunzmann, V.; Schroll, S.; et al. Perioperative chemotherapy with or without epidermal growth factor receptor blockade in unselected patients with locally advanced oesophagogastric adenocarcinoma: Randomized phase II study with advanced biomarker program of the German Cancer Society (AIO/CAO STO-0801). *Eur. J. Cancer* **2018**, *93*, 119–126.
53. Satoh, T.; Lee, K.H.; Rha, S.Y.; Sasaki, Y.; Park, S.H.; Komatsu, Y.; Yasui, H.; Kim, T.-Y.; Yamaguchi, K.; Fuse, N.; et al. Randomized phase II trial of nimotuzumab plus irinotecan versus irinotecan alone as second-line therapy for patients with advanced gastric cancer. *Gastric Cancer* **2015**, *18*, 824–832. [CrossRef] [PubMed]
54. Lordick, F.; Luber, B.; Lorenzen, S.; Hegewisch-Becker, S.; Folprecht, G.; Wöll, E.; Decker, T.; Endlicher, E.; Röthling, N.; Schuster, T.; et al. Cetuximab plus oxaliplatin/leucovorin/5-fluorouracil in first-line metastatic gastric cancer: A phase II study of the Arbeitsgemeinschaft Internistische Onkologie (AIO). *Br. J. Cancer* **2010**, *102*, 500–505. [CrossRef] [PubMed]
55. Moehler, M.; Mueller, A.; Trarbach, T.; Lordick, F.; Seufferlein, T.; Kubicka, S.; Geißler, M.; Schwarz, S.; Galle, P.R.; Kanzler, S. Cetuximab with irinotecan, folinic acid and 5-fluorouracil as first-line treatment in advanced gastroesophageal cancer: A prospective multi-center biomarker-oriented phase II study. *Ann. Oncol.* **2011**, *22*, 1358–1366. [CrossRef] [PubMed]
56. Lordick, F.; Kang, Y.K.; Chung, H.C.; Salman, P.; Oh, S.C.; Bodoky, G.; Kurteva, G.; Volovat, C.; Moiseyenko, V.M.; Gorbunova, V.; et al. Capecitabine and cisplatin with or without cetuximab for patients with previously untreated advanced gastric cancer (EXPAND): A randomised, open-label phase 3 trial. *Lancet Oncol.* **2013**, *14*, 490–499. [CrossRef]

57. Zhang, X.; Xu, J.; Liu, H.; Yang, L.; Liang, J.; Xu, N.; Bai, Y.; Wang, J.; Shen, L. Predictive biomarkers for the efficacy of cetuximab combined with cisplatin and capecitabine in advanced gastric or esophagogastric junction adenocarcinoma: A prospective multicenter phase 2 trial. *Med. Oncol.* **2014**, *31*, 226. [CrossRef]
58. Liu, X.; Guo, W.; Zhang, W.; Yin, J.; Zhang, J.; Zhu, X.; Liu, T.; Chen, Z.; Wang, B.; Chang, J.; et al. A multi-center phase II study and biomarker analysis of combined cetuximab and modified FOLFIRI as second-line treatment in patients with metastatic gastric cancer. *BMC Cancer* **2017**, *17*, 188. [CrossRef]
59. Wilke, H.; Muro, K.; Van Cutsem, E.; Oh, S.C.; Bodoky, G.; Shimada, Y.; Hironaka, S.; Sugimoto, N.; Lipatov, O.; Kim, T.Y.; et al. Ramucirumab plus paclitaxel versus placebo plus paclitaxel in patients with previously treated advanced gastric or gastro-oesophageal junction adenocarcinoma (RAINBOW): A double-blind, randomised phase 3 trial. *Lancet Oncol.* **2014**, *15*, 1224–1235. [CrossRef]
60. Ohtsu, A.; Shah, M.A.; Van Cutsem, E.; Rha, S.Y.; Sawaki, A.; Park, S.R.; Lim, H.Y.; Yamada, Y.; Wu, J.; Langer, B.; et al. Bevacizumab in combination with chemotherapy as first-line therapy in advanced gastric cancer: A randomized, double-blind, placebo-controlled phase III study. *J. Clin. Oncol.* **2011**, *29*, 3968–3976. [CrossRef]
61. Meulendijks, D.; de Groot, J.W.; Los, M.; Boers, J.E.; Beerepoot, L.V.; Polee, M.N.; Beeker, A.; Portielje, J.E.; Goey, S.H.; de Jong, R.S.; et al. Bevacizumab combined with docetaxel, oxaliplatin, and capecitabine, followed by maintenance with capecitabine and bevacizumab, as first-line treatment of patients with advanced HER2-negative gastric cancer: A multicenter phase 2 study. *Cancer* **2016**, *122*, 1434–1443. [CrossRef]
62. Meulendijks, D.; Beerepoot, L.V.; Boot, H.; de Groot, J.W.; Los, M.; Boers, J.E.; Vanhoutvin, S.A.; Polee, M.B.; Beeker, A.; Portielje, J.E.; et al. Trastuzumab and bevacizumab combined with docetaxel, oxaliplatin and capecitabine as first-line treatment of advanced HER2-positive gastric cancer: A multicenter phase II study. *Investig. New Drugs* **2016**, *34*, 119–128. [CrossRef]
63. Moehler, M.; Mueller, A.; Hartmann, J.T.; Ebert, M.P.; Al-Batran, S.E.; Reimer, P.; Weihrauch, M.; Lordick, F.; Trarbach, T.; Biesterfeld, S.; et al. An open-label, multicentre biomarker-oriented AIO phase II trial of sunitinib for patients with chemo-refractory advanced gastric cancer. *Eur. J. Cancer* **2011**, *47*, 1511–1520. [CrossRef]
64. Moehler, M.; Gepfner-Tuma, I.; Maderer, A.; Thuss-Patience, P.C.; Ruessel, J.; Hegewisch-Becker, S.; Wilke, H.; Al-Batran, S.E.; Rafiyan, M.-R.; Weißinger, F.; et al. Sunitinib added to FOLFIRI versus FOLFIRI in patients with chemorefractory advanced adenocarcinoma of the stomach or lower esophagus: A randomized, placebo-controlled phase II AIO trial with serum biomarker program. *BMC Cancer* **2016**, *16*, 699. [CrossRef] [PubMed]
65. Won, E.; Basunia, A.; Chatila, W.K.; Hechtman, J.F.; Chou, J.F.; Ku, G.Y.; Chalasani, S.B.; Boyar, M.S.; Goldberg, Z.; Desai, A.M.; et al. Efficacy of Combined VEGFR1-3, PDGFα/β, and FGFR1-3 Blockade Using Nintedanib for Esophagogastric Cancer. *Clin. Cancer Res.* **2019**, *25*, 3811–3817. [CrossRef]
66. Van Cutsem, E.; Bang, Y.J.; Mansoor, W.; Petty, R.D.; Chao, Y.; Cunningham, D.; Ferry, D.R.; Smith, N.R.; Frewer, P.; Ratnayake, J.; et al. A randomized, open-label study of the efficacy and safety of AZD4547 monotherapy versus paclitaxel for the treatment of advanced gastric adenocarcinoma with FGFR2 polysomy or gene amplification. *Ann. Oncol.* **2017**, *28*, 1316–1324. [CrossRef] [PubMed]
67. Iveson, T.; Donehower, R.C.; Davidenko, I.; Tjulandin, S.; Deptala, A.; Harrison, M.; Nirni, S.; Lakshmaiah, K.; Thomas, A.; Jiang, Y.; et al. Rilotumumab in combination with epirubicin, cisplatin, and capecitabine as first-line treatment for gastric or oesophagogastric junction adenocarcinoma: An open-label, dose de-escalation phase 1b study and a double-blind, randomised phase 2 study. *Lancet Oncol.* **2014**, *15*, 1007–1018. [CrossRef]
68. Zhu, M.; Tang, R.; Doshi, S.; Oliner, K.S.; Dubey, S.; Jiang, Y.; Donehower, R.C.; Iveson, T.; Loh, E.Y.; Zhang, Y. Exposure-response analysis of rilotumumab in gastric cancer: The role of tumour MET expression. *Br. J. Cancer* **2015**, *112*, 429–437. [CrossRef]
69. Catenacci, D.V.; Tebbutt, N.C.; Davidenko, I.; Murad, A.M.; Al-Batran, S.E.; Ilson, D.H.; Tjulandin, S.; Gotovkin, E.; Karaszewska, B.; Bondarenko, I.; et al. Rilotumumab plus epirubicin, cisplatin, and capecitabine as first-line therapy in advanced MET-positive gastric or gastro-oesophageal junction cancer (RILOMET-1): A randomised, double-blind, placebo-controlled, phase 3 trial. *Lancet Oncol.* **2017**, *18*, 1467–1482. [CrossRef]
70. Shah, M.A.; Bang, Y.J.; Lordick, F.; Alsina, M.; Chen, M.; Hack, S.P.; Bruey, J.M.; Smith, D.; McCaffery, I.; Shames, D.S.; et al. Effect of Fluorouracil, Leucovorin, and Oxaliplatin With or Without Onartuzumab in HER2-Negative, MET-Positive Gastroesophageal Adenocarcinoma: The METGastric Randomized Clinical Trial. *JAMA Oncol.* **2017**, *3*, 620–627. [CrossRef]
71. Sahin, U.; Türeci, Ö.; Manikhas, G.; Lordick, F.; Rusyn, A.; Vynnychenko, I.; Dudov, A.; Bazin, I.; Bondarenko, I.; Melichar, B.; et al. FAST: A randomised phase II study of zolbetuximab (IMAB362) plus EOX versus EOX alone for first-line treatment of advanced CLDN18.2-positive gastric and gastro-oesophageal adenocarcinoma. *Ann. Oncol.* **2021**, *32*, 609–619. [CrossRef]
72. Bang, Y.J.; Im, S.A.; Lee, K.W.; Cho, J.Y.; Song, E.K.; Kyung, H.L.; Kim, Y.H.; Park, J.O.; Chun, H.G.; Zang, D.Y.; et al. Randomized, Double-Blind Phase II Trial With Prospective Classification by ATM Protein Level to Evaluate the Efficacy and Tolerability of Olaparib Plus Paclitaxel in Patients With Recurrent or Metastatic Gastric Cancer. *J. Clin. Oncol.* **2015**, *33*, 3858–3865. [CrossRef] [PubMed]
73. Bang, Y.J.; Kang, Y.K.; Ng, M.; Chung, H.C.; Wainberg, Z.A.; Gendreau, S.; Chan, W.Y.; Xu, N.; Maslyar, D.; Meng, R.; et al. A phase II, randomised study of mFOLFOX6 with or without the Akt inhibitor ipatasertib in patients with locally advanced or metastatic gastric or gastroesophageal junction cancer. *Eur. J. Cancer* **2019**, *108*, 17–24. [CrossRef] [PubMed]

74. Yoo, C.; Ryu, M.H.; Na, Y.S.; Ryoo, B.Y.; Lee, C.W.; Kang, Y.K. Vorinostat in combination with capecitabine plus cisplatin as a first-line chemotherapy for patients with metastatic or unresectable gastric cancer: Phase II study and biomarker analysis. *Br. J. Cancer* **2016**, *114*, 1185–1190. [CrossRef] [PubMed]
75. Shah, M.A.; Starodub, A.; Sharma, S.; Berlin, J.; Patel, M.; Wainberg, Z.A.; Chaves, J.; Gordon, M.; Windsor, K.; Brachmann, C.B.; et al. Andecaliximab/GS-5745 Alone and Combined with mFOLFOX6 in Advanced Gastric and Gastroesophageal Junction Adenocarcinoma: Results from a Phase I Study. *Clin. Cancer Res.* **2018**, *24*, 3829–3837. [CrossRef]
76. Shah, M.A.; Bodoky, G.; Starodub, A.; Cunningham, D.; Yip, D.; Wainberg, Z.A.; Bendell, J.; Thai, D.; He, J.; Bhargava, P.; et al. Phase III Study to Evaluate Efficacy and Safety of Andecaliximab with mFOLFOX6 as First-Line Treatment in Patients With Advanced Gastric or GEJ Adenocarcinoma (GAMMA-1). *J. Clin. Oncol.* **2021**, *39*, 990–1000. [CrossRef]
77. Muro, K.; Chung, H.C.; Shankaran, V.; Geva, R.; Catenacci, D.; Gupta, S.; Eder, J.P.; Golan, T.; Le, D.T.; Burtness, B.; et al. Pembrolizumab for patients with PD-L1-positive advanced gastric cancer (KEYNOTE-012): A multicentre, open-label, phase 1b trial. *Lancet Oncol.* **2016**, *17*, 717–726. [CrossRef]
78. Fuchs, C.S.; Doi, T.; Jang, R.W.; Muro, K.; Satoh, T.; Machado, M.; Sun, W.; Jalal, S.I.; Shah, M.A.; Metges, J.-P.; et al. Safety and Efficacy of Pembrolizumab Monotherapy in Patients with Previously Treated Advanced Gastric and Gastroesophageal Junction Cancer: Phase 2 Clinical KEYNOTE-059 Trial. *JAMA Oncol.* **2018**, *4*, e180013. [CrossRef]
79. Kim, S.T.; Cristescu, R.; Bass, A.J.; Kim, K.M.; Odegaard, J.I.; Kim, K.; Liu, X.Q.; Sher, X.; Jung, H.; Lee, M.; et al. Comprehensive molecular characterization of clinical responses to PD-1 inhibition in metastatic gastric cancer. *Nat. Med.* **2018**, *24*, 1449–1458. [CrossRef]
80. Kawazoe, A.; Yamaguchi, K.; Yasui, H.; Negoro, Y.; Azuma, M.; Amagai, K.; Hara, H.; Baba, H.; Tsuda, M.; Hosaka, H.; et al. Safety and efficacy of pembrolizumab in combination with S-1 plus oxaliplatin as a first-line treatment in patients with advanced gastric/gastroesophageal junction cancer: Cohort 1 data from the KEYNOTE-659 phase IIb study. *Eur. J. Cancer* **2020**, *129*, 97–106. [CrossRef]
81. Wang, F.; Wei, X.L.; Wang, F.H.; Xu, N.; Shen, L.; Dai, G.H.; Yuan, X.L.; Chen, Y.; Yang, S.J.; Shi, J.H.; et al. Safety, efficacy and tumor mutational burden as a biomarker of overall survival benefit in chemo-refractory gastric cancer treated with toripalimab, a PD-1 antibody in phase Ib/II clinical trial NCT02915432. *Ann. Oncol.* **2019**, *30*, 1479–1486. [CrossRef]
82. Kang, Y.K.; Boku, N.; Satoh, T.; Ryu, M.H.; Chao, Y.; Kato, K.; Chung, H.C.; Chen, J.S.; Muro, K.; Kang, W.K.; et al. Nivolumab in patients with advanced gastric or gastro-oesophageal junction cancer refractory to, or intolerant of, at least two previous chemotherapy regimens (ONO-4538-12, ATTRACTION-2): A randomised, double-blind, placebo-controlled, phase 3 trial. *Lancet* **2017**, *390*, 2461–2471. [CrossRef]
83. Huang, J.; Mo, H.; Zhang, W.; Chen, X.; Qu, D.; Wang, X.; Wu, D.; Wang, X.; Lan, B.; Yang, B.; et al. Promising efficacy of SHR-1210, a novel anti-programmed cell death 1 antibody, in patients with advanced gastric and gastroesophageal junction cancer in China. *Cancer* **2019**, *125*, 742–749. [CrossRef] [PubMed]
84. Moehler, M.; Dvorkin, M.; Boku, N.; Özgüroglu, M.; Ryu, M.H.; Muntean, A.S.; Lonardi, S.; Nechaeva, M.; Bragagnoli, A.C.; Coskun, H.S.; et al. Phase III Trial of Avelumab Maintenance After First-Line Induction Chemotherapy Versus Continuation of Chemotherapy in Patients with Gastric Cancers: Results from JAVELIN Gastric 100. *J. Clin. Oncol.* **2020**, *39*, 966–977. [CrossRef]
85. Janjigian, Y.Y.; Maron, S.B.; Chatila, W.K.; Millang, B.; Chavan, S.S.; Alterman, C.; Chou, J.K.; Segal, M.F.; Simmons, M.Z.; Momtaz, P.; et al. First-line pembrolizumab and trastuzumab in HER2-positive oesophageal, gastric, or gastro-oesophageal junction cancer: An open-label, single-arm, phase 2 trial. *Lancet Oncol.* **2020**, *21*, 821–831. [CrossRef]
86. Catenacci, D.V.; Kang, Y.K.; Park, H.; Uronis, H.E.; Lee, K.W.; Ng, M.C.; Enzinger, P.C.; Park, S.H.; Gold, P.J.; Lacy, J.; et al. Margetuximab plus pembrolizumab in patients with previously treated, HER2-positive gastro-oesophageal adenocarcinoma (CP-MGAH22-05): A single-arm, phase 1b–2 trial. *Lancet Oncol.* **2020**, *21*, 1066–1076. [CrossRef]
87. Kelly, R.J.; Lee, J.; Bang, Y.J.; Almhanna, K.; Blum-Murphy, M.; Catenacci, D.V.; Chung, H.C.; Wainberg, Z.A.; Gibson, M.K.; Lee, K.W.; et al. Safety and Efficacy of Durvalumab and Tremelimumab Alone or in Combination in Patients with Advanced Gastric and Gastroesophageal Junction Adenocarcinoma. *Clin. Cancer Res.* **2020**, *26*, 846–854. [CrossRef]
88. Shi, L.; Zhou, Q.; Wu, J.; Ji, M.; Li, G.; Jiang, J.; Wu, C. Efficacy of adjuvant immunotherapy with cytokine-induced killer cells in patients with locally advanced gastric cancer. *Cancer Immunol. Immunother.* **2012**, *61*, 2251–2259. [CrossRef]
89. Kim, S.T.; Banks, K.C.; Pectasides, E.; Kim, S.Y.; Kim, K.; Lanman, R.B.; Talasaz, A.; An, J.; Choi, M.G.; Lee, J.H.; et al. Impact of genomic alterations on lapatinib treatment outcome and cell-free genomic landscape during HER2 therapy in HER2+ gastric cancer patients. *Ann. Oncol.* **2018**, *29*, 1037–1048. [CrossRef]
90. Luber, B.; Deplazes, J.; Keller, G.; Walch, A.; Rauser, S.; Eichmann, M.; Langer, R.; Höfler, H.; Hegewisch-Becker, S.; Folprecht, G.; et al. Biomarker analysis of cetuximab plus oxaliplatin/leucovorin/5-fluorouracil in first-line metastatic gastric and oesophago-gastric junction cancer: Results from a phase II trial of the Arbeitsgemeinschaft Internistische Onkologie (AIO). *BMC Cancer* **2011**, *11*, 509. [CrossRef]
91. Van Cutsem, E.; de Haas, S.; Kang, Y.K.; Ohtsu, A.; Tebbutt, N.C.; Xu, J.M.; Yong, W.P.; Langer, B.; Delmar, P.; Scherer, S.J.; et al. Bevacizumab in combination with chemotherapy as first-line therapy in advanced gastric cancer: A biomarker evaluation from the AVAGAST randomized phase III trial. *J. Clin. Oncol.* **2012**, *30*, 2119–2127. [CrossRef] [PubMed]
92. Van Cutsem, E.; Muro, K.; Cunningham, D.; Bodoky, G.; Sobrero, A.; Cascinu, S.; Ajani, A.; Oh, S.C.; Al-Batran, S.E.; Wainberg, Z.A.; et al. Biomarker analyses of second-line ramucirumab in patients with advanced gastric cancer from RAINBOW, a global, randomized, double-blind, phase 3 study. *Eur. J. Cancer* **2020**, *127*, 150–157. [CrossRef]

93. Kim, S.T.; Ahn, S.; Lee, J.; Lee, S.J.; Park, S.H.; Park, Y.S.; Lim, H.Y.; Kang, W.K.; Kim, K.M.; Park, J.O. Value of FGFR2 expression for advanced gastric cancer patients receiving pazopanib plus CapeOX (capecitabine and oxaliplatin). *J. Cancer Res. Clin. Oncol.* **2016**, *142*, 1231–1237. [CrossRef]
94. Choi, Y.Y.; Kim, H.; Shin, S.J.; Kim, H.Y.; Lee, J.; Yang, H.K.; Kim, W.H.; Kim, Y.W.; Kook, M.C.; Park, Y.K.; et al. Microsatellite Instability and Programmed Cell Death-Ligand 1 Expression in Stage II/III Gastric Cancer: Post Hoc Analysis of the CLASSIC Randomized Controlled study. *Ann. Surg.* **2019**, *270*, 309–316. [CrossRef] [PubMed]
95. Shah, M.A.; Wainberg, Z.A.; Catenacci, D.V.; Hochster, H.S.; Ford, J.; Kunz, P.; Lee, F.C.; Kallender, H.; Cecchi, F.; Rabe, D.C.; et al. Phase II study evaluating 2 dosing schedules of oral foretinib (GSK1363089), cMET/VEGFR2 inhibitor, in patients with metastatic gastric cancer. *PLoS ONE* **2013**, *8*, e54014. [CrossRef] [PubMed]
96. Choi, J.; Lee, H.E.; Lee, H.S.; Han, N.; Kim, M.A.; Kim, W.H. Evaluation of Intratumoral and Intertumoral Heterogeneity of MET Protein Expression in Gastric Cancer. *Appl. Immunohistochem. Mol. Morphol.* **2018**, *26*, 445–453. [CrossRef]
97. El Darsa, H.; El Sayed, R.; Abdel-Rahman, O. MET Inhibitors for the Treatment of Gastric Cancer: What's Their Potential? *J. Exp. Pharmacol.* **2020**, *12*, 349–361. [CrossRef] [PubMed]
98. Sahin, U.; Koslowski, M.; Dhaene, K.; Usener, D.; Brandenburg, G.; Seitz, G.; Huber, C.; Türeci, Ö. Claudin-18 splice variant 2 is a pan-cancer target suitable for therapeutic antibody development. *Clin. Cancer Res.* **2008**, *14*, 7624–7634. [CrossRef]
99. Rohde, C.; Yamaguchi, R.; Mukhina, S.; Sahin, U.; Itoh, K.; Türeci, Ö. Comparison of Claudin 18.2 expression in primary tumors and lymph node metastases in Japanese patients with gastric adenocarcinoma. *Jpn. J. Clin. Oncol.* **2019**, *49*, 870–876. [CrossRef] [PubMed]
100. Yamaguchi, K.; Shitara, K.; Al-Batran, S.E.; Bang, Y.-J.; Catenacci, D.; Enzinger, P.; Ilson, D.; Kim, S.; Lordick, F.; Shah, M.; et al. SPOTLIGHT: Comparison of zolbetuximab or placebo + mFOLFOX6 as first-line treatment in patients with claudin18.2+/HER2- locally advanced unresectable or metastatic gastric or gastroesophageal junction adenocarcinoma (GEJ): A randomized phase III study. *Ann. Oncol.* **2019**, *30*, IX66–IX67. [CrossRef]
101. Freeman, G.J.; Long, A.J.; Iwai, Y.; Bourque, K.; Chernova, T.; Nishimura, H.; Fitz, L.J.; Malenkovich, O.T.; Byrne, M.C. Engagement of the PD-1 immunoinhibitory receptor by a novel B7 family member leads to negative regulation of lymphocyte activation. *J. Exp. Med.* **2000**, *192*, 1027–1034. [CrossRef]
102. Liu, X.; Choi, M.G.; Kim, K.; Kim, K.-M.; Kim, S.T.; Park, S.H.; Cristescu, R.; Peter, S.; Lee, J. High PD-L1 expression in gastric cancer (GC) patients and correlation with molecular features. *Pathol. Res. Pract.* **2020**, *216*, 152881. [CrossRef]
103. Garcia, C.; Ring, K.L. The Role of PD-1 Checkpoint Inhibitions in Gynecologic Malignancies. *Curr. Treat. Options Oncol.* **2018**, *19*, 70. [CrossRef]
104. Chung, H.C.; Bang, Y.J.; Fuchs, C.S.; Qin, S.K.; Satoh, T.; Shitara, K.; Tabernero, J.; Van Cutsem, E.; Alsina, M.; Cao, Z.A.; et al. First-line pembrolizumab/placebo plus trastuzumab and chemotherapy in HER2-positive advanced gastric cancer: KEYNOTE-811. *Future Oncol.* **2021**, *17*, 491–501. [CrossRef]
105. Kelly, R.J.; Ajani, J.A.; Kuzdzal, J.; Zander, T.; Van Cutsem, E.; Piessen, G.; Mendez, G.; Feliciano, J.; Motoyama, S.; Lièvre, A.; et al. Adjuvant Nivolumab in Resected Esophageal or Gastroesophageal Junction Cancer. *N. Engl. J. Med.* **2021**, *384*, 1191–1203. [CrossRef]
106. Fashoyin-Aje, L.; Donoghue, M.; Chen, H.; He, K.; Veeraraghavan, J.; Goldberg, K.B.; Keegan, P.; McKee, A.E.; Pazdur, R. FDA Approval Summary: Pembrolizumab for Recurrent Locally Advanced or Metastatic Gastric or Gastroesophageal Junction Adenocarcinoma Expressing PD-L1. *Oncologist* **2019**, *24*, 103–109. [CrossRef] [PubMed]
107. Puneet Kazmi, H.R.; Kumari, S.; Tiwari, S.; Khanna, A.; Narayan, G. Epigenetic Mechanisms and Events in Gastric Cancer-Emerging Novel Biomarkers. *Pathol. Oncol. Res.* **2018**, *24*, 757–770. [CrossRef] [PubMed]
108. Pirini, F.; Noazin, S.; Jahuira-Arias, M.H.; Rodriguez-Torres, S.; Friess, L.; Michailidi, C.; Cok, J.; Combe, J.; Vargas, G.; Prado, W.; et al. Early detection of gastric cancer using global, genome-wide and IRF4, ELMO1, CLIP4 and MSC DNA methylation in endoscopic biopsies. *Oncotarget* **2017**, *8*, 38501–38516. [CrossRef] [PubMed]
109. Shigaki, H.; Baba, M.; Watanabe, M.; Murata, A.; Iwagami, S.; Miyake, K.; Ishimoto, T.; Iwatsuki, M.; Baba, H. LINE-1 hypomethylation in gastric cancer, detected by bisulfite pyrosequencing, is associated with poor prognosis. *Gastric Cancer* **2013**, *16*, 480–487. [CrossRef]
110. Alarcon, M.A.; Olivares, W.; Cordova-Delgado, M.; Munoz-Medel, M.; de Mayo, T.; Carrasco-Avino, G.; Wichmann, I.; Landeros, N.; Amigo, J.; Norero, E.; et al. The Reprimo-Like Gene Is an Epigenetic-Mediated Tumor Suppressor and a Candidate Biomarker for the Non-Invasive Detection of Gastric Cancer. *Int. J. Mol. Sci.* **2020**, *21*, 9472. [CrossRef]
111. Amigo, J.D.; Opazo, J.C.; Jorquera, R.; Wichmann, I.A.; Garcia-Bloj, B.A.; Alarcon, M.A.; Owen, G.I.; Corvalan, A.H. The Reprimo Gene Family: A Novel Gene Lineage in Gastric Cancer with Tumor Suppressive Properties. *Int. J. Mol. Sci.* **2018**, *19*, 1862. [CrossRef] [PubMed]
112. Kubo, T.; Kawano, Y.; Himuro, N.; Sugita, S.; Sato, Y.; Ishikawa, K.; Takada, K.; Murase, K.; Miyanishi, K.; Sato, T.; et al. BAK is a predictive and prognostic biomarker for the therapeutic effect of docetaxel treatment in patients with advanced gastric cancer. *Gastric Cancer* **2016**, *19*, 827–838. [CrossRef] [PubMed]
113. You, Y.; Bai, F.; Ye, Z.; Zhang, N.; Yao, L.; Tang, Y.; Li, X. Downregulated CDK10 expression in gastric cancer: Association with tumor progression and poor prognosis. *Mol. Med. Rep.* **2018**, *17*, 6812–6818. [CrossRef] [PubMed]

114. Kim, J.W.; Cho, H.J.; Kim, M.; Lee, K.H.; Kim, M.A.; Han, S.W.; Oh, D.Y.; Lee, H.J.; Im, S.A.; Kim, T.Y.; et al. Differing effects of adjuvant chemotherapy according to BRCA1 nuclear expression in gastric cancer. *Cancer Chemother. Pharmacol.* **2013**, *71*, 1435–1443. [CrossRef]
115. Li, P.; He, C.Y.; Xu, Q.; Sun, L.P.; Ha, M.W.; Yuan, Y. Effect of the -2081G/A polymorphism of the TLR4 gene and its interaction with Helicobacter pylori infection on the risk of gastric cancer in Chinese individuals. *Genet. Test. Mol. Biomarkers* **2014**, *18*, 610–615. [CrossRef]
116. Hou, K.; Zhu, Z.; Wang, Y.; Zhang, C.; Yu, S.; Zhu, Q.; Yan, B. Overexpression and Biological Function of Ubiquitin-Specific Protease 42 in Gastric Cancer. *PLoS ONE* **2016**, *11*, e0152997. [CrossRef] [PubMed]
117. Arpalahti, L.; Laitinen, A.; Hagström, J.; Mustonen, H.; Kokkola, A.; Böckelman, C.; Haglund, C.; Homberg, C.I. Positive cytoplasmic UCHL5 tumor expression in gastric cancer is linked to improved prognosis. *PLoS ONE* **2018**, *13*, e0193125. [CrossRef] [PubMed]
118. Yoon, D.H.; Ryu, M.H.; Park, Y.S.; Lee, H.J.; Lee, C.; Ryoo, B.Y.; Lee, J.L.; Chang, H.M.; Kim, T.W.; Kang, Y.K. Phase II study of everolimus with biomarker exploration in patients with advanced gastric cancer refractory to chemotherapy including fluoropyrimidine and platinum. *Br. J. Cancer* **2012**, *106*, 1039–1044. [CrossRef] [PubMed]
119. Wainberg, Z.A.; Soares, H.P.; Patel, R.; DiCarlo, B.; Park, D.J.; Liem, A.; Wang, H.-J.; Yonemoto, L.; Martinez, D.; Laux, I.; et al. Phase II trial of everolimus in patients with refractory metastatic adenocarcinoma of the esophagus, gastroesophageal junction and stomach: Possible role for predictive biomarkers. *Cancer Chemother. Pharmacol.* **2015**, *76*, 61–67. [CrossRef]
120. Yamada, Y.; Boku, N.; Nishina, T.; Yamaguchi, K.; Denda, T.; Tsuji, A.; Hamamoto, Y.; Konishi, K.; Tsuji, Y.; Amagai, K.; et al. Impact of excision repair cross-complementing gene 1 (ERCC1) on the outcomes of patients with advanced gastric cancer: Correlative study in Japan Clinical Oncology Group Trial JCOG9912. *Ann. Oncol.* **2013**, *24*, 2560–2565. [CrossRef]
121. Tsuburaya, A.; Sugimoto, N.; Imamura, H.; Nishikawa, K.; Imamoto, H.; Tsujinaka, T.; Esaki, T.; Horita, Y.; Kimura, Y.; Fujiya, T.; et al. Molecular Biomarker Study in a Randomised Phase III Trial of Irinotecan Plus S-1 versus S-1 for Advanced Gastric Cancer (GC0301/TOP-002). *Clin. Oncol.* **2016**, *28*, e45–e51. [CrossRef]
122. Sasako, M.; Terashima, M.; Ichikawa, W.; Ochiai, A.; Kitada, K.; Kurahashi, I.; Sakuramoto, S.; Katai, H.; Sano, T.; Imamura, H. Impact of the expression of thymidylate synthase and dihydropyrimidine dehydrogenase genes on survival in stage II/III gastric cancer. *Gastric Cancer* **2015**, *18*, 538–548. [CrossRef]
123. Hirakawa, M.; Sato, Y.; Ohnuma, H.; Takayama, T.; Sagawa, T.; Nobuoka, T.; Harada, K.; Miyamoto, H.; Sato, Y.; Takahashi, Y.; et al. A phase II study of neoadjuvant combination chemotherapy with docetaxel, cisplatin, and S-1 for locally advanced resectable gastric cancer: Nucleotide excision repair (NER) as potential chemoresistance marker. *Cancer Chemother. Pharmacol.* **2013**, *71*, 789–797. [CrossRef]
124. Shi, X.J.; Wei, Y.; Ji, B. Systems Biology of Gastric Cancer: Perspectives on the Omics-Based Diagnosis and Treatment. *Front. Mol. Biosci.* **2020**, *7*, 203. [CrossRef] [PubMed]
125. Bang, Y.J.; Kim, Y.W.; Yang, H.K.; Chung, H.C.; Park, Y.K.; Lee, K.H.; Lee, K.W.; Kim, Y.H.; Noh, S.I.; Cho, J.Y.; et al. Adjuvant capecitabine and oxaliplatin for gastric cancer after D2 gastrectomy (CLASSIC): A phase 3 open-label, randomised controlled trial. *Lancet* **2012**, *379*, 315–321. [CrossRef]
126. Cheong, J.H.; Yang, H.K.; Kim, H.; Kim, W.H.; Kim, Y.W.; Kook, M.C.; Park, Y.K.; Kim, H.H.; Lee, H.S.; Lee, K.H.; et al. Predictive test for chemotherapy response in resectable gastric cancer: A multi-cohort, retrospective analysis. *Lancet Oncol.* **2018**, *19*, 629–638. [CrossRef]
127. Roh, C.K.; Choi, Y.Y.; Choi, S.; Seo, W.J.; Cho, M.; Jang, E.; Son, T.; Kim, H.I.; Kim, H.; Hyung, W.J.; et al. Single Patient Classifier Assay, Microsatellite Instability, and Epstein-Barr Virus Status Predict Clinical Outcomes in Stage II/III Gastric Cancer: Results from CLASSIC Trial. *Yonsei Med. J.* **2019**, *60*, 132–139. [CrossRef] [PubMed]
128. Cunningham, D.; Allum, W.H.; Stenning, S.P.; Thompson, J.N.; Van de Velde, C.J.; Nicolson, M.; Scarffe, J.H.; Lofts, F.J.; Falk, S.J.; Iveson, T.J.; et al. Perioperative chemotherapy versus surgery alone for resectable gastroesophageal cancer. *N. Engl. J. Med.* **2006**, *355*, 11–20. [CrossRef]
129. Smyth, E.C.; Nyamundanda, G.; Cunningham, D.; Fontana, E.; Ragulan, C.; Tan, I.B.; Lin, S.J.; Wotherspoon, A.; Ninkivell, M.; Fassan, M.; et al. A seven-Gene Signature assay improves prognostic risk stratification of perioperative chemotherapy treated gastroesophageal cancer patients from the MAGIC trial. *Ann. Oncol.* **2018**, *29*, 2356–2362. [CrossRef]
130. Sundar, R.; Huang, K.K.; Qamra, A.; Kim, K.M.; Kim, S.T.; Kang, W.K.; Tan, A.L.; Lee, J.; Tan, P. Epigenomic promoter alterations predict for benefit from immune checkpoint inhibition in metastatic gastric cancer. *Ann. Oncol.* **2019**, *30*, 424–430. [CrossRef]
131. Li, Z.; Gao, X.; Peng, X.; Chen, M.-J.; Li, Z.; Wei, B.; Wen, X.; Wei, B.; Dong, Y.; Bu, Z.; et al. Multi-omics characterization of molecular features of gastric cancer correlated with response to neoadjuvant chemotherapy. *Sci. Adv.* **2020**, *6*, eaay4211. [CrossRef]
132. Smyth, E.C.; Wotherspoon, A.; Peckitt, C.; Gonzalez, D.; Hulkki-Wilson, S.; Eltahir, Z.; Fassan, M.; Rugge, M.; Valeri, N.; Okines, A.; et al. Mismatch Repair Deficiency, Microsatellite Instability, and Survival: An Exploratory Analysis of the Medical Research Council Adjuvant Gastric Infusional Chemotherapy (MAGIC) Trial. *JAMA Oncol.* **2017**, *3*, 1197–1203. [CrossRef] [PubMed]
133. Ratti, M.; Lampis, A.; Hahne, J.C.; Passalacqua, R.; Valeri, N. Microsatellite instability in gastric cancer: Molecular bases, clinical perspectives, and new treatment approaches. *Cell Mol. Life Sci.* **2018**, *75*, 4151–4162. [CrossRef] [PubMed]

134. Okines, A.F.; Gonzales de Castro, D.; Cunningham, D.; Chau, I.; Langley, R.E.; Thompson, L.C.; Stenning, S.P.; Saffery, C.; Barbachano, Y.; Coxon, F.; et al. Biomarker analysis in oesophagogastric cancer: Results from the REAL3 and TransMAGIC trials. *Eur. J. Cancer* **2013**, *49*, 2116–2125. [CrossRef]
135. Geiss, G.K.; Bumgarner, R.E.; Birditt, B.; Dahl, T.; Dowidar, N.; Dunaway, D.L.; Fell, H.P.; Ferree, S.; George, R.D.; Grogan, T.; et al. Direct multiplexed measurement of gene expression with color-coded probe pairs. *Nat. Biotechnol.* **2008**, *26*, 317–325. [CrossRef] [PubMed]
136. Das, K.; Taguri, M.; Imamura, H.; Sugimoto, N.; Nishikawa, K.; Yoshida, K.; Tan, P.; Tsuburaya, A. Genomic predictors of chemotherapy efficacy in advanced or recurrent gastric cancer in the GC0301/TOP002 phase III clinical trial. *Cancer Lett.* **2018**, *412*, 208–215. [CrossRef]
137. Kitamura, S.; Tanahashi, T.; Aoyagi, E.; Nakagawa, T.; Okamoto, K.; Kimura, T.; Miyamoto, H.; Mitsui, Y.; Rokutan, K.; Muguruma, N.; et al. Response Predictors of S-1, Cisplatin, and Docetaxel Combination Chemotherapy for Metastatic Gastric Cancer: Microarray Analysis of Whole Human Genes. *Oncology* **2017**, *93*, 127–135. [CrossRef] [PubMed]
138. Wei, L.; Sun, J.; Zhang, N.; Zheng, Y.; Wang, X.; Lv, L.; Liu, J.; Xu, Y.; Shen, Y.; Yang, M. Noncoding RNAs in gastric cancer: Implications for drug resistance. *Mol. Cancer* **2020**, *19*, 62. [CrossRef] [PubMed]
139. Endo, H.; Shiroki, T.; Nakagawa, T.; Yokoyama, M.; Tamai, K.; Yamanami, H.; Fujiya, T.; Sato, I.; Yamaguchi, K.; Tanaka, N.; et al. Enhanced Expression of Long Non-Coding RNA HOTAIR Is Associated with the Development of Gastric Cancer. *PLoS ONE* **2013**, *8*, e77070. [CrossRef]
140. Du, M.; Wang, W.; Jin, H.; Wang, Q.; Ge, Y.; Lu, J.; Ma, G.; Chu, H.; Tong, N.; Zhu, H.; et al. The association analysis of lncRNA HOTAIR genetic variants and gastric cancer risk in a Chinese population. *Oncotarget* **2015**, *6*, 31255–31262. [CrossRef]
141. Hao, N.B.; He, Y.F.; Li, X.Q.; Wang, K.; Wang, R.L. The role of miRNA and lncRNA in gastric cancer. *Oncotarget* **2017**, *8*, 81572–81582. [CrossRef]
142. Xiong, S.; Hu, M.; Li, C.; Zhou, X.; Chen, H. Role of miR-34 in gastric cancer: From bench to bedside (Review). *Oncol. Rep.* **2019**, *42*, 1635–1646. [CrossRef]
143. Pan, X.M.; Sun, R.F.; Li, Z.H.; Guo, X.M.; Qin, H.J.; Gao, L.B. Pri-miR-34b/c rs4938723 polymorphism is associated with a decreased risk of gastric cancer. *Genet. Test. Mol. Biomarkers* **2015**, *19*, 198–202. [CrossRef]
144. Mu, Y.P.; Tang, S.; Sun, W.J.; Gao, W.M.; Wang, M.; Su, X.L. Association of miR-193b down-regulation and miR-196a up-regulation with clinicopathological features and prognosis in gastric cancer. *Asian Pac. J. Cancer Prev.* **2014**, *15*, 8893–8900. [CrossRef] [PubMed]
145. Deng, M.; Tang, H.L.; Lu, X.H.; Liu, M.Y.; Lu, X.M.; Gu, Y.X.; Liu, J.F.; He, Z.M. miR-26a suppresses tumor growth and metastasis by targeting FGF9 in gastric cancer. *PLoS ONE* **2013**, *8*, e72662. [CrossRef] [PubMed]
146. Malhotra, U.; Mukherjee, S.; Fountzilas, C.; Boland, P.; Miller, A.; Patnaik, S.; Attwood, K.; Yendamuri, S.; Adjei, A.; Kannisto, E.; et al. Pralatrexate in Combination with Oxaliplatin in Advanced Esophagogastric Cancer: A Phase II Trial with Predictive Molecular Correlates. *Mol. Cancer Ther.* **2020**, *19*, 304–311. [CrossRef]
147. Ahn, D.H.; Rah, H.; Choi, Y.K.; Jeon, Y.J.; Min, K.T.; Kwack, K.; Hong, S.P.; Hwang, S.G.; Kim, N.K. Association of the miR-146aC>G, miR-149T>C, miR-196a2T>C, and miR-499A>G polymorphisms with gastric cancer risk and survival in the Korean population. *Mol. Carcinog.* **2013**, *52*, E39–E51. [CrossRef]
148. Ahadi, A. A systematic review of microRNAs as potential biomarkers for diagnosis and prognosis of gastric cancer. *Immunogenetics* **2021**, *73*, 155–161. [CrossRef]
149. Huang, M.; He, Y.R.; Liang, L.C.; Huang, Q.; Zhu, Z.Q. Circular RNA hsa_circ_0000745 may serve as a diagnostic marker for gastric cancer. *World J. Gastroenterol.* **2017**, *23*, 6330–6338. [CrossRef]
150. Qiu, H.B.; Zhang, L.Y.; Ren, C.; Zeng, Z.L.; Wu, W.J.; Luo, H.Y.; Zhou, Z.W.; Xu, R.H. Targeting CDH17 suppresses tumor progression in gastric cancer by downregulating Wnt/β-catenin signaling. *PLoS ONE* **2013**, *8*, e56959. [CrossRef]
151. Tuncel, T.; Karagoz, B.; Haholu, A.; Ozgun, A.; Emirzeoglu, L.; Bilgi, O.; Kandemir, E.G. Immunoregulatory function of HLA-G in gastric cancer. *Asian Pac. J. Cancer Prev.* **2013**, *14*, 7681–7684. [CrossRef] [PubMed]
152. Di Bartolomeo, M.; Pietrantonio, F.; Pellegrinelli, A.; Martinetti, A.; Mariani, L.; Daidone, M.G.; Bajetta, E.; Pelosi, G.; de Braud, F.; Floriani, I.; et al. Osteopontin, E-cadherin, and β-catenin expression as prognostic biomarkers in patients with radically resected gastric cancer. *Gastric Cancer* **2016**, *19*, 412–420. [CrossRef] [PubMed]
153. Seker, M.; Aydin, D.; Bilici, A.; Yavuzer, D.; Ozgun, M.G.; Ozcelik, M.; Aydin, O.; Aliustaoglu, M. Correlation of Caveolin-1 Expression with Prognosis in Patients with Gastric Cancer after Gastrectomy. *Oncol. Res. Treat.* **2017**, *40*, 185–190. [CrossRef] [PubMed]
154. Liu, H.; Shen, Z.; Wang, Z.; Wang, X.; Zhang, H.; Qin, J.; Qin, X.; Xu, J.; Sun, Y. Increased expression of IDO associates with poor postoperative clinical outcome of patients with gastric adenocarcinoma. *Sci. Rep.* **2016**, *6*, 21319. [CrossRef] [PubMed]
155. Yan, P.; Li, Y.H.; Tang, Z.J.; Shu, X.; Liu, X. High monocarboxylate transporter 4 protein expression in stromal cells predicts adverse survival in gastric cancer. *Asian Pac. J. Cancer Prev.* **2014**, *15*, 8923–8929. [CrossRef] [PubMed]
156. Romiti, A.; Di Rocco, R.; Milione, M.; Ruco, L.; Ziparo, V.; Zullo, A.; Duranti, E.; Sarcina, I.; Barucca, V.; D'Antonio, C.; et al. Somatostatin receptor subtype 2 A (SSTR2A) and HER2 expression in gastric adenocarcinoma. *Anticancer Res.* **2012**, *32*, 115–119.
157. Huang, Z.; Zhang, N.; Zha, L.; Mao, H.C.; Chen, X.; Xiang, J.F.; Zhang, H.; Wang, Z.W. Aberrant expression of the autocrine motility factor receptor correlates with poor prognosis and promotes metastasis in gastric carcinoma. *Asian Pac. J. Cancer Prev.* **2014**, *15*, 989–997. [CrossRef]

158. Thomaidis, T.; Maderer, A.; Al-Batran, S.E.; Kany, J.; Pauligk, C.; Steinmetz, K.; Schad, A.; Hofheinz, R.; Schmalenberg, H.; Homann, N.; et al. VEGFR-3 and CXCR4 as predictive markers for treatment with fluorouracil, leucovorin plus either oxaliplatin or cisplatin in patients with advanced esophagogastric cancer: A comparative study of the Arbeitsgemeinschaft Internistische Onkologie (AIO). *BMC Cancer* 2014, *14*, 476. [CrossRef] [PubMed]
159. Zhang, C.X.; Wu, C.T.; Xiao, L.; Tang, S.H. The diagnostic and clinicopathological value of trefoil factor 3 in patients with gastric cancer: A systsematic review and meta-analysis. *Biomarkers* 2021, *26*, 95–102. [CrossRef]
160. He, L.J.; Xie, D.; Hu, P.J.; Liao, Y.J.; Deng, H.X.; Kung, H.F.; Zhu, S.L. Macrophage migration inhibitory factor as a potential prognostic factor in gastric cancer. *World J. Gastroenterol.* 2015, *21*, 9916–9926. [CrossRef]
161. Hu, R.; Sou, K.; Takeoka, S. A rapid and highly sensitive biomarker detection platform based on a temperature-responsive liposome-linked immunosorbent assay. *Sci. Rep.* 2020, *10*, 18086. [CrossRef]
162. Hacker, U.T.; Escalona-Espinosa, L.; Consalvo, N.; Goede, V.; Schiffmann, L.; Scherer, S.J.; Hedge, P.; Van Cutsem, E.; Coutelle, O.; Büning, H. Evaluation of Angiopoietin-2 as a biomarker in gastric cancer: Results from the randomised phase III AVAGAST trial. *Br. J. Cancer* 2016, *114*, 855–862. [CrossRef]
163. Shikata, K.; Ninomiya, T.; Yonemoto, K.; Ikeda, F.; Hata, J.; Doi, Y.; Fukuhara, M.; Matsumoto, T.; Iida, M.; Kitazono, T.; et al. Optimal cutoff value of the serum pepsinogen level for prediction of gastric cancer incidence: The Hisayama Study. *Scand. J. Gastroenterol.* 2012, *47*, 669–675. [CrossRef]
164. Bang, C.S.; Lee, J.J.; Baik, G.H. Prediction of Chronic Atrophic Gastritis and Gastric Neoplasms by Serum Pepsinogen Assay: A Systematic Review and Meta-Analysis of Diagnostic Test Accuracy. *J. Clin. Med.* 2019, *8*, 657. [CrossRef]
165. Nagel, M.; Schulz, J.; Maderer, A.; Goepfert, K.; Gehrke, N.; Thomaidis, T.; Thuss-Patience, P.C.; Al-Batran, S.E.; Hegewisch-Becker, S.; Grimminger, P.; et al. Cytokeratin-18 fragments predict treatment response and overall survival in gastric cancer in a randomized controlled trial. *Tumor Biol.* 2018, *40*, 1–8. [CrossRef] [PubMed]
166. Kaplan, M.A.; Kucukoner, M.; Inal, A.; Urakci, Z.; Evliyaoglu, O.; Firat, U.; Kaya, M.; Isikdogan, A. Relationship between serum soluble vascular adhesion protein-1 level and gastric cancer prognosis. *Oncol. Res. Treat.* 2014, *37*, 340–344. [CrossRef]
167. Zhang, J.; Jin, H.C.; Zhu, A.K.; Ying, R.C.; Wei, W.; Zhang, F.J. Prognostic significance of plasma chemerin levels in patients with gastric cancer. *Peptides* 2014, *61*, 7–11. [CrossRef] [PubMed]
168. Wei, Y.; Wang, T.; Song, H.; Tian, L.; Lyu, G.; Zhao, L.; Xue, Y. C-C motif chemokine 22 ligand (CCL22) concentrations in sera of gastric cancer patients are related to peritoneal metastasis and predict recurrence within one year after radical gastrectomy. *J. Surg. Res.* 2017, *211*, 266–278. [CrossRef] [PubMed]
169. Xu, B.B.; Lu, J.; Zheng, Z.F.; Xie, J.W.; Wang, J.B.; Lin, J.X.; Chen, Q.Y.; Cao, L.L.; Lin, M.; Tu, R.H.; et al. The predictive value of the preoperative C-reactive protein-albumin ratio for early recurrence and chemotherapy benefit in patients with gastric cancer after radical gastrectomy: Using randomized phase III trial data. *Gastric Cancer* 2019, *22*, 1016–1028. [CrossRef]
170. Lu, J.; Xu, B.B.; Zheng, Z.F.; Xie, J.W.; Wang, J.B.; Lin, J.X.; Chen, Q.Y.; Cao, L.L.; Lin, M.; Tu, R.H.; et al. CRP/prealbumin, a novel inflammatory index for predicting recurrence after radical resection in gastric cancer patients: Post hoc analysis of a randomized phase III trial. *Gastric Cancer* 2019, *22*, 536–545. [CrossRef]
171. Lin, T.C. The role of visfatin in cancer proliferation, angiogenesis, metastasis, drug resistance and clinical prognosis. *Cancer Manag. Res.* 2019, *11*, 3481–3491. [CrossRef]
172. Lu, G.W.; Wang, Q.J.; Xia, M.M.; Qian, J. Elevated plasma visfatin levels correlate with poor prognosis of gastric cancer patients. *Peptides* 2014, *58*, 60–64. [CrossRef]
173. Fujiwara, Y.; Okada, K.; Hanada, H.; Tamura, S.; Kimura, Y.; Fujita, J.; Imamura, H.; Kishi, K.; Yano, M.; Miki, H.; et al. The clinical importance of a transcription reverse-transcription concerted (TRC) diagnosis using peritoneal lavage fluids in gastric cancer with clinical serosal invasion: A prospective, multicenter study. *Surgery* 2014, *155*, 417–423. [CrossRef]
174. Tamura, S.; Fujiwara, Y.; Kimura, Y.; Fujita, J.; Imamura, H.; Kinuta, M.; Yano, M.; Hiratsuka, M.; Kobayashi, K.; Okada, K.; et al. Prognostic information derived from RT-PCR analysis of peritoneal fluid in gastric cancer patients: Results from a prospective multicenter clinical trial. *J. Surg. Oncol.* 2014, *109*, 75–80. [CrossRef] [PubMed]
175. Xie, D.; Wang, Y.; Shen, J.; Hu, J.; Yin, P.; Gong, J. Detection of carcinoembryonic antigen in peritoneal fluid of patients undergoing laparoscopic distal gastrectomy with complete mesogastric excision. *Br. J. Surg.* 2018, *105*, 1471–1479. [CrossRef] [PubMed]
176. Lee, M.W.; Kim, G.H.; Jeon, H.K.; Park, S.J. Clinical Application of Circulating Tumor Cells in Gastric Cancer. *Gut Liver* 2019, *13*, 394–401. [CrossRef] [PubMed]
177. Pernot, S.; Badouel, C.; Terme, M.; Castan, F.; Cazes, A.; Bouche, O.; Bennouna, J.; Francois, E.; Ghiringhelli, F.; De La Fouchardiere, C.; et al. Dynamic evaluation of circulating tumour cells in patients with advanced gastric and oesogastric junction adenocarcinoma: Prognostic value and early assessment of therapeutic effects. *Eur. J. Cancer* 2017, *79*, 15–22. [CrossRef]
178. Sclafani, F.; Smyth, E.; Cunningham, D.; Chau, I.; Turner, A.; Watkins, D. A pilot study assessing the incidence and clinical significance of circulating tumor cells in esophagogastric cancers. *Clin. Colorectal. Cancer* 2014, *13*, 94–99. [CrossRef]
179. Li, M.; Zhang, B.; Zhang, Z.; Liu, X.; Qi, X.; Zhao, J.; Jiang, Y.; Zhai, H.; Ji, Y.; Luo, D. Stem cell-like circulating tumor cells indicate poor prognosis in gastric cancer. *Biomed. Res. Int.* 2014, *2014*, 981261. [CrossRef] [PubMed]
180. Kim, J.; Bae, J.-S. Tumor-Associated Macrophages and Neutrophils in Tumor Microenvironment. *Mediators Inflamm.* 2016, *2016*, 6058147. [CrossRef]

181. Tada, Y.; Togashi, Y.; Kotani, D.; Kuwata, T.; Sato, E.; Kawazoe, A.; Doi, T.; Wada, H.; Nishikawa, H.; Shitara, K. Targeting VEGFR2 with Ramucirumab strongly impacts effector/ activated regulatory T cells and CD8(+) T cells in the tumor microenvironment. *J. Immunother. Cancer* **2018**, *6*, 106. [CrossRef]
182. Pernot, S.; Terme, M.; Radosevic-Robin, N.; Castan, F.; Badoual, C.; Marcheteau, E.; Penault-Llorca, F.; Bouche, O.; Bennouna, J.; Francois, E.; et al. Infiltrating and peripheral immune cell analysis in advanced gastric cancer according to the Lauren classification and its prognostic significance. *Gastric Cancer* **2020**, *23*, 73–81. [CrossRef]
183. Zeng, D.; Li, M.; Zhou, R.; Zhang, J.; Sun, H.; Shi, M.; Bin, J.; Liao, Y.; Rao, J.; Liao, W. Tumor Microenvironment Characterization in Gastric Cancer Identifies Prognostic and Immunotherapeutically Relevant Gene Signatures. *Cancer Immunol. Res.* **2019**, *7*, 737–750. [CrossRef]
184. Li, B.; Jiang, Y.; Li, G.; Fisher, G.A., Jr.; Li, R. Natural killer cell and stroma abundance are independently prognostic and predict gastric cancer chemotherapy benefit. *JCI Insight.* **2020**, *5*, e136570. [CrossRef]
185. Zhang, C.; Li, D.; Yu, R.; Li, C.; Song, Y.; Chen, X.; Fan, Y.; Liu, Y.; Qu, X. Immune Landscape of Gastric Carcinoma Tumor Microenvironment Identifies a Peritoneal Relapse Relevant Immune Signature. *Front. Immunol.* **2021**, *12*, 651033. [CrossRef] [PubMed]
186. Li, W.; Song, D.; Li, H.; Liang, L.; Zhao, N.; Liu, T. Reduction in Peripheral CD19+CD24hCD27+ B Cell Frequency Predicts Favourable Clinical Course in XELOX-Treated Patients with Advanced Gastric Cancer. *Cell Physiol. Biochem.* **2017**, *41*, 2045–2052. [CrossRef] [PubMed]
187. Gu, X.; Gao, X.S.; Cui, M.; Xie, M.; Peng, C.; Bai, Y.; Guo, W.; Han, L.; Gu, X.; Xiong, W. Clinicopathological and prognostic significance of platelet to lymphocyte ratio in patients with gastric cancer. *Oncotarget* **2016**, *7*, 49878–49887. [CrossRef]
188. Chen, L.; Hao, Y.; Cong, X.; Zou, M.; Li, S.; Zhu, L.; Song, H.; Xue, Y. Peripheral Venous Blood Platelet-to-Lymphocyte Ratio (PLR) for Predicting the Survival of Patients With Gastric Cancer Treated With SOX or XELOX Regimen Neoadjuvant Chemotherapy. *Technol. Cancer Res. Treat.* **2019**, *18*, 1–13. [CrossRef] [PubMed]
189. Shimada, H.; Takiguchi, N.; Kainuma, O.; Soda, H.; Ikeda, A.; Cho, A.; Miyazaki, A.; Gunji, H.; Yamamoto, H.; Nagata, M. High preoperative neutrophil-lymphocyte ratio predicts poor survival in patients with gastric cancer. *Gastric Cancer* **2010**, *13*, 170–176. [CrossRef] [PubMed]
190. Kim, H.S.; Lee, H.; Shin, S.J.; Beom, S.H.; Jung, M.; Bae, S.; Lee, E.Y.; Park, K.H.; Choi, Y.Y.; Son, T.; et al. Complementary utility of targeted next-generation sequencing and immunohistochemistry panels as a screening platform to select targeted therapy for advanced gastric cancer. *Oncotarget* **2017**, *8*, 38389–38398. [CrossRef]
191. Park, J.J.; Hsu, G.; Siden, E.G.; Thorlund, K.; Mills, E.J. An overview of precision oncology basket and umbrella trials for clinicians. *CA Cancer J. Clin.* **2020**, *70*, 125–137. [CrossRef]
192. Malone, E.R.; Oliva, M.; Sabatini, P.J.; Stockley, T.L.; Siu, L.L. Molecular profiling for precision cancer therapies. *Genome Med.* **2020**, *12*, 8. [CrossRef] [PubMed]

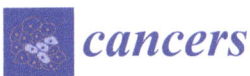

Review

Challenges for Better Diagnosis and Management of Pancreatic and Biliary Tract Cancers Focusing on Blood Biomarkers: A Systematic Review

Hiroto Tominaga [1], Juntaro Matsuzaki [1,*], Chihiro Oikawa [1], Kensho Toyoshima [1], Haruki Manabe [1], Eriko Ozawa [1], Atsushi Shimamura [1], Riko Yokoyama [1], Yusuke Serizawa [1], Takahiro Ochiya [2] and Yoshimasa Saito [1,*]

1 Division of Pharmacotherapeutics, Keio University Faculty of Pharmacy, 1-5-30 Shibakoen, Minato-ku, Tokyo 105-8512, Japan; tominagahiroto@keio.jp (H.T.); 0808oocc@keio.jp (C.O.); toyoken724@keio.jp (K.T.); haruki.may19@keio.jp (H.M.); eriko.ozw@gmail.com (E.O.); btw.orz.321427@keio.jp (A.S.); rikoy@keio.jp (R.Y.); serizawa.y29@keio.jp (Y.S.)
2 Department of Molecular and Cellular Medicine, Institute of Medical Science, Tokyo Medical University, 6-7-1 Nishishinjuku, Shinjuku-ku, Tokyo 160-0023, Japan; tochiya@tokyo-med.ac.jp
* Correspondence: juntaro.matsuzaki@keio.jp (J.M.); saito-ys@pha.keio.ac.jp (Y.S.)

Simple Summary: Pancreatic and biliary tract cancers are malignant tumors that have a very poor prognosis and are resistant to chemotherapy. The later a cancer is detected, the worse the prognosis becomes; therefore, early detection is important. Biomarkers are physiological indices that serve as a guide to indicate the presence or absence of a certain disease, or its progression. The purpose of our research is to summarize previously reported biomarkers for the diagnosis and prognosis of pancreatic and biliary tract cancers.

Abstract: Background: pancreatic cancer (PCa) and biliary tract cancer (BTC) are cancers with a poor prognosis and few effective treatments. One of the reasons for this is late detection. Many researchers are tackling to develop non-invasive biomarkers for cancer, but few are specific for PCa or BTC. In addition, genetic abnormalities occur in cancer tissues, which ultimately affect the expression of various molecules. Therefore, it is important to identify molecules that are altered in PCa and BTC. For this systematic review, a systematic review of Medline and Embase to select biomarker studies of PCa and BTC patients was conducted. Results: after reviewing 72 studies, 79 biomarker candidates were identified, including 22 nucleic acids, 43 proteins, and 14 immune cell types. Of the 72 studies, 61 examined PCa, and 11 examined BTC. Conclusion: PCa and BTC are characterized by nucleic acid, protein, and immune cell profiles that are markedly different from those of healthy subjects. These altered molecules and cell subsets may serve as cancer-specific biomarkers, particularly in blood. Further studies are needed to better understand the diagnosis and prognosis of PCa and BTC.

Keywords: biomarker; chemoresistance; liquid biopsy; microRNA; long non-coding RNA

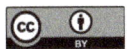

1. Introduction

Pancreatic cancer (PCa) is the fourth most common cause of death in Japan. Indeed, there were an estimated 496,000 (234,000 in Asia) new cases annually worldwide in 2020, and the number of new cases is estimated to be 802,000 (424,000 in Asia) in 2040 [1]. Despite the rapid evolution of cancer treatments in recent years, the 5-year survival rate for PCa is only 5–6% [2]. Biliary tract cancer (BTC), which includes cholangiocarcinoma (both intrahepatic cholangiocarcinoma (ICC) and extrahepatic cholangiocarcinoma (ECC)) and gallbladder cancer, also has a poor prognosis [3]. BTC has a low incidence, accounting for about 3% of all adult cancers [4]. Most cases are unresectable [3], and even if they could be found in the resectable stage, recurrence rates are very high [5,6]. The 5-year survival rate for BTC is about 5–15% [7,8]. Since PCa and BTC are less symptomatic, these cancers are generally hard to detect at an early stage. Furthermore, PCa and BTC have similar pathological characteristics, which makes it difficult to discriminate them just by blood biomarkers. Therefore, identifying good biomarkers for the diagnosis and prognosis of PCa and BTC is important for both early diagnosis and treatment. This review comprehensively summarized the current state of blood biomarker studies for PCa and BTC, which may lead to early detection and improved prognosis.

2. Methods

A systematic electronic search of the Medline (https://pubmed.ncbi.nlm.nih.gov, accessed on 10 February 2021) and Embase (https://www.embase.com, accessed on 10 February 2021) databases was performed to identify studies reporting the characteristics of PCa and BTC patients (Figure 1). The search was performed using the following terms with Boolean operators: (biliary OR bile OR cholangiocarcinoma OR pancreatic OR pancreas) AND biomarker AND (checkpoint OR chemoresistance) AND (blood OR serum OR plasma). The same terms were used on Medline and Embase, and duplicated articles were deleted. Articles that were not written in English, review articles, conference abstracts, and articles about cancer types other than PCa or BTC were excluded. A systematic review of articles that met the selection criteria was performed. Abstract and in-text reviews were performed by a single reviewer (H.T.). The selected research articles were cross-searched to identify additional relevant studies. This review also introduces tissue biomarkers and other biomarkers that can be applied as blood biomarkers.

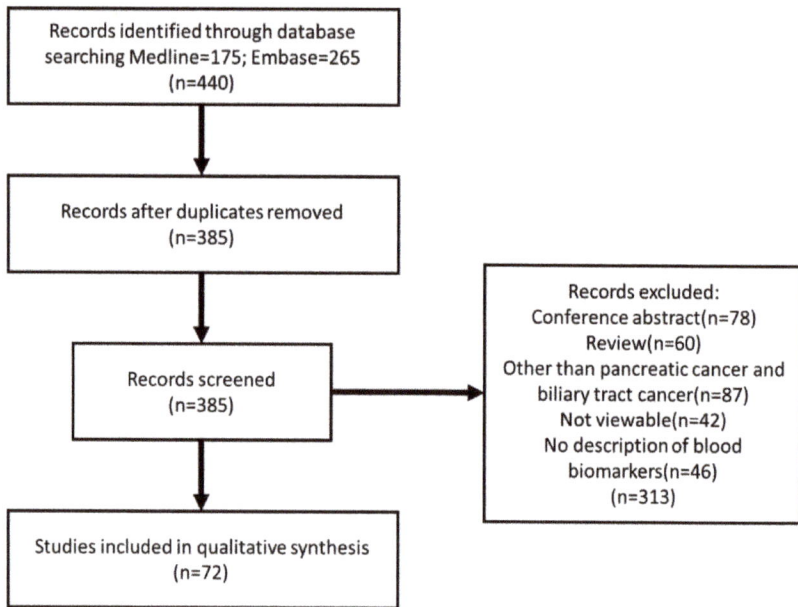

Figure 1. Flow diagram of literature search.

3. Results

3.1. Characteristics of PCa

3.1.1. Non-Coding RNA

Many circulating microRNAs were reported as biomarkers for PCa patients (Table 1). Meta-analysis revealed that, compared with healthy controls, elevated plasma miR-744 levels in PCa patients were a poor prognostic factor, contributing to reduced progression-free survival [9]. Serum miR-21 levels were also elevated and were even higher in patients with gemcitabine-resistant PCa; these elevated levels correlated with poor survival [10,11].

Serum miR-7 expression was lower in PCa patients than in controls and had an adverse effect on prognosis [12]. In addition, plasma miR-34a and miR-150 levels, and expression of miR-34a and miR-150 in tumor tissue, were lower in PCa patients than in healthy controls [13]. Plasma miR-107, miR-126, miR-451, miR-145, miR-491-5p, and miR-146b-5p levels decreased in PCa patients, with miR-107 being the most decreased miRNA [14]. PCa patients showed high amounts of miR-191, miR-21, and miR-451a in serum exosomes, and high miR-21 was associated with overall survival and resistance to chemotherapy [15]. MiR-200b and miR-200c were overexpressed in serum exosomes from PCa patients, and high expression of miR-200c in total serum exosomes and miR-200b in EpCAM-positive serum exosomes correlated with shorter overall survival (OS). In PCa patients, nucleic acids other than mRNA were also altered; for example, serum LINC01559 expression was markedly increased than in healthy controls and correlated with survival [16]. Expression of let-7 family members (especially let-7d) in the plasma of PCa patients correlated inversely with overall survival [11].

Table 1. Biomarker candidates for non-coding RNA identified in the present systematic review.

Cancer Type	Biomarker	Diagnosis	Prognosis	Chemoresistance	Species	Plasma	Serum	Serum Exosome	Tissue	Ref.
PCa	miR-205	X		X	Human, Mouse				Y	[17]
	miR-7	X	X		Human		Y			[12]
	miR-200b, miR-200c	X			Human			Y		[18]
	miR-191, miR-21, miR-451a	X	X		Human			Y		[15]
	miR-744	X	X		Human	Y				[9]
	LINC01559	X		X	Human		Y			[16]
	miR-34a, miR-150	X	X		Human	Y			Y	[13]
	miR-21			X	Human		Y			[10,11]
	let-7	X	X		Human	Y	Y			[11]
	miR-107	X	X		Human	Y				[14]
BTC	miR-155HG	X		X	Human				Y	[19]

PCa, pancreatic cancer; BTC, biliary tract cancer.

3.1.2. Protein Expression

A very large number of protein biomarker candidates were extracted (Table 2). High expression of colon carcinoma-1 (MACC1) oncogene in serum of PCa patients correlated with lymph node metastasis, distant metastasis, and a later TNM stage [20]. Plasma IL-8 was the circulating factor that correlated most significantly with the overall survival of PCa patients [21]. PIM-1 expression was upregulated significantly in PCa tissues compared with normal tissues. In addition, plasma PIM-1 levels were significantly increased and were associated with TNM stage (II/III/IV) [22]. Although protein levels in the blood are unknown, many proteins that can be tissue biomarkers for PCa were also identified by our search algorithm. 72% of PCa patients expressed activated insulin/IGF receptors on tumor cells [23]. Expression of CD133, Notch1, Notch2, and Notch4 receptors was significantly higher in PCa tissues than in pancreatic tissues from patients with benign lesions [13]. Patients with lower levels of lactate and higher levels of human equilibrium nucleoside transporter (hENT1) in PCa tissue had better survival rates [24]. Disheveled-axin (DIX) domain (DIXDC1), a protein containing a coiled-coil domain and a DIX domain, was also highly expressed in PCa tissues and correlated with worse OS [25]. By contrast, expression of the V-domain Ig suppressor of T cell activation (VISTA) in PCa tissues was significantly associated with prolonged OS [26], and while expression of PD-1 or PD-L1 in pancreatic neuroendocrine tumors was rare, expression of PD-L2 was common in neuroendocrine tumor subtypes. Expression of immune-related proteins was also altered, with well-differentiated pancreatic neuroendocrine tumors expressing low levels of PD-1 and PD-L1 [27]. Cancer-associated pancreatic fibroblasts isolated from the tumors of PCa patients showed higher expression of PD-L1 than primary dermal fibroblasts from healthy subjects [28]. Low HLA class I expression in PCa tissues was the only risk factor for poor survival; PD-L1-negative and HLA class I high-expressing PCa was significantly associated with an increased number of infiltrating CD8+ T cells in the TME, and with improved prognosis [29]. The spindle and kinetochore-associated genes SKA1-3 were highly expressed in PCa tissues; high expression of SKA1 and SKA3 was associated with a poor prognosis [30].

Table 2. Biomarker candidates for proteins identified in the present systematic review.

Cancer Type	Biomarker	Diagnosis	Prognosis	Chemoresistance	Species	Plasma	Serum	Tissue	Cell	Cell Exosome	Ref.
PCa	EphA2			X	Human					Y	[31]
	Galectin-9	X	X		Human			Y			[32]
	FAK	X		X	Mouse			Y			[33]
	CD11b	X		X	Human			Y			[34]
	MLL1			X	Human, Mouse			Y			[35]
	CD47		X		Human			Y			[32]
	Granulin			X	Human, Mouse			Y	Y		[36]
	EHF			X	Mouse			Y			[37]
	IFNγ			X	Human			Y			[38]
	PDL-2	X			Human			Y			[27]
	CD38/CD101	X	X		Human	Y		Y			[39]
	ATP, HMGB1			X	Mouse			Y			[40]
	Gastrin		X		Mouse			Y			[41]
	IL8	X	X		Human	Y					[21]
	PD-L1, PD-L2	X			Human			Y			[28]
	CDH3, PLAU, LFNG		X		Human	Y					[42]
	CD16	X			Human			Y			[43]
	PIM-1	X	X		Human	Y					[22]
	IL3			X	Mouse			Y			[44]
	Lactic acid	X	X		Human			Y			[24]
	CD171			X	Mouse			Y			[45]
	EpCAM, CD3			X	Human				Y		[46]
	DIXDC1	X	X		Human			Y			[25]
	sVCAM-1		X		Human, Mouse	Y		Y			[47]
	VISTA	X	X		Human			Y			[26]
	IGF	X			Human			Y			[23]
	LOX family			X	Human, Mouse			Y			[48]
	MACC1	X		X	Human		Y				[20]
	ETF			X	Mouse			Y			[37]
	IRE1α	X			Human, Mouse			Y	Y		[49]
	Slug			X	Human				Y		[50]
	ADAM family	X		X	Human			Y			[51]
	HLA class I		X		Human			Y			[29]
	SKA1, SKA3	X	X		Human			Y			[30]
BTC	GITR, CTLA4	X		X	Human			Y			[52]
	HHLA2	X	X		Human			Y			[53]
	PD-1	X		X	Human			Y			[52,54]
	FasL, MCP-1, IFNγ		X		Human		Y				[55]
	C24-Ceramide	X	X		Human			Y			[56]
	Csk2	X	X	X	Human			Y			[57]
	BUB1B		X		Human			Y			[58]
	MFAP5	X	X		Human	Y		Y			[59]
	PD-1/PD-L1	X	X		Human			Y			[60]

PCa, pancreatic cancer; BTC, biliary tract cancer.

3.1.3. Immune Cell Types

Several biomarker candidates were also extracted for immune cells (Table 3). High CD38/CD101 co-expression by PD-1+ CD8+ T cells in the peripheral blood of PCa patients or tumor-infiltrating lymphocytes (TILs) in PCa tissues correlated significantly with tumor/node/metastasis (T/N/M) classification, and with clinical stage and survival [39]. Immune cell changes were more common in tumor tissue. Cytokines and chemokines associated with immune cells that were altered in tumor tissues may be potential biomarkers in blood. In PCa, the paraneoplastic stroma containing cancer cells harbored fewer CD8+ T cells than stroma without cancer cells [61]. By contrast, the number of tumor-infiltrating

CD68+M, CD163+M2, and CD47 cells was higher, and these cells were significantly associated with decreased OS [32]. Expression of tumor antigens MYPT1, PSMC5, and TRFR was also significantly higher in PCa tissues than in healthy controls; patients with antibodies specific for these antigens showed improved disease-free survival after granulocyte macrophage colony-stimulating factor-secreting pancreatic cancer vaccine (GVAX) therapy [62]. Tumor-infiltrating T cells showed higher expression of galectin 9 than normal T cells [63].

Table 3. Biomarker candidates for immune cells identified in the present systematic review.

Cancer Type	Biomarker	Diagnosis	Prognosis	Chemoresistance	Species	Serum	Tissue	Cell	Ref.
PCa	ILC2			X	Human, Mouse		Y	Y	[64]
	CD8(+) T cells	X		X	Human, Mouse		Y		[61,65,66]
	Myeloid cells	X			Mouse		Y		[67]
	Mesothelin-specific cells		X		Human	Y			[68]
	M2-type macrophages			X	Mouse		Y		[69]
	MYPT1, PSMC5, TRFR	X			Human		Y		[62]
	TAM		X		Mouse		Y		[70]
	CD4+ T cells			X	Mouse		Y		[66]
	Treg	X			Human		Y		[71]
	T cells, NK cells		X		Mouse		Y		[72]
BTC	PD-1(+)/CD8(+) TILs		X		Human		Y		[73]

PCa, pancreatic cancer.

3.2. Characteristics of BTC

3.2.1. Non-Coding RNA

No candidate blood biomarkers for BTC were extracted. Cholangiocarcinoma (CCA) tissues showed lower expression of the lncRNA miR-155 host gene (miR-155HG). In addition, miR-155HG was closely associated with improved OS [19].

3.2.2. Protein Expression

MFAP5 levels in the serum of ICC patients and expression of MFAP5 in the ECC tissues was lower than in healthy controls [59]. The co-stimulatory receptor GITR, and co-inhibitory receptors PD-1 and CTLA4, were overexpressed by TILs when compared with T cells in blood and normal tissues [52]. Some candidate biomarkers in blood that had been altered in the tissue were also extracted. In GBC tissues, elevated expression of SPTLC1 and CERS2, and that of their product C24-ceramide, was associated with tumor stage, distal metastasis, and poor prognosis [56]. Expression of BUB1B was increased in CCA tissues, and ECC patients with high expression of BUB1B showed worse OS and recurrence-free survival than those with low expression of BUB1B [58]. Cks2 was significantly elevated in BTC tissues, and its overexpression was associated with poor differentiation, CA19-9, and a poor prognosis [57].

3.2.3. Immune Cell Types

Serum soluble FasL, MCP-1, and interferon-γ also correlated with poor prognosis in BTC patients [55]. Some immune cells that had been altered in the tissue were extracted. The percentage of cytotoxic T cells and natural killer cells was lower in CCA tissues than in normal tissues; however, the percentage of regulatory T cells was higher [52]. In ECC patients, a higher ratio of PD-1(+)/CD8(+) TILs meant lower OS, recurrence-free survival, and distant metastasis-free survival [73]. The number of PD-1+ T cells and expression of PD-L1 in the tumor tissues of ICC patients were elevated, which had a negative impact on prognosis. By contrast, high numbers of PD-1+ T cells or high expression of PD-L1 in normal tissues had no effect on prognosis [60]. Furthermore, expression of HHLA2 in ICC tissues was more common than that of PD-L1 (49.0% vs. 28.1%, respectively); overexpression of HHLA2 was associated with decreased CD3 + TIL and CD8 + TIL numbers and higher CD4+ Foxp3+/CD8 + TIL ratios, which affected OS. By contrast, infiltration of the tumor by PD-L1-expressing T cells and CD163+ tumor-associated macrophages were not associated with OS [53].

3.3. Treatment of PCa and BTC

3.3.1. PCa, BTC, and Immune Checkpoint Inhibition

In recent years, immune checkpoint inhibitors have been used to treat cancer. CD8+ cytotoxic T cells are important effectors of the immune response against cancer. Immune checkpoint inhibitors are effective only when CD8+ T cells infiltrate the tumor; thus, immune checkpoint inhibitors alone are ineffective against PCa because CD8+ T cells do not infiltrate the tumor [74,75]. Many factors regulate the movement of CD8+ T cells, including activation of the tumor endothelium by T cell-derived IL-3, which triggers T cell infiltration [44], and deficiency of tumor ETS homology factor, which causes a decrease in the number of regulatory T cells, myeloid-derived suppressor cells, and tumor-infiltrating CD8+ T cells [37]. Although metastatic PCa tumors are largely resistant to anti-PD-1 therapy, blockade of PD-1 in granulin-depleted tumors restores anti-tumor immunity [36]. PD-1/PD-L1 and CD8 T cells are closely related, as PD-1 blockade can increase CD8 T cell and tumor-specific interferon-γ production in the tumor microenvironment [38] or produce anti-tumor effects by increasing KLRG1 + LAG3 - TNFα+ tumor-specific T cells in tumors [76]. Bone marrow cells inhibit CD8+ T cell anti-tumor activity by inducing expression of PD-L1 by tumor cells in an epidermal growth factor receptor (EGFR)/mitogen-activated protein kinase (MAPK)-dependent manner [67]. In addition, there are many pathways that alter immune cells, such as when gastrin is stimulated concurrently with PD-1 AB administration, tumors have less fibrosis, inhibitory Treg lymphocytes, and tumor-associated macrophages [41]. The combination of an anti-PD-L1 mouse monoclonal (MAb) and a TGF-β type I receptor small molecule kinase inhibitor (LY364947) results in the long-term survival of mice due to the influx of CD8α T cells into the TME [77]. Moreover, the combination of entinostat (ENT), a histone deacetylase inhibitor, and immune checkpoint inhibition significantly alter the infiltration and function of innate immune cells, allowing for a more potent adaptive immune response [65]. Inhibition of MLL1, a PD-L1 transcriptional activator, in combination with an anti-PD-L1 or an anti-PD-1 antibody, effectively suppresses pancreatic tumor growth in a FasL- and CTL-dependent manner [35]. In addition, immune checkpoint inhibitors are important in combination with other drugs, as inhibition of over-activated focal adhesion kinase (FAK) greatly reduces tumor fibrosis and the number of tumor-infiltrating immunosuppressive cells, making them sensitive to T-cell immunotherapy and PD-1 antagonists [33]. The role of CD8+ T cells in immune checkpoint inhibition is very important; for example, treatment with a small glutamine analog (6-diazo-5-oxo-L-norleucine [DON]) reduces the amount of hyaluronan and collagen in the TME, leading to extensive remodeling of the extracellular matrix and increased infiltration by CD8+ T cells [78]. On the other hand, other immune cells have also been implicated in anti-tumor effects, such as CD4+-dependent anti-tumor effects [66] and innate lymphocytes (ILC2), which are anticancer immune cells in PCa immunotherapy and emerge as tissue-specific enhancers of cancer immunity that amplify the efficacy of anti-PD-1 immunotherapy [64]. Partial activation of CD11b leads to repolarization of tumor-associated macrophages, reduced numbers of tumor-infiltrating immunosuppressive myeloid cells, and enhanced dendritic cell responses, all of which improve anti-tumor T cell-mediated immunity and make checkpoint inhibitors effective in previously unresponsive PCa models [34]. Targeting immune cells is important; indeed, the combination of a CD40 agonist and a PD-1 antagonist MAb exerts anti-tumor effects, which are manifested through tumor infiltration by IFNγ-, Granzyme B-, and TNFα-secreting effector T cells [79]. The combination of agonist antibodies (ABS) targeting the immunostimulatory CD40 receptor plus MEK inhibitors suppressing M2 macrophages, bone marrow-derived suppressor cells, and T regulatory cells generates a potent synergistic anti-tumor effect [69]. Mice with EHF-overexpressing tumors responded significantly better to anti-PD-1 therapy than those with control tumors [37]. In addition, anti-PD-L1 therapy sensitized pancreatic cancer cells to antiangiogenic therapy and, conversely, antiangiogenic therapy improved anti-PD-L1 therapy [80].

3.3.2. Resistance of PCa and BTC to Chemotherapy

Although gemcitabine is used as a drug to treat PCa, cancer often becomes resistant; this is one of the reasons PCa is difficult to treat [81]. Cancer stem-like cells (CSLC), which can differentiate into a variety of mature cell types, have a high rate of metastasis and are implicated in resistance to chemotherapy [82]. Chemoresistant cancer cells possess stem-like characteristics, such as the ability to form spheres and high expression of cancer stem cell-like surface markers CD44/CD133 [83]. Therefore, it is important to target CSLCs. The combination of activated T cells and cutamaxomab eliminates CSLCs [46]. Soluble vascular cell adhesion molecule-1 (SVCAM-1) increases tumor resistance to gemcitabine [47]; however, combining gemcitabine with inhibition of the adhesion molecule L1CAM (CD171) reduces VEGF expression and the number of CD31-positive vessels, resulting in a stronger anti-tumor effect [45]. Cell adhesion molecules are also implicated in chemotherapy resistance. Knockdown of Slug, which regulates epithelial-mesenchymal transition (EMT), makes cells sensitive to gemcitabine [50]. Increased activity of LOX family proteins promotes chemoresistance because LOX proteins mediate collagen cross-linking and reinforce the tumor stroma and extracellular matrix (ECM), thereby promoting resistance to chemotherapy [48]. In addition, miRNAs are involved. MiR-205 reduces the expression of chemoresistance markers and re-sensitizes cells to gemcitabine [17]. In addition, the combination of ursolic acid and gemcitabine decreases Ki67 and miR-29A expression, thereby inhibiting tumor cell proliferation [84]. Expression of exosomal ephrin A receptor 2 (EphA2) may induce chemoresistance [31], whereas suppression of the NF-κB pathway may make cells sensitive to gemcitabine [85].

4. Discussion

There were many more studies of PCa (n = 61) than of BTC (n = 11), which may reflect the overwhelmingly larger numbers of PCa patients compared with BTC patients. However, such as PCa, BTC is a cancer that is difficult to diagnose/treat and has a poor prognosis; therefore, it is important to identify biomarkers for this cancer type. In addition, for clinical application, it is important to clarify whether PCa biomarkers can be used as BTC biomarkers in PCa and BTC, which have similar characteristics. We found differential expression of many miRNAs in PCa and BTC patients compared with healthy individuals. MiRNAs are small non-coding RNAs that negatively regulate the expression of most of the mRNAs in cells and have unique and diverse expression patterns in cancers [86]. Because miRNAs expression is altered not only in cancer tissues but also in plasma, blood-borne miRNAs such as miR-21 and miR-107 are promising biomarkers for diagnosis and prognosis of PCa and BTC. Protein expressions and immune cell compositions are also different in cancer tissues and normal tissues. Usually, tissue biomarkers are useful for predicting cancer prognosis and resistance to treatment but cannot be used for diagnosis. However, we found that many biomarkers in tissue also appeared in the blood. Thus, it is important to investigate the expression of tissue biomarkers in blood. In addition, there are many therapeutic targets for PCa and BTC, which can be useful biomarkers in blood. For example, the number of immune cells, such as cytotoxic T cells and natural killer cells, was low in PCa and BTC, whereas expression of immune checkpoint molecules, such as PD-1/PD-L1 and PD2/PDL2, was high. Immune checkpoint inhibitors are promising cancer drugs, but they are only effective when CD8+ T cells can infiltrate the tumor [74]. Hence, disease prognosis and sensitivity to immune checkpoint inhibitors can be predicted by examining immune checkpoint molecules, such as PD-1/PD-L1, and immune cells, such as CD8 + T cells, in the blood. In addition, stem cell markers may be useful biomarkers of chemotherapy resistance. Currently, cell-free DNA sequencing is in progress in the US, and miRNA testing technology is being developed in Japan. Especially, the methylation status of cell-free DNA is one of the most promising circulating biomarkers for various cancer detection [87].

5. Conclusions

A large number of miRNAs were extracted as candidate biomarkers in blood for the diagnosis and prognosis of PCa and BTC. A total of 37 biomarkers for diagnosis, 22 biomarkers for prognosis, and 23 biomarkers for treatment resistance were detected. Thus far, it is hard to predict which markers would be better than the others, thus that we should keep on investigating and verifying many kinds of biomarkers in parallel. Ultimately, some combinations of several different types of biomarkers will be applied to future clinical practice. Further research for biomarkers in the blood is warranted for early detection and proper management of PCa and BTC.

Author Contributions: Study design, H.T., J.M.; data collection, H.T., C.O., K.T., H.M., E.O., A.S., R.Y. and Y.S. (Yusuke Serizawa); writing—original draft preparation, H.T.; writing—review and editing, J.M., T.O. and Y.S. (Yoshimasa Saito). All authors have read and agreed to the published version of the manuscript.

Funding: This research was supported by a Grant-in-Aid for Scientific Research C (17K09471, to J.M.) from the Japan Society for the Promotion of Science (JSPS).

Institutional Review Board Statement: Not applicable.

Conflicts of Interest: The authors declare no conflict of interest.

References

1. Sung, H.; Ferlay, J.; Siegel, R.L.; Laversanne, M.; Soerjomataram, I.; Jemal, A.; Bray, F. Global Cancer Statistics 2020: GLOBOCAN Estimates of Incidence and Mortality Worldwide for 36 Cancers in 185 Countries. *CA Cancer J. Clin.* **2021**, *71*, 209–249. [CrossRef]
2. Seufferlein, T.; Mayerle, J. Pancreatic cancer in 2015: Precision medicine in pancreatic cancer—Fact or fiction? *Nat. Rev. Gastroen-terol. Hepatol.* **2016**, *13*, 74–75. [CrossRef]
3. Jansen, H.; Pape, U.-F.; Utku, N. A review of systemic therapy in biliary tract carcinoma. *J. Gastrointest. Oncol.* **2020**, *11*, 770–789. [CrossRef]
4. Banales, J.M.; Cardinale, V.; Carpino, G.; Marzioni, M.; Andersen, J.B.; Invernizzi, P.; Lind, G.E.; Folseraas, T.; Forbes, S.J.; Fouassier, L.; et al. Expert consensus document: Cholangiocarcinoma: Current knowledge and future perspectives consensus statement from the European Network for the Study of Cholangiocarcinoma (ENS-CCA). *Nat. Rev. Gastroenterol. Hepatol.* **2016**, *13*, 261–280. [CrossRef]
5. Wang, Y.; Li, J.; Xia, Y.; Gong, R.; Wang, K.; Yan, Z.; Wan, X.; Liu, G.; Wu, D.; Shi, L.; et al. Prognostic nomogram for intrahepatic cholangiocarcinoma after partial hepatectomy. *J. Clin. Oncol.* **2013**, *31*, 1188–1195. [CrossRef] [PubMed]
6. Wang, S.J.; Lemieux, A.; Kalpathy-Cramer, J.; Ord, C.B.; Walker, G.V.; Fuller, C.; Kim, J.-S.; Thomas, C.R., Jr. Nomogram for predicting the benefit of adjuvant chemoradiotherapy for resected gallbladder cancer. *J. Clin. Oncol.* **2011**, *29*, 4627–4632. [CrossRef]
7. Anderson, C.; Kim, R. Adjuvant therapy for resected extrahepatic cholangiocarcinoma: A review of the literature and future directions. *Cancer Treat. Rev.* **2009**, *35*, 322–327. [CrossRef]
8. De Oliveira, M.L.; Cunningham, S.C.; Cameron, J.L.; Kamangar, F.; Winter, J.M.; Lillemoe, K.D.; Choti, M.A.; Yeo, C.J.; Schulick, R.D. Cholangiocarcinoma: Thirty-one-year experience with 564 patients at a single institution. *Ann. Surg.* **2007**, *245*, 755–762. [CrossRef]
9. Miyamae, M.; Komatsu, S.; Ichikawa, D.; Kawaguchi, T.; Hirajima, S.; Okajima, W.; Ohashi, T.; Imamura, T.; Konishi, H.; Shiozaki, A.; et al. Plasma microRNA profiles: Identification of miR-744 as a novel diagnostic and prognostic biomarker in pancreatic cancer. *Br. J. Cancer* **2015**, *113*, 1467–1476. [CrossRef] [PubMed]
10. Song, W.-F.; Wang, L.; Huang, W.-Y.; Cai, X.; Cui, J.-J.; Wang, L.-W. MiR-21 upregulation induced by promoter zone histone acetylation is associated with chemoresistance to gemcitabine and enhanced malignancy of pancreatic cancer cells. *Asian Pac. J. Cancer Prev.* **2013**, *14*, 7529–7536. [CrossRef] [PubMed]
11. Ali, S.; Almhanna, K.; Chen, W.; Philip, P.A.; Sarkar, F.H. Differentially expressed miRNAs in the plasma may provide a molecular signature for aggressive pancreatic cancer. *Am. J. Transl. Res.* **2010**, *3*, 28–47.
12. Ye, Z.-Q.; Zou, C.-L.; Chen, H.-B.; Jiang, M.-J.; Mei, Z.; Gu, D.-N. MicroRNA-7 as a Potential Biomarker for Prognosis in Pancreatic Cancer. *Dis. Markers* **2020**, *2020*, 1–13. [CrossRef] [PubMed]

13. Long, L.-M.; Zhan, J.-K.; Wang, H.-Q.; Li, S.; Chen, Y.-Y.; Liu, Y.-S. The Clinical Significance of miR-34a in Pancreatic Ductal Carcinoma and Associated Molecular and Cellular Mechanisms. *Pathobiology* **2017**, *84*, 38–48. [CrossRef] [PubMed]
14. Imamura, T.; Komatsu, S.; Ichikawa, D.; Miyamae, M.; Okajima, W.; Ohashi, T.; Kiuchi, J.; Nishibeppu, K.; Konishi, H.; Shiozaki, A.; et al. Depleted tumor suppressor miR-107 in plasma relates to tumor progression and is a novel therapeutic target in pancreatic cancer. *Sci. Rep.* **2017**, *7*, 1–14. [CrossRef]
15. Goto, T.; Fujiya, M.; Konishi, H.; Sasajima, J.; Fujibayashi, S.; Hayashi, A.; Utsumi, T.; Sato, H.; Iwama, T.; Ijiri, M.; et al. An elevated expression of serum exosomal microRNA-191, -21, -451a of pancreatic neoplasm is considered to be efficient diagnostic marker. *BMC Cancer* **2018**, *18*, 1–11. [CrossRef]
16. Deng, Z.; Li, X.; Shi, Y.; Lu, Y.; Yao, W.; Wang, J. A Novel Autophagy-Related lncRNAs Signature for Prognostic Prediction and Clinical Value in Patients With Pancreatic Cancer. *Front. Cell Dev. Biol.* **2020**, *8*, 606817. [CrossRef] [PubMed]
17. Chaudhary, A.K.; Mondal, G.; Kumar, V.; Kattel, K.; Mahato, R.I. Chemosensitization and inhibition of pancreatic cancer stem cell proliferation by overexpression of mi-croRNA-205. *Cancer Lett.* **2017**, *402*, 1–8. [CrossRef] [PubMed]
18. Reese, M.; Flammang, I.; Yang, Z.; Dhayat, S.A.; Yang, Z. Potential of Exosomal microRNA-200b as Liquid Biopsy Marker in Pancreatic Ductal Adenocarcinoma. *Cancers* **2020**, *12*, 197. [CrossRef]
19. Peng, L.; Chen, Z.; Chen, Y.; Wang, X.; Tang, N. MIR155HG is a prognostic biomarker and associated with immune infiltration and immune checkpoint molecules expression in multiple cancers. *Cancer Med.* **2019**, *8*, 7161–7173. [CrossRef]
20. Wang, G.; Kang, M.-X.; Lu, W.-J.; Chen, Y.; Zhang, B.; Wu, Y.-L. MACC1: A potential molecule associated with pancreatic cancer metastasis and chemoresistance. *Oncol. Lett.* **2012**, *4*, 783–791. [CrossRef]
21. Merz, V.; Zecchetto, C.; Santoro, R.; Simionato, F.; Sabbadini, F.; Mangiameli, D.; Piro, G.; Cavaliere, A.; Deiana, M.; Valenti, M.T.; et al. Plasma IL8 Is a Biomarker for TAK1 Activation and Predicts Resistance to Nanoliposomal Irinotecan in Patients with Gemcitabine-Refractory Pancreatic Cancer. *Clin. Cancer Res.* **2020**, *26*, 4661–4669. [CrossRef] [PubMed]
22. Xu, J.; Xiong, G.; Cao, Z.; Huang, H.; Wang, T.; You, L.; Zhou, L.; Zheng, L.; Hu, Y.; Zhang, T.; et al. PIM-1 contributes to the malignancy of pancreatic cancer and displays diagnostic and prognostic value. *J. Exp. Clin. Cancer Res.* **2016**, *35*, 133. [CrossRef] [PubMed]
23. Ireland, L.; Santos, A.; Ahmed, M.S.; Rainer, C.; Nielsen, S.R.; Quaranta, V.; Weyer-Czernilofsky, U.; Engle, D.D.; Perez-Mancera, P.A.; Coupland, S.E.; et al. Chemoresistance in Pancreatic Cancer Is Driven by Stroma-Derived Insulin-Like Growth Factors. *Cancer Res.* **2016**, *76*, 6851–6863. [CrossRef]
24. Phua, L.C.; Goh, S.; Tai, D.W.M.; Leow, W.Q.; Alkaff, S.M.F.; Chan, C.Y.; Kam, J.H.; Lim, T.K.H.; Chan, E.C.Y. Metabolomic prediction of treatment outcome in pancreatic ductal adenocarcinoma patients receiving gemcitabine. *Cancer Chemother. Pharmacol.* **2018**, *81*, 277–289. [CrossRef]
25. Li, X.; Xiao, Y.; Fan, S.; Xiao, M.; Wang, X.; Zhu, X.; Chen, X.; Li, C.; Zong, G.; Zhou, G.; et al. Overexpression of DIXDC1 correlates with enhanced cell growth and poor prognosis in human pancreatic ductal adenocarcinoma. *Hum. Pathol.* **2016**, *57*, 182–192. [CrossRef] [PubMed]
26. Hou, Z.; Pan, Y.; Fei, Q.; Lin, Y.; Zhou, Y.; Liu, Y.; Guan, H.; Yu, X.; Lin, X.; Lu, F.; et al. Prognostic significance and therapeutic potential of the immune checkpoint VISTA in pancreatic cancer. *J. Cancer Res. Clin. Oncol.* **2021**, *147*, 517–531. [CrossRef]
27. da Silva, A.; Bowden, M.; Zhang, S.; Masugi, Y.; Thorner, A.R.; Herbert, Z.T.; Zhou, C.W.; Brais, L.; Chan, J.A.; Hodi, S.; et al. Characterization of the Neuroendocrine Tumor Immune Microenvironment. *Pancreas* **2018**, *47*, 1123–1129. [CrossRef]
28. Gorchs, L.; Moro, C.F.; Bankhead, P.; Kern, K.P.; Sadeak, I.; Meng, Q.; Rangelova, E.; Kaipe, H. Human Pancreatic Carcinoma-Associated Fibroblasts Promote Expression of Co-inhibitory Markers on CD4(+) and CD8(+) T-Cells. *Front. Immunol.* **2019**, *10*, 847. [CrossRef]
29. Imai, D.; Yoshizumi, T.; Okano, S.; Uchiyama, H.; Ikegami, T.; Harimoto, N.; Itoh, S.; Soejima, Y.; Aishima, S.; Oda, Y.; et al. The prognostic impact of programmed cell death ligand 1 and human leukocyte antigen class I in pancreatic cancer. *Cancer Med.* **2017**, *6*, 1614–1626. [CrossRef]
30. Liu, Y.; Jin, Z.-R.; Huang, X.; Che, Y.-C.; Liu, Q. Identification of Spindle and Kinetochore-Associated Family Genes as Therapeutic Targets and Prognostic Biomarkers in Pancreas Ductal Adenocarcinoma Microenvironment. *Front. Oncol.* **2020**, *10*, 553536. [CrossRef] [PubMed]
31. Fan, J.; Wei, Q.; Koay, E.J.; Liu, Y.; Ning, B.; Bernard, P.W.; Zhang, N.; Han, H.; Katz, M.H.; Zhao, Z.; et al. Chemoresistance Transmission via Exosome-Mediated EphA2 Transfer in Pancreatic Cancer. *Theranostics* **2018**, *8*, 5986–5994. [CrossRef] [PubMed]
32. Pan, Y.; Lu, F.; Fei, Q.; Yu, X.; Xiong, P.; Yu, X.; Dang, Y.; Hou, Z.; Lin, W.; Lin, X.; et al. Single-cell RNA sequencing reveals compartmental remodeling of tumor-infiltrating immune cells induced by anti-CD47 targeting in pancreatic cancer. *J. Hematol. Oncol.* **2019**, *12*, 1–18. [CrossRef]
33. Jiang, H.; Hegde, S.; Knolhoff, B.L.; Zhu, Y.; Herndon, J.M.; Meyer, M.; Nywening, T.M.; Hawkins, T.G.; Shapiro, I.M.; Weaver, D.T.; et al. Targeting focal adhesion kinase renders pancreatic cancers responsive to checkpoint immunotherapy. *Nat. Med.* **2016**, *22*, 851–860. [CrossRef] [PubMed]
34. Panni, R.Z.; Herndon, J.M.; Zuo, C.; Hegde, S.; Hogg, G.D.; Knolhoff, B.L.; Breden, M.A.; Li, X.; Krisnawan, V.E.; Khan, S.Q.; et al. Agonism of CD11b reprograms innate immunity to sensitize pancreatic cancer to immunotherapies. *Sci. Transl. Med.* **2019**, *11*, eaau9240. [CrossRef]
35. Lu, C.; Paschall, A.V.; Shi, H.; Savage, N.; Waller, J.L.; Sabbatini, M.E.; Oberlies, N.; Pearce, C.; Liu, K. The MLL1-H3K4me3 Axis-Mediated PD-L1 Expression and Pancreatic Cancer Immune Evasion. *J. Natl. Cancer Inst.* **2017**, *109*, djw283. [CrossRef]

36. Quaranta, V.; Rainer, C.; Nielsen, S.R.; Raymant, M.L.; Ahmed, M.S.; Engle, D.D.; Taylor, A.; Murray, T.; Campbell, F.; Palmer, D.H.; et al. Macrophage-Derived Granulin Drives Resistance to Immune Checkpoint Inhibition in Metastatic Pancreatic Cancer. *Cancer Res.* **2018**, *78*, 4253–4269. [CrossRef]
37. Liu, J.; Jiang, W.; Zhao, K.; Wang, H.; Zhou, T.; Bai, W.; Wang, X.; Zhao, T.; Huang, C.; Gao, S.; et al. Tumoral EHF predicts the efficacy of anti-PD1 therapy in pancreatic ductal adenocarcinoma. *J. Exp. Med.* **2019**, *216*, 656–673. [CrossRef]
38. Soares, K.C.; Rucki, A.A.; Wu, A.; Olino, K.; Xiao, Q.; Chai, Y.; Wamwea, A.; Bigelow, E.; Lutz, E.; Liu, L.; et al. PD-1/PD-L1 blockade together with vaccine therapy facilitates effector t-cell infiltration into pancreatic tumors. *J. Immunother.* **2015**, *38*, 1–11. [CrossRef]
39. Zhang, M.; Yang, J.; Zhou, J.; Gao, W.; Zhang, Y.; Lin, Y.; Wang, H.; Ruan, Z.; Ni, B. Prognostic Values of CD38(+)CD101(+)PD1(+)CD8(+) T Cells in Pancreatic Cancer. *Immunol. Investig.* **2019**, *48*, 466–479. [CrossRef]
40. Kanaya, N.; Kuroda, S.; Kakiuchi, Y.; Kumon, K.; Tsumura, T.; Hashimoto, M.; Morihiro, T.; Kubota, T.; Aoyama, K.; Kikuchi, S.; et al. Immune Modulation by Telomerase-Specific Oncolytic Adenovirus Synergistically Enhances Antitumor Efficacy with Anti-PD1 Antibody. *Mol. Ther.* **2020**, *28*, 794–804. [CrossRef]
41. Osborne, N.; Sundseth, R.; Burks, J.; Cao, H.; Liu, X.; Kroemer, A.H.; Sutton, L.; Cato, A.; Smith, J.P. Gastrin vaccine improves response to immune checkpoint antibody in murine pancreatic cancer by altering the tu-mor microenvironment. *Cancer Immunol. Immunother.* **2019**, *68*, 1635–1648. [CrossRef]
42. Liu, P.; Weng, Y.; Sui, Z.; Wu, Y.; Meng, X.; Wu, M.; Jin, H.; Tan, X.; Zhang, L.; Zhang, Y. Quantitative secretomic analysis of pancreatic cancer cells in serum-containing conditioned medium. *Sci. Rep.* **2016**, *6*, 37606. [CrossRef]
43. Oberg, H.-H.; Kellner, C.; Gonnermann, D.; Sebens, S.; Bauerschlag, D.; Gramatzki, M.; Kabelitz, D.; Peipp, M.; Wesch, D.; Kellner, C.; et al. Tribody [(HER2)(2)×CD16] Is More Effective Than Trastuzumab in Enhancing γδ T Cell and Natural Killer Cell Cytotoxicity Against HER2-Expressing Cancer Cells. *Front. Immunol.* **2018**, *9*, 814. [CrossRef]
44. Zaidi, N.; Quezada, S.A.; Kuroiwa, J.M.Y.; Zhang, L.; Jaffee, E.M.; Steinman, R.M.; Wang, B. Anti-CTLA-4 synergizes with dendritic cell-targeted vaccine to promote IL-3-dependent CD4(+) effector T cell infiltration into murine pancreatic tumors. *Ann. N. Y. Acad. Sci.* **2019**, *1445*, 62–73. [CrossRef]
45. Schäfer, H.; Dieckmann, C.; Korniienko, O.; Moldenhauer, G.; Kiefel, H.; Salnikov, A.; Krüger, A.; Altevogt, P.; Sebens, S. Combined treatment of L1CAM antibodies and cytostatic drugs improve the therapeutic response of pancreatic and ovarian carcinoma. *Cancer Lett.* **2012**, *319*, 6–82. [CrossRef]
46. Umebayashi, M.; Kiyota, A.; Koya, N.; Tanaka, H.; Onishi, H.; Katano, M.; Morisaki, T. An epithelial cell adhesion molecule- and CD3-bispecific antibody plus activated T-cells can eradicate chemo-resistant cancer stem-like pancreatic carcinoma cells in vitro. *Anticancer. Res.* **2014**, *34*, 4509–4519.
47. Takahashi, R.; Ijichi, H.; Sano, M.; Miyabayashi, K.; Mohri, D.; Kim, J.; Kimura, G.; Nakatsuka, T.; Fujiwara, H.; Yamamoto, K.; et al. Soluble VCAM-1 promotes gemcitabine resistance via macrophage infiltration and predicts therapeutic response in pancreatic cancer. *Sci. Rep.* **2020**, *10*, 1–13. [CrossRef]
48. Le Calvé, B.; Griveau, A.; Vindrieux, D.; Maréchal, R.; Wiel, C.; Svrcek, M.; Gout, J.; Azzi-Martin, L.; Payen, L.; Cros, J.; et al. Lysyl oxidase family activity promotes resistance of pancreatic ductal adenocarcinoma to chemotherapy by limiting the intratumoral anticancer drug distribution. *Oncotarget* **2016**, *7*, 32100–32112. [CrossRef]
49. Thakur, P.C.; Miller-Ocuin, J.L.; Nguyen, K.; Matsuda, R.; Singhi, A.D.; Zeh, H.J.; Bahary, N. Inhibition of endoplasmic-reticulum-stress-mediated autophagy enhances the effectiveness of chemotherapeutics on pancreatic cancer. *J. Transl. Med.* **2018**, *16*, 190. [CrossRef] [PubMed]
50. Tsukasa, K.; Ding, Q.; Yoshimitsu, M.; Miyazaki, Y.; Matsubara, S.; Takao, S. Slug contributes to gemcitabine resistance through epithelial-mesenchymal transition in CD133(+) pancreatic cancer cells. *Hum. Cell* **2015**, *28*, 167–174. [CrossRef]
51. Qi, B.; Liu, H.; Dong, Y.; Shi, X.; Zhou, Q.; Zeng, F.; Bao, N.; Li, Q.; Yuan, Y.; Yao, L.; et al. The nine ADAMs family members serve as potential biomarkers for immune infiltration in pancreatic adenocarcinoma. *PeerJ* **2020**, *8*, e9736. [CrossRef]
52. Zhou, G.; Sprengers, D.; Mancham, S.; Erkens, R.; Boor, P.P.C.; van Beek, A.A.; Doukas, M.; Noordam, L.; Carrascosa, L.C.; Ruiter, V.; et al. Reduction of immunosuppressive tumor microenvironment in cholangiocarcinoma by ex vivo targeting immune check-point molecules. *J. Hepatol.* **2019**, *71*, 753–762. [CrossRef] [PubMed]
53. Jing, C.-Y.; Fu, Y.-P.; Yi, Y.; Zhang, M.-X.; Zheng, S.-S.; Huang, J.-L.; Gan, W.; Xu, X.; Lin, J.-J.; Zhang, J.; et al. HHLA2 in intrahepatic cholangiocarcinoma: An immune checkpoint with prognostic significance and wider expression compared with PD-L1. *J. Immunother. Cancer* **2019**, *7*, 77. [CrossRef] [PubMed]
54. Liu, Y.; Cheng, Y.; Xu, Y.; Wang, Z.; Du, X.; Li, C.; Peng, J.; Gao, L.; Liang, X.; Ma, C. Increased expression of programmed cell death protein 1 on NK cells inhibits NK-cell-mediated anti-tumor function and indicates poor prognosis in digestive cancers. *Oncogene* **2017**, *36*, 6143–6153. [CrossRef]
55. Feng, K.; Liu, Y.; Zhao, Y.; Yang, Q.; Dong, L.; Liu, J.; Li, X.; Zhao, Z.; Mei, Q.; Han, W. Efficacy and biomarker analysis of nivolumab plus gemcitabine and cisplatin in patients with unresectable or metastatic biliary tract cancers: Results from a phase II study. *J. Immunother. Cancer* **2020**, *8*, e000367. [CrossRef] [PubMed]
56. Zhang, Y.; Wang, H.; Chen, T.; Wang, H.; Liang, X.; Zhang, Y.; Duan, J.; Qian, S.; Qiao, K.; Zhang, L.; et al. C24-Ceramide Drives Gallbladder Cancer Progression Through Directly Targeting Phosphatidylinositol 5-Phosphate 4-Kinase Type-2 Gamma to Facilitate Mammalian Target of Rapamycin Signaling Activation. *Hepatology* **2021**, *73*, 692–712. [CrossRef]

57. Shen, D.-Y.; Zhan, Y.-H.; Wang, Q.-M.; Rui, G.; Zhang, Z.-M. Oncogenic potential of Cyclin Kinase Subunit-2 in cholangiocarcinoma. *Liver Int.* **2013**, *33*, 137–148. [CrossRef] [PubMed]
58. Jiao, C.Y.; Feng, Q.C.; Li, C.X.; Wang, D.; Han, S.; Zhang, Y.D.; Jiang, W.J.; Chang, J.; Wang, X.; Li, X.C. BUB1B promotes extrahepatic cholangiocarcinoma progression via JNK/c-Jun pathways. *Cell Death Dis.* **2021**, *12*, 1–13. [CrossRef]
59. Li, J.-H.; Zhu, X.-X.; Li, F.-X.; Huang, C.-S.; Huang, X.-T.; Wang, J.-Q.; Gao, Z.-X.; Li, S.-J.; Xu, Q.-C.; Zhao, W.; et al. MFAP5 facilitates the aggressiveness of intrahepatic Cholangiocarcinoma by activating the Notch1 signaling pathway. *J. Exp. Clin. Cancer Res.* **2019**, *38*, 1–15. [CrossRef]
60. Lu, J.-C.; Zeng, H.-Y.; Sun, Q.-M.; Meng, Q.-N.; Huang, X.-Y.; Zhang, P.-F.; Yang, X.; Peng, R.; Gao, C.; Wei, C.-Y.; et al. Distinct PD-L1/PD1 Profiles and Clinical Implications in Intrahepatic Cholangiocarcinoma Patients with Different Risk Factors. *Theranostics* **2019**, *9*, 4678–4687. [CrossRef] [PubMed]
61. Seo, Y.D.; Jiang, X.; Sullivan, K.M.; Jalikis, F.G.; Smythe, K.S.; Abbasi, A.; Vignali, M.; Park, J.O.; Daniel, S.K.; Pollack, S.M.; et al. Mobilization of CD8(+) T Cells via CXCR4 Blockade Facilitates PD-1 Checkpoint Therapy in Human Pancreatic Cancer. *Clin. Cancer Res.* **2019**, *25*, 3934–3945. [CrossRef]
62. Yuan, J. Circulating protein and antibody biomarker for personalized cancer immunotherapy. *J. Immunother. Cancer* **2016**, *4*, 46. [CrossRef] [PubMed]
63. Seifert, A.M.; Reiche, C.; Heiduk, M.; Tannert, A.; Meinecke, A.-C.; Baier, S.; von Renesse, J.; Kahlert, C.; Distler, M.; Welsch, T.; et al. Detection of pancreatic ductal adenocarcinoma with galectin-9 serum levels. *Oncogene* **2020**, *39*, 3102–3113. [CrossRef]
64. Moral, J.A.; Leung, J.; Rojas, L.A.; Ruan, J.; Zhao, J.; Sethna, Z.; Ramnarain, A.; Gasmi, B.; Gururajan, M.; Redmond, D.; et al. ILC2s amplify PD-1 blockade by activating tissue-specific cancer immunity. *Nature* **2020**, *579*, 130–135. [CrossRef]
65. Christmas, B.J.; Rafie, C.I.; Hopkins, A.C.; Scott, B.A.; Ma, H.S.; Cruz, K.A.; Woolman, S.; Armstrong, T.D.; Connolly, R.M.; Azad, N.A.; et al. Entinostat Converts Immune-Resistant Breast and Pancreatic Cancers into Checkpoint-Responsive Tumors by Reprogramming Tumor-Infiltrating MDSCs. *Cancer Immunol. Res.* **2018**, *6*, 1561–1577. [CrossRef]
66. Patel, J.M.; Cui, Z.; Wen, Z.-F.; Dinh, C.T.; Hu, H.-M. Peritumoral administration of DRibbles-pulsed antigen-presenting cells enhances the antitumor efficacy of anti-GITR and anti-PD-1 antibodies via an antigen presenting independent mechanism. *J. Immunother. Cancer* **2019**, *7*, 311. [CrossRef] [PubMed]
67. Zhang, Y.; Velez-Delgado, A.; Mathew, E.; Li, D.; Mendez, F.M.; Flannagan, K.; Rhim, A.D.; Simeone, D.M.; Beatty, G.L.; di Magliano, M.P. Myeloid cells are required for PD-1/PD-L1 checkpoint activation and the establishment of an immunosuppressive environment in pancreatic cancer. *Gut* **2017**, *66*, 124–136. [CrossRef]
68. Le, D.T.; Lutz, E.; Uram, J.N.; Sugar, E.A.; Onners, B.; Solt, S.; Zheng, L.; Diaz, L.A., Jr.; Donehower, R.C.; Jaffee, E.M.; et al. Evaluation of ipilimumab in combination with allogeneic pancreatic tumor cells transfected with a GM-CSF gene in previously treated pancreatic cancer. *J. Immunother.* **2013**, *36*, 382–389. [CrossRef] [PubMed]
69. Baumann, D.; Hägele, T.; Mochayedi, J.; Drebant, J.; Vent, C.; Blobner, S.; Noll, J.H.; Nickel, I.; Schumacher, C.; Boos, S.L.; et al. Proimmunogenic impact of MEK inhibition synergizes with agonist anti-CD40 immunostimulatory antibodies in tumor therapy. *Nat. Commun.* **2020**, *11*, 1–18. [CrossRef]
70. Stromnes, I.M.; Burrack, A.L.; Hulbert, A.; Bonson, P.; Black, C.; Brockenbrough, J.S.; Raynor, J.F.; Spartz, E.; Pierce, R.H.; Greenberg, P.D.; et al. Differential Effects of Depleting versus Programming Tumor-Associated Macrophages on Engineered T Cells in Pancreatic Ductal Adenocarcinoma. *Cancer Immunol. Res.* **2019**, *7*, 977–989. [CrossRef] [PubMed]
71. Bengsch, F.; Knoblock, D.M.; Liu, A.; McAllister, F.; Beatty, G.L. CTLA-4/CD80 pathway regulates T cell infiltration into pancreatic cancer. *Cancer Immunol. Immunother.* **2017**, *66*, 1609–1617. [CrossRef]
72. Brooks, J.; Fleischmann-Mundt, B.; Woller, N.; Niemann, J.; Ribback, S.; Peters, K.; Demir, I.E.; Armbrecht, N.; Ceyhan, G.O.; Manns, M.P.; et al. Perioperative, Spatiotemporally Coordinated Activation of T and NK Cells Prevents Recurrence of Pancreatic Cancer. *Cancer Res.* **2017**, *78*, 475–488. [CrossRef]
73. Lim, Y.-J.; Koh, J.; Kim, K.; Chie, E.-K.; Kim, B.; Lee, K.-B.; Jang, J.-Y.; Kim, S.-W.; Oh, D.-Y.; Bang, Y.-J.; et al. High ratio of programmed cell death protein 1 (PD-1)(+)/CD8(+) tumor-infiltrating lymphocytes identifies a poor prog-nostic subset of extrahepatic bile duct cancer undergoing surgery plus adjuvant chemoradiotherapy. *Radiother. Oncol.* **2015**, *117*, 165–170. [CrossRef] [PubMed]
74. Royal, R.E.; Levy, C.; Turner, K.; Mathur, A.; Hughes, M.; Kammula, U.S.; Sherry, R.M.; Topalian, S.L.; Yang, J.C.; Lowy, I.; et al. Phase 2 Trial of Single Agent Ipilimumab (Anti-CTLA-4) for Locally Advanced or Metastatic Pancreatic Adenocarcinoma. *J. Immunother.* **2010**, *33*, 828–833. [CrossRef] [PubMed]
75. Brahmer, J.R.; Tykodi, S.S.; Chow, L.Q.M.; Hwu, W.-J.; Topalian, S.L.; Hwu, P.; Drake, C.G.; Camacho, L.H.; Kauh, J.; Odunsi, K.; et al. Safety and Activity of Anti–PD-L1 Antibody in Patients with Advanced Cancer. *N. Engl. J. Med.* **2012**, *366*, 2455–2465. [CrossRef] [PubMed]
76. Burrack, A.L.; Spartz, E.J.; Raynor, J.F.; Wang, I.; Olson, M.; Stromnes, I.M. Combination PD-1 and PD-L1 Blockade Promotes Durable Neoantigen-Specific T Cell-Mediated Immunity in Pancreatic Ductal Adenocarcinoma. *Cell Rep.* **2019**, *28*, 2140–2155. [CrossRef] [PubMed]
77. Sow, H.S.; Ren, J.; Camps, M.; Ossendorp, F.; ten Dijke, P. Combined Inhibition of TGF-β Signaling and the PD-L1 Immune Checkpoint Is Differentially Effective in Tumor Models. *Cells* **2019**, *8*, 320. [CrossRef]

78. Sharma, N.; Gupta, V.K.; Garrido, V.T.; Hadad, R.; Durden, B.C.; Kesh, K.; Giri, B.; Ferrantella, A.; Dudeja, V.; Saluja, A.; et al. Targeting tumor-intrinsic hexosamine biosynthesis sensitizes pancreatic cancer to anti-PD1 therapy. *J. Clin. Investig.* **2020**, *130*, 451–465. [CrossRef]
79. Ma, H.S.; Poudel, B.; Torres, E.R.; Sidhom, J.-W.; Robinson, T.M.; Christmas, B.; Scott, B.; Cruz, K.; Woolman, S.; Wall, V.Z.; et al. A CD40 Agonist and PD-1 Antagonist Antibody Reprogram the Microenvironment of Nonimmunogenic Tumors to Allow T-cell–Mediated Anticancer Activity. *Cancer Immunol. Res.* **2019**, *7*, 428–442. [CrossRef] [PubMed]
80. Allen, E.; Jabouille, A.; Rivera, L.B.; Lodewijckx, I.; Missiaen, R.; Steri, V.; Feyen, K.; Tawney, J.; Hanahan, D.; Michael, I.P.; et al. Combined antiangiogenic and anti–PD-L1 therapy stimulates tumor immunity through HEV formation. *Sci. Transl. Med.* **2017**, *9*, eaak9679. [CrossRef]
81. Sergeant, G.; Vankelecom, H.; Gremeaux, L.; Topal, B. Role of cancer stem cells in pancreatic ductal adenocarcinoma. *Nat. Rev. Clin. Oncol.* **2009**, *6*, 580–586. [CrossRef]
82. Singh, A.; Settleman, J. EMT, cancer stem cells and drug resistance: An emerging axis of evil in the war on cancer. *Oncogene* **2010**, *29*, 4741–4751. [CrossRef] [PubMed]
83. Dallas, N.A.; Xia, L.; Fan, F.; Gray, M.J.; Gaur, P.; Van Buren, G.; Samuel, S.; Kim, M.P.; Lim, S.J.; Ellis, L.M. Chemoresistant colorectal cancer cells, the cancer stem cell phenotype, and increased sensitivity to insulin-like growth factor-i receptor inhibition. *Cancer Res.* **2009**, *69*, 1951–1957. [CrossRef]
84. Prasad, S.; Yadav, V.R.; Sung, B.; Gupta, S.C.; Tyagi, A.K.; Aggarwal, B.B. Ursolic acid inhibits the growth of human pancreatic cancer and enhances the antitumor potential of gemcitabine in an orthotopic mouse model through suppression of the inflammatory microenvironment. *Oncotarget* **2016**, *7*, 13182–13196. [CrossRef] [PubMed]
85. Waters, J.A.; Matos, J.; Yip-Schneider, M.; Aguilar-Saavedra, J.R.; Crean, C.D.; Beane, J.D.; Dumas, R.P.; Suvannasankha, A.; Schmidt, C.M. Targeted nuclear factor-kappaB suppression enhances gemcitabine response in human pancreatic tumor cell line murine xenografts. *Surgery* **2015**, *158*, 881–889. [CrossRef] [PubMed]
86. Landgraf, P.; Rusu, M.; Sheridan, R.; Sewer, A.; Iovino, N.; Aravin, A.; Pfeffer, S.; Rice, A.; Kamphorst, A.O.; Landthaler, M.; et al. A mammalian microrna expression atlas based on small rna library sequencing. *Cell* **2007**, *129*, 1401–1414. [CrossRef] [PubMed]
87. Liu, M.; Oxnard, G.; Klein, E.; Swanton, C.; Seiden, M.; Smith, D.; Richards, D.; Yeatman, T.J.; Cohn, A.L.; Lapham, R.; et al. Sensitive and specific multi-cancer detection and localization using methylation signatures in cell-free DNA. *Ann. Oncol.* **2020**, *31*, 745–759. [CrossRef]

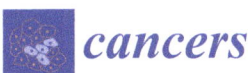

Review

Experimental and Clinical Evidence Supports the Use of Urokinase Plasminogen Activation System Components as Clinically Relevant Biomarkers in Gastroesophageal Adenocarcinoma

Gary Tincknell [1,2,3], Ann-Katrin Piper [1,4], Morteza Aghmesheh [1,2,4], Therese Becker [5,6,7], Kara Lea Vine [1,3], Daniel Brungs [1,2,4] and Marie Ranson [1,3,*]

1 Illawarra Health and Medical Research Institute, Wollongong, NSW 2522, Australia; gwt714@uowmail.edu.au (G.T.); akpiper@uow.edu.au (A.-K.P.); morteza@uow.edu.au (M.A.); kara@uow.edu.au (K.L.V.); Daniel.Brungs@health.nsw.gov.au (D.B.)
2 Illawarra Cancer Care Centre, Illawarra Shoalhaven Local Health District, Wollongong, NSW 2500, Australia
3 School of Chemistry and Molecular Biosciences, University of Wollongong, Wollongong, NSW 2522, Australia
4 School of Medicine, University of Wollongong, Wollongong, NSW 2522, Australia
5 Ingham Institute for Applied Medical Research, Liverpool, NSW 2170, Australia; Therese.Becker@inghaminstitute.org.au
6 UNSW Medicine, University of New South Wales, Kensington, NSW 2052, Australia
7 School of Medicine, Western Sydney University, Sydney, NSW 2560, Australia
* Correspondence: mranson@uow.edu.au

Simple Summary: Patients with gastric and oesophageal adenocarcinomas (GOCs) have short life expectancies as their tumours spread to other sites early. This is facilitated by the increased expression of the urokinase plasminogen activation system (uPAS); a feature of the majority of GOCs. There is increasing appreciation of the importance of uPAS expression in a range of cell types within the tumour microenvironment. Abundant clinical evidence indicates that altered expression of uPAS proteins is associated with worse outcomes, including time to tumour recurrence and patient survival. Emerging technologies, including liquid biopsy, suggest a role of uPAS for the detection of circulating tumour cells, which are responsible for the dissemination of cancers. We review and summarise pre-clinical and clinical data that supports the use of uPAS as a biomarker in GOC.

Abstract: Gastric and oesophageal cancers (GOCs) are lethal cancers which metastasise early and recur frequently, even after definitive surgery. The urokinase plasminogen activator system (uPAS) is strongly implicated in the invasion and metastasis of many aggressive tumours including GOCs. Urokinase plasminogen activator (uPA) interaction with its receptor, urokinase plasminogen activator receptor (uPAR), leads to proteolytic activation of plasminogen to plasmin, a broad-spectrum protease which enables tumour cell invasion and dissemination to distant sites. uPA, uPAR and the plasminogen activator inhibitor type 1 (PAI-1) are overexpressed in some GOCs. Accumulating evidence points to a causal role of activated receptor tyrosine kinase pathways enhancing uPAS expression in GOCs. Expression of these components are associated with poorer clinicopathological features and patient survival. Stromal cells, including tumour-associated macrophages and myofibroblasts, also express the key uPAS proteins, supporting the argument of stromal involvement in GOC progression and adverse effect on patient survival. uPAS proteins can be detected on circulating leucocytes, circulating tumour cells and within the serum; all have the potential to be developed into circulating biomarkers of GOC. Herein, we review the experimental and clinical evidence supporting uPAS expression as clinical biomarker in GOC, with the goal of developing targeted therapeutics against the uPAS.

Keywords: urokinase plasminogen activator (uPA); urokinase plasminogen activator receptor (uPAR); plasminogen activator inhibitor type 1 (PAI-1); circulating tumour cell (CTC); biomarkers; gastric cancer; oesophageal cancer; serine proteases; tumour microenvironment; serpins

Citation: Tincknell, G.; Piper, A.-K.; Aghmesheh, M.; Becker, T.; Vine, K.L.; Brungs, D.; Ranson, M. Experimental and Clinical Evidence Supports the Use of Urokinase Plasminogen Activation System Components as Clinically Relevant Biomarkers in Gastroesophageal Adenocarcinoma. *Cancers* 2021, 13, 4097. https://doi.org/10.3390/cancers13164097

Academic Editor: Takaya Shimura

Received: 21 June 2021
Accepted: 9 August 2021
Published: 14 August 2021

Publisher's Note: MDPI stays neutral with regard to jurisdictional claims in published maps and institutional affiliations.

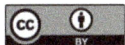

Copyright: © 2021 by the authors. Licensee MDPI, Basel, Switzerland. This article is an open access article distributed under the terms and conditions of the Creative Commons Attribution (CC BY) license (https://creativecommons.org/licenses/by/4.0/).

1. Introduction

Gastroesophageal cancers (GOC) are amongst the leading causes of cancer related morbidity and mortality worldwide [1]. Gastric cancers are ranked fifth for incidence and third for deaths worldwide [1]. Oesophageal carcinomas join gastric cancers in the global top 10 for both incidence (9th) and mortality (6th) [1]. GOCs often present at an advanced stage owing to its aggressiveness and early metastasis formation, with 25–50% of GOC presenting as metastatic at diagnosis [2–4]. Henceforth, *GOC* will refer to adenocarcinomas arising from any location within the oesophagus or stomach, otherwise individual locations will be identified.

The plasminogen activation system is a multi-component regulatory system that, under normal conditions, functions in the clearance of blood clots and degradation of the extracellular matrix (ECM) and basement membranes (BM) during tissue remodelling processes such as wound healing [5–10]. However, unregulated plasminogen activation via the urokinase plasminogen activator (uPA) is implicated in key events in tumour progression, specifically solid tumour invasion and metastasis [5–10]. Through binding of uPA to the uPA receptor (uPAR), which is typically cell-surface-bound, co-localised plasminogen is converted to plasmin [6,11]. As a broad-spectrum serine protease, plasmin then directly and indirectly (via the activation of pro-metalloproteinases) degrades a wide range of proteins in the ECM and BMs. This process enables tumour cell dissemination around the body, a key step required for the seeding of tumour cells at distant sites to form metastases [6,7,11–15]. Tissue plasminogen activator (tPA) is the intra-vascular counterpart to uPA, involved in fibrin degradation to prevent blood clot formation [13]. However, tPA does not appear to play a significant role in the development of solid tumours [16].

Overexpression of components of the uPA system (uPAS) in GOCs, on tumour cells and/or associated stromal cells in the tumour microenvironment (TME), is strongly associated with worse tumour staging [17–20], clinicopathological features [21–27] and reduced patient survival [12,17,18]. Here we review the important role the uPAS plays in the development and progression of GOC and summarise the available evidence of its role as a biomarker in GOC.

2. Major Components and Function of the uPAS

The key components of the uPAS include uPA, uPAR, plasminogen and specific uPA and plasmin inhibitors. uPA is a single stranded extracellular protein, secreted as an inactive double stranded zymogen (pro-urokinase), which is produced by leucocytes, fibroblasts and the urogenital system in normal physiological conditions [7]. Upon binding to its receptor uPAR, pro-uPA is converted to active uPA by proteolytic cleavage via plasmin and potentially cathepsin, plasma kallikrein or mast cell tryptase in the TME, resulting in the conversion of co-localised plasminogen to plasmin (via a number of potential cell-surface localised proteins containing c-terminal lysins) (reviewed by Ranson and Andronicos [6]). This positive feedback loop of plasmin-mediated pro-uPA activation and uPA-mediated plasminogen activation, results in increased proteolytic activity at the cell surface which is protected from inhibition by plasmin-specific inhibitors (e.g., α2-antiplasmin) [6,13,28]. Bound plasmin then also cleaves a range of multiple downstream extracellular targets, including ECM proteins such as fibrin, fibronectin and laminin and pro-metalloproteinases (pro-MMPs) (reviewed by Deryugina and Quigley [29]). Plasmin and MMP activity can also regulate cellular growth and migration through cleavage of extracellular components to release or activate chemokines, cytokines and growth factors (e.g., hepatocyte growth factor (HGF)/scatter factor, macrophage-stimulating protein, transforming growth factor (TGF) and basic fibroblast growth factor) [30,31] (Figure 1).

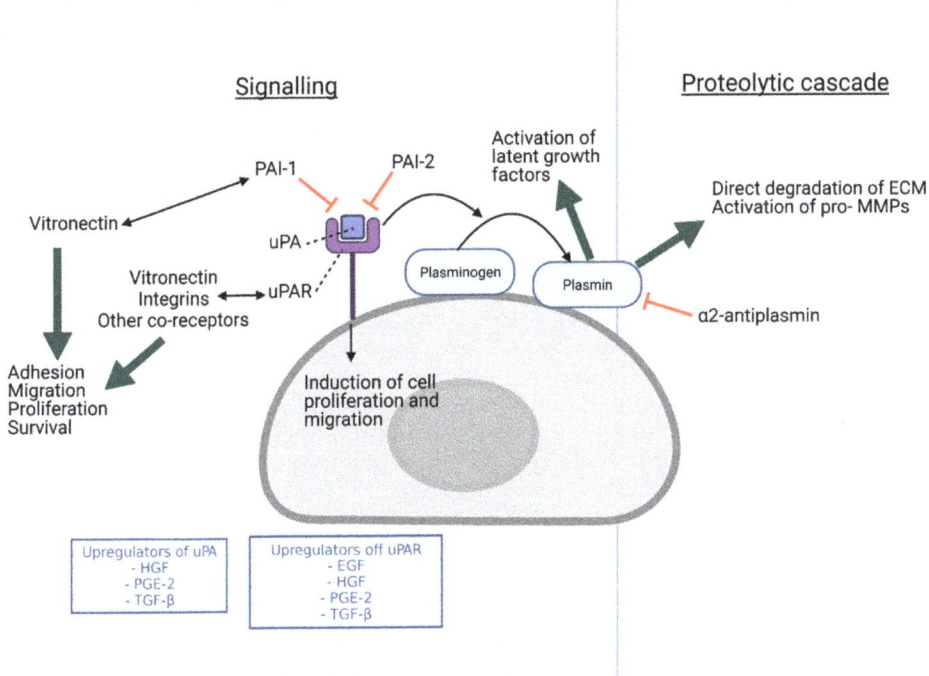

Figure 1. Overview of the urokinase plasminogen activation system. The binding of urokinase plasminogen activator (uPA) to its receptor, urokinase plasminogen activator receptor (uPAR) and generation of cell surface localised plasmin (which is protected from inhibition by α2-antiplasmin) instigates multiple extracellular and intracellular (signaling) effects resulting in tissue remodeling and cellular proliferation, cell survival as well as altered cellular adhesion and migration. In cancer, uPAS components including uPA, uPAR and plasminogen activator inhibitor-1 (PAI-1) are upregulated in an uncontrolled fashion and contribute to inappropriate cell signaling and proteolysis. Upregulators of the plasminogen activation system include, but are not limited to, the Epidermal Growth Factor (EGF), Hepatocyte Growth Factor (HGF), Prostaglandin-E2 (PGE-2) and Tumour Growth Factor-beta (TGF-β). See text for details. Created with BioRender.com (accessed on 17 June 2021).

uPAR is a heavily glycosylated protein and is either membrane-bound via a glycosyl-phosphatidylinositol anchor or found in its soluble forms [7]. uPAR consists of three similarly structured domains, made up of approximately 90 residues each, with domain 1 (D1) responsible for uPA binding leading to plasmin generation at the cell surface. Through complex direct and indirect interactions with a range of binding partners (including vitronectin, integrins, growth factor receptors and others), uPA-bound uPAR can also modulate downstream cell signalling pathways (Figure 1) [31–33]. Thus, the combined proteolytic and signalling outputs of the uPAS activate many downstream events driving ECM degradation, cell proliferation, adhesion and migration.

Soluble uPAR (suPAR) is produced through cleavage of the membrane bound uPAR; this cleavage occurs between the glycosylphosphatidylinositol (GPI)-anchor molecule and domain 3 of uPAR facilitated by plasmin, cathepsin G and GPI-specific phospholipase-D and can be identified in plasma, ascites and urine [34]. Vascular endothelial cells, monocytes and neutrophils are all known producers of suPAR [35]. Three detectable subgroups of suPAR have been identified: intact suPAR (I-III), domain 1 (D1)-suPAR(I) and intact and cleaved domains 2 (D2) and 3 (D3)-suPAR (I-III)+(II-III) [36]. suPAR (I-III) competes with membrane-bound uPAR for binding to uPA through its D2 and D3 domains and maintains its cell adhesion role through vitronectin binding with the D1 domain [37,38]. Fragmented suPAR (suPAR (I) and suPAR (II-III)) lose their ability to bind with vitronectin, resulting in reduced cell adhesion [38]. D1 is required for uPA binding, however suPAR (I) alone has low affinity for uPAR in the absence of D2 and D3 [39]. suPAR (II-III) has been shown to be a chemotactic molecule through 7TM receptor FPR-like receptor 1, attracting immune cells to cancers [40–42].

A key level of control in the regulation of plasmin activity arises through inhibition of uPA (and tPA) via the serine proteinase inhibitors (serpins) plasminogen activator inhibitor (PAI)-1 and PAI-2 (Figure 1). While the expression of both PAI proteins can be stimulated by various factors, including inflammatory conditions, under normal physiological conditions PAI-1 is mainly produced by endothelial cells and PAI-2 by synciotrophoblasts of the placenta in late pregnancy [13]. Activation of uPAS, such as infection and inflammation, results in increased PAI-1 expression in fibroblasts, adipocytes, smooth muscle cells and macrophage cells, whereas increased PAI-2 expression is detected in endothelial cells, macrophages, monocytes and platelets [11,43]. Both PAI-1 and PAI-2 irreversibly bind to and inhibit uPAR-bound uPA [11]. The uPA-PAI/uPAR complex is then taken up into the cell via low density lipoprotein receptor-related protein-mediated endocytosis [44–46]. uPAR is then recycled to the cell surface for further uPA interaction [44–46]. The two PAI proteins bestow different effects on cancer: cancers with high PAI-1 expression have been consistently demonstrated to have poorer clinical outcomes, whereas the effect of elevated PAI-2 expression levels are less well defined and the impact on clinical outcomes less pronounced [11,47]. Even though both PAI proteins mediate uPA/uPAR endocytosis, there are clear differences in functional outcomes from these interactions with endocytosis receptors [46,48]. For example, PAI-2 inhibits and clears cell surface uPA (and hence proteolytic activity) without influencing the promitogenic signalling pathways activated via PAI-1 [48]; this has been explained by distinct structural elements that underlie the interactions of these serpins with endocytic receptors [46]. PAI-1 also has established roles in various other cancer-promoting activities including resisting tumour cell death, increased cell migration and angiogenesis, via a variety of mechanisms that affect cell adhesion and signalling pathways (reviewed in detail by Kubala and Declerck 2019 [47]). Thus, while both serpins have anti-plasminogen activation activity, and loss or gain of PAI-2 expression has been shown in a cancer context-specific manner to be associated with worse or improved outcomes, respectively [11]; the clinical data showing that increased PAI-1 expression is strongly correlated with poor cancer outcome is highly convincing [47]. Moreover, PAI-1 levels can predict a response to chemotherapy in breast cancer, with increased PAI-1 levels associated with improved outcomes following administration of chemotherapy [49]. PAI-1 is thus also considered an important cancer biomarker.

3. Regulation of the uPAS

The expression and activity of the uPAS is tightly regulated during physiological processes to prevent unnecessary ECM remodelling through the production of excessive plasmin at the cell surface and dysregulated downstream signalling [11,50,51]. Certain cells secrete uPA and express uPAR at low levels [52] however, hormones [53–56], growth factors [55,57–59], cytokines [60,61] and tumour promoters [62–64], which also affect cellular proliferation and differentiation, induce overexpression of these components [65] in a variety of cancer cell lines.

Key cancer signalling pathways also alter uPAS mRNA and protein expression in GOC cell lines and xenografts. uPAS expression can be modulated by targeting key pathways with drug blockade [66,67], transfection of interfering or promoting RNA [68–71] and exposure to exogenous stimulating proteins [72–77]. Table 1 summarises the molecules and pathways linked to the regulation of uPAS in GOC cell lines.

Table 1. Molecules and pathways linked to regulation of the urokinase plasminogen activation system (uPAS) in gastroesophageal adenocarcinoma cell lines.

Molecule, Pathway	Derived Cell Line [1]	Effect on uPAS	Reference
		Upregulators	
Epidermal Growth Factor (EGF) Extracellular cell signalling transducer	SGC-7901	Exogenous EGF increased uPAR mRNA. Blockade of ERK1/2 reduced uPAR mRNA expression	Wang, P., et al., 2017 [72]
	BGC-823	Reduced uPA mRNA seen in ERK blockade	Wang, J., et al., 2016 [68]
Osteopontin Linked to PI3K/NFκB/IKK pathways	SGC-7901 BGC-823	siRNA against Osteopontin resulted in reduced uPA mRNA levels. Xenograft model showing reduced tumour growth	Gong, M., et al., 2008 [69]
Hepatocyte Growth Factor (HGF)/cMET pathway Extracellular cell signalling transducer		Exogenous HGF exposure increased uPA and uPAR protein levels. Blockade of uPAR with antibody or siRNA resulted in reduced wound invasion, which could not be overcome with exogenous HGF.	Kyung Hee, L., et al., 2006 [73]
		HGF signal transduction occurs via JunB/survivin pathway. Survivin inhibition resulted in reduced uPA protein expression and reduced cell invasion.	Kyung Hee, L., et al., 2011 [78]
	NUGC-3 MKN-28	MEK inhibition resulted in reduced uPA protein levels, whilst PI3K inhibition showed no change in uPA level. Suggesting uPA activation by HGF via ERK pathway.	Lee, K., et al., 2014 [70]
		HGF signal transduction via PKC/PKD pathway can release HDAC5; HDAC5 increased uPA and MMP-9 activity. Blockade of HDAC5 (even in presence of exogenous HGF) resulted in reduced uPA protein levels. HDAC5-inhibited cells showed reduced cell invasion.	Lee, K., et al., 2010 [66]
COX-PGE2 pathway	AGS	Exogenous prostaglandin E2 resulted in increased levels of uPA and uPAR (protein and mRNA).	Lian, S., et al., 2017 [74]
		Nicotine exposure increased PGE2 resulting in increased uPA and uPAR protein expression	Shin, V., et al., 2005 [75]
Laminin receptor (67LR)	SGC-7901 MKN-45	Downregulation of 67LR resulted in reduced cell line uPA protein expression.	Liu, L., et al., 2010 [79]
TGF-β pathway	SNU-216	Exogenous macrophage inhibitory cytokine 1 (MIC-1; a member of the TGF-β superfamily) resulted in increased uPA and uPAR (mRNA and protein); PAI-1 (mRNA) unaltered.	Lee, D., et al., 2003 [76]
		Interferon gamma inhibition resulted in TGF-B downregulation via smad 2/3 pathway with downregulation of uPA protein expression.	Kuga, H., et al., 2003 [67]
	OE33 FLOW	Increased PAI-1 mRNA levels on exposure via downstream activation of PI3K, ERK and JNK pathways on TGF-β activation.	Onwuegbusi, B., et al., 2007 [71]

Table 1. *Cont.*

Molecule, Pathway	Derived Cell Line [1]	Effect on uPAS	Reference
		Downregulators	
p75NTR, NF-κB signalling pathway	SGC7901 MKN45	Upregulation of p75NTR protein caused reduced protein levels of uPA.	Jin, H., et al., 2005 [80]
Tspan9, ERK1/2 pathway	SGC7901	Reduced protein levels of uPA through ERK1/2 blockade.	Li, P. et al., 2016 [77]

[1] Gastric cancer cell lines: SGC7901 (metastatic, human papilloma virus+), BGC-823 (metastatic, human papilloma virus+), NUGC-3 (metastatic, microsatellite instable, TP53 mutation), MKN-28 (metastatic, microsatellite stable, TP53 mutation), AGS (primary, HPV negative, microsatellite stable) and SNU-216 (metastatic, TP53 mutation). Oesophageal cell lines: OE33 (primary cancer, TP53 mutation) and FLOW (primary, TP53 mutation). Key: uPAS = urokinase plasminogen activation system; uPAR = urokinase plasminogen activator receptor; uPA = urokinase plasminogen activator; PAI-1 = plasminogen activator inhibitor-1; ERK = extracellular signal-regulated kinase; PI3K = phosphoinositide 3-kinase; NFkB = nuclear factor kB; IKK = inhibitor of NFkB kinase; siRNA = small interfering RNA; cMET = mesenchymal epithelial transition factor; MEK = mitogen-activated protein kinase kinase; PKC = protein kinase C; PKD = protein kinase D; HDAC5 = histone deacetylase 5; MMP = matrix metalloproteinase; COX = cyclooxygenase; TGF-β = transforming growth factor-beta; MIC = macrophage inhibitory cytokine; JNK = Jun-N-terminal kinases.

Exposure to exogenous growth factors such as epidermal growth factor increases uPAR mRNA expression, and this appears to occur through the mitogen-activated protein kinase (MAPK)/extracellular signal-related kinases (ERK) signalling pathway [72]. uPA and uPAR are both also upregulated upon HGF exposure, again, uPAS expression is reportedly linked to the MAPK/ERK pathway rather than phosphoinositide 3-kinase (PI3K) pathway [70]. Increased prostaglandin E2 levels (including as a result of nicotine exposure) resulted in increased uPA and uPAR levels via the cyclooxygenase-prostaglandin pathway [74,75]. Upregulation of transforming growth factor-beta (TGF-β) pathway also results in increased uPA and uPAR expression via the MAPK/ERK but also via the PI3K and Jun-N-terminal kinases pathways [67,71,76].

4. The Clinical Relevance of uPAS Expression in GOCs

The expression of uPAS in tumour tissue, stroma and liquid biopsies correlates to both clinicopathological features of tumours [18–20] and patient survival data [12,17,18,27]. In general, the assessment of the uPAS relies on protein or mRNA expression and levels, opposed to assessment of the function (or activity) of the individual proteins of the system. Immunohistochemistry (IHC) and enzyme-linked immunosorbent assay (ELISA) are the most used methods for protein assessment.

4.1. Tumour Expression and Association with Clinicopathological Features

A meta-analysis by Brungs et al. evaluated uPAS expression in GOCs, which demonstrated the following expression levels: uPA 52.8%, uPAR 56.8%, PAI-1 53.3% and PAI-2 57.5% of all patients with GOC [17]. Reporting of PAI-2 expression in oesophageal adenocarcinomas (via ELISA) is variable with some studies showing reduced levels and downregulation [81,82].

Activation of the uPAS system is a requirement for tumour cells to invade deeper into the ECM or seed at distant metastatic sites [83]. Therefore, it is not unexpected to find that increased expression of the uPAS proteins in GOC is associated with worse clinicopathological features including depth of invasion (T score), presence of metastasis (N score-lymph nodes, M score-distant metastasis) and histological grade of disease (Table 2).

Table 2. Key references demonstrating the association of overexpression of each uPAS protein with clinicopathological features.

Clinicopathological Feature	uPA	uPAR	PAI-1
		Key References	
T stage	[22–24]	[21,23,26]	[21,23–26]
Lymph nodes	[22–24]	[21,23,26]	[21,23–26]
Distant metastasis	[22–24]		[24]
Vascular invasion	[22–24]	[21,23,26]	[21,23,25,26]
Lymphatic invasion	[22–24]	[21,23,26]	[21,23,25,26]
Peritoneal disease [1]	[22,23]		
Serosal involvement [1]	[22,23]		
Depth of invasion		[21,23,26]	[21,23–26]
Histological grade		[21,23,26]	[24]

Empty boxes demonstrate no reported evidence found. [1] Gastric cancer only. Key: T stage = tumour invasion stage.

Relative uPA expression levels are biologically important: where >20% of primary tumour cells stained positive for uPA, higher tumour staging and histological grading was seen [84]. As will be discussed below, the combination of uPA and PAI-1 has been shown to be useful as biomarkers of worse prognosis, however one study found that PAI-1 negative, highly uPA-expressing gastric adenocarcinomas were associated with increased volume and number of metastases [22]. Comparison of high nodal and low nodal stage III gastric adenocarcinomas confirmed *SERPINE1* gene expression (encoding for PAI-1) was higher in those patients with increased nodal disease (>2x compared to healthy tissue) [85]. It can thus be concluded that upregulated PAI-1 expression is an important regulator of malignant lymph node development [85].

To date, PAI-2 alone has not been associated with any clinicopathological features as described in Table 2 [22,86]. However, advanced clinical staging of GOCs is associated with high uPA protein expression but absence of PAI-2 [86]. Gastric adenocarcinoma patients with a higher nodal status (>5 involved lymph nodes) was seen with low PAI-2 protein expression [87]. A lack of PAI-2 is therefore likely to be associated with worse tumour staging in combination with other uPAS protein dysregulation.

The peritoneum of patients with GOC peritoneal metastases shows generalised uPAS upregulation compared to uninvolved peritoneum of patients with GOC metastases at other sites [88]. uPAS expression (uPA, uPAR, PAI-1), however, did not alter between malignant and non-malignant peritoneum within the patients with peritoneal metastases [88]. Translational investigations confirm the role of altered uPAS expressing cell lines in the development of peritoneal metastasis [89] and increased ascites formation [90].

Retrospective analysis of GOCs with lymph node metastases showed uPAS protein expression in the primary tumour was correlated with lymph nodal metastases [19]. 82% of patients with malignant lymph nodes had strong uPA expression in the primary gastric cancer (IHC $\geq$ 50%), while in lymph node-negative disease, the primary cancer only showed uPA expression in 52% of cases [19]. uPAS expression in malignant lymph nodes demonstrates the critical role of uPAS in tumour invasion at secondary sites [18,20].

4.2. Tumour Expression and Association with Clinical Outcomes

uPAS overexpression is associated with poorer disease-free and overall survival (OS) of patients with GOCs (meta-analysis results of IHC, ISH and ELISA shown in Table 3) [17]. In individual studies, uPAS expression showed variable strength of association with prognosis (reviewed by Brungs et al., 2017 [17]).

Table 3. Urokinase plasminogen activation system association with relapse-free- and overall survival (combined immunohistochemistry, in situ hybridisation and enzyme-linked immunosorbent assay data).

	Recurrence-Free Survival HR (95% CI)	Overall Survival HR (95% CI)
uPA	1.90 (1.16–3.11, p = 0.01) 3 studies, 467 patients	2.21 (1.74–2.80, p < 0.0001) 12 studies, 1094 patients
uPAR	2.69 (NR, p = 0.03) 1 study, 203 patients	2.19 (1.80–2.66, p < 0.0001) 11 studies, 1036 patients
PAI-1	1.96 (1.07–3.58, p = 0.03) 3 studies, 467 patients	1.84 (1.28–2.64, p < 0.0001) 10 studies, 839 patients
PAI-2	NR no studies	0.97 (0.48–1.94, p = 0.92) 2 studies, 145 patients

CI = Confidence intervals, HR = Hazard Ratio, NR = not reported. Brungs et al. [17].

Subgroup analysis of uPAS expression in intestinal and diffuse gastric adenocarcinomas was assessed by Heiss et al. [91]. In this study uPA and uPAR were assessed on intestinal-type gastric adenocarcinomas and could not be associated with prognosis or recurrence-free survival; however, PAI-1 overexpression was an independent factor for recurrence-free survival [91]. In diffuse-type gastric adenocarcinoma, overexpression of uPA, uPAR and PAI-1 was associated with poorer overall- and recurrence-free survivals [91]; PAI-2 showed association with OS but not recurrence-free survival [91]. These subgroup findings may not be truly representative due to possible under powering with reduced numbers in the subgroup analysis.

Oesophageal adenocarcinomas that show uPAS overexpression are associated with poorer prognosis with elevated uPA protein levels shown to be associated with reduced median OS [24].

4.3. Intra-Tumoural Heterogeneity

uPAS expression shows significant intra-tumoural heterogeneity in GOC and can vary widely within patients, within the same tumour, between the primary tumour and its metastatic tumour or between different tumour histology types. For example, Alpízar-Alpízar et al. demonstrated uPAR overexpression at the invading front of gastric adenocarcinomas but not the tumour core [12]. This expression pattern was significantly associated with poorer OS in multivariate analysis (Hazard ratio (HR) = 2.39; 95% confidence interval (CI): 1.22–4.69; p = 0.011) [12].

We have investigated uPAR expression at the tumour core and invasion front in an Australian cohort of GOC patients [92]. uPAR IHC was assessed by an experienced anatomical pathologist with the following cut off values: 0—no uPAR positive cells, 1—less than 1% uPAR positive cells, 2—1–5% uPAR positive cells, 3—5–10% uPAR positive cells and 4—more than 10% uPAR positive cells. We found that increased uPAR expression at the invasion front (uPAR IHC 0–1 vs. >2) was significantly associated with worse patient survival (Figure 2a). uPAR expression within the tumour core was not significantly associated with OS (Figure 2b).

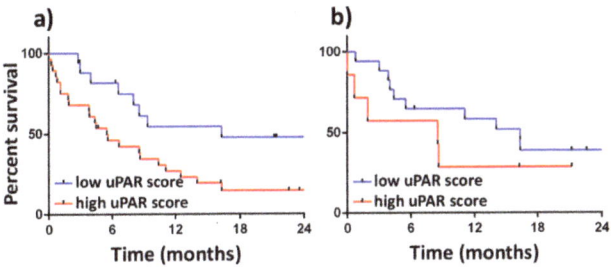

Figure 2. Kaplan-Meier curve showing association of GOC tumour uPAR score and overall survival (OS). Low uPAR (0–1) and high uPAR expression (>2) on tumour cells assessed by immunohistochemistry (IHC) at (**a**) tumour invasion front (n = 43; p = 0.02) and (**b**) tumour core (n = 24; p = 0.2).

uPAR overexpression at the invading front of tumours has been supported in a number of other studies [18,21]. Increased uPA [22] and PAI-1 [21] expression at the leading edge of the cancer is also recognised. The higher uPAS expression at the invasion front is critical to facilitate tumour progression through the surrounding stroma.

4.4. Expression in Tumour-Associated Stromal Cells

The invasion of cancer cells into normal tissues relies on interactions between the tumour and the surrounding stroma. There is increasing evidence of the importance of stroma in initiating and regulating the speed of invasion [93–95]. The stromal cells within the TME of particular interest are immune cells such as leucocytes and tumour-associated macrophages, as well as fibroblasts, blood- and lymphatic endothelial cells [96]. uPAS overexpression is seen in the immediate adjacent stromal cells where it assists in the degradation of the stromal laminin and fibronectin [12].

As expected, the most critical tumour region for uPAS expression in the stroma is at the advancing tumour front. Macrophages and myofibroblasts at the invading front of GOCs express increased uPAR compared to the tumour core [12,18]. In adenocarcinomas arising from the oesophagus, gastroesophageal junction and cardia, strongly uPAR-expressing macrophages at the invasion front are inversely correlated to OS when compared to those with lower expressing macrophages (multivariate, HR 6.26, 95%CI 2.37–16; p = 0.0002) [18]. This was not replicated in distal gastric adenocarcinomas [12]. Conflicting results may be due to the dual role of macrophages in tumours as either pro-tumourigenic or anti-tumourigenic; thus, assessment of uPAR alone may be insufficient to describe the role of macrophages in cancer progression [97]. In addition, intra-observer variability in assessing uPAR expression was high which may have confounded results [18].

uPAR-expressing myofibroblasts (defined by expression of α-smooth actin) are not significantly associated with patient outcomes in GOC [12,18]. However, further work is needed to clarify if uPAR expression on the population of so-called cancer-associated fibroblasts, a fibroblast subpopulation which are more likely to be involved in cancer modification, is prognostic.

Similarly, in other solid tumours, stromal uPAS expression is significantly linked with tumour-associated stromal cells, and in the case of colon cancer poorer clinical outcomes [27]. There is evidence in breast-, colon- and lung cancer of strong association of uPAS expression on both macrophages and fibroblasts (Table 4). In colon cancer, there is further supporting evidence of stromal uPAS expression being inversely associated with disease free survival times (multivariate HR 1.71, 95%CI 1.05–2.80; p = 0.002), and a tendency to worse OS (p = 0.07) [27].

Table 4. Urokinase plasminogen activation system expression in the tumour microenvironment of other solid tumours.

Tissue	Cell Type	uPA	uPAR	PAI-1	PAI-2
Breast, ductal	Macrophages	+ [98]	+ [99,100]	+ [101]	
	Fibroblasts	+ [98,102]	Weak [102]	Weak [102]	
Colon	Macrophages		+ [103]		
	Fibroblasts	+ [104]	+ [103]		
Lung	Macrophages	+ [105]		+ [105]	+ [105]
	Fibroblasts				

Key references noted in each positive box. Boxes unfilled demonstrate no available evidence. Abbreviations: uPA = urokinase plasminogen activator; uPAR = urokinase plasminogen activator receptor; PAI-1 = plasminogen activator inhibitor 1; PAI-2 = plasminogen activator inhibitor 2; + = medium to strong positivity.

4.5. Interactions of the uPAS with Other Proteolytic Enzymes

There are many MMPs with different functional roles, with variable association with cancer occurrence and progression [106]. In one study of gastric adenocarcinoma, both uPA and MMP-9 mRNAs were shown to be expressed in 58% of tumours, but co-expression was not explored [107]. However, both uPA and MMP-9 were shown to be independent prognostic factors, in addition to standard prognostic tumour features [107]. Co-expression of MMP-2 with uPA, uPAR, PAI-1 or PAI-2 is seen in gastric cancer, with co-expression of MMP-2 and uPAR associated with worse OS [108]. Gastric adenocarcinoma tissues overexpressing MMP-2 mRNA are associated with lymph node metastases, histological differentiation and diffused or mixed Lauren's classification when compared to normal adjacent tissues [109].

Cathepsin B is a cysteine protease which has indirect proteolytic activity through interactions with pro-uPA, pro-MMPs, TGF-β and toll-like receptor 3, therefore it has an important role in cell proliferation, differentiation and angiogenesis [110,111]. Cathepsin B is localised in mitochondria and here it initiates apoptosis [111]. Cathepsin B helps catalyse pro-uPA to its active form urokinase [112]. Serum Cathepsin B and soluble uPA levels were shown to be higher in gastric cancer patients when compared to patients with premalignant adenomas, which were higher again than normal controls [113]. Increased serum levels of both Cathepsin B and uPA were also seen in metastatic compared to localised GOCs [113].

5. uPAS Assessment in Blood

Peripheral blood sampling allows for minimally invasive assessment of patient's tumour and immune response. The uPAS has been assessed in serum [35,36,114–117], immune cells [118] and circulating tumour cells (CTCs) [92]. However, assessment of peripheral circulating uPAS proteins in serum or plasma can be complicated by elevated uPAS expression levels seen in non-malignant conditions including renal failure, sepsis, inflammatory arthritis and cardiovascular disease [119,120]. Overall, there is poor correlation of each individual uPAS protein assessed in the plasma and primary cancer tissue samples in patients with gastric adenocarcinoma, with plasma uPAS levels not associated with cancer staging or severity [121]. However, higher uPAR mRNA levels were seen in the peripheral blood of patients with gastric cancer compared to those with benign gastric diseases and the mRNA levels were also associated with more advanced tumour stages [114].

5.1. Soluble uPAS Proteins in the Serum

To date, only two studies have investigated the role of serum uPA levels in GOC with inconsistent findings. Herszényi, et al. showed serum uPA levels were associated with a diagnosis of GOC and the severity of disease [113]. However, Vidal, et al. showed serum uPA levels in surgically curative gastric adenocarcinoma patients compared to healthy controls were comparable, with no significant associations seen with pathological features or clinical outcomes [115]. The lack of serum uPA discrimination may be due to the early stage of these cancers or participant selection. The prognostic role of blood uPA levels were however reported in advanced and metastatic breast cancer [122].

ELISA [35] and time-resolved fluoroimmunoassay [123] are both methods which are available for detection of suPAR. However, neither of these techniques are used routinely in clinical practice and would currently be considered for research use only. In GOC patients, levels of all suPAR subunits were reported at almost double that of aged-matched healthy individuals ([ng/mL] 5.74 ± 5.3 vs. 2.77 ± 0.77; $p < 0.0001$), and significantly higher in those with metastatic disease compared to non-metastatic disease ([ng/mL] 7.00 ± 6.13 vs. 4.75 ± 4.43; $p > 0.05$) [35,36]. In vitro models have shown that tumour-associated suPAR can direct migration, promote mitosis and angiogenesis of human umbilical vein endothelial cells demonstrating the potential role of suPAR in the progression of tumours [116].

suPAR has been better characterised in other gastrointestinal cancers. In colon cancer, increased pre-operative suPAR levels are significantly associated with poorer prognosis [117]. Interestingly, the dynamics of suPAR also appear important. In patients with paired pre-operative and six-month post-operative suPAR recordings, a rising suPAR level was associated with shorter survivals, while the converse was seen for those with a falling post-operative suPAR [124]. Those patients with highest suPAR levels following liver metastases had worse prognosis [124]. Increased levels of suPAR are postulated to be a product of more aggressive cancer and demonstrating non-radiological invasive disease, hence it has potential as a prognostic biomarker.

5.2. uPAS Expression on Peripheral Blood Mononuclear Cells in GOC

Peripheral blood mononuclear cells (PBMCs), identified by gradient centrifugation of blood, includes the majority of leukocytes. In malignancy, monocytes may display both pro-tumoural and anti-tumoural effects on cancers [118]. As such, assessment may be able to aid prognostic decision making.

uPA mRNA assessed in peripheral blood monocytes in treatment naïve patients, following gastrectomy, demonstrated that patients with more advanced disease showed higher relative levels prior to adjuvant chemotherapy (stage III vs. I or II; $p = 0.014$) [125]. OS was also significantly reduced in patients with uPA mRNA expression above the median value ($p = 0.014$) [125].

5.3. Evidence of uPAS on Circulating Tumour Cells

In addition to leukocytes, the PBMC layer also contains CTCs, which are a critical link in the development of distant metastases. High CTCs numbers in GOCs show worse prognosis and poor response to therapy [126,127].

Current food and drug administration agency approved CTC isolation utilises epithelial cell adhesion molecule (EpCAM) expression as a positive marker for CTCs [128]. EpCAM is a marker of the epithelial phenotype and, as such, may not capture CTCs that have undergone epithelial to mesenchymal transition (EMT) [128]. uPAR is a known translocator of cells to the mesenchymal phenotype [129]. Given the propensity of cells at the invasive front in GOC to overexpress uPAR (Figure 2) and likely give rise to CTCs that have undergone EMT, uPAR has the potential to be utilised as an alternate CTC capture target molecule.

Brungs et al. assessed 43 patients from whom CTCs were isolated using the standard EpCAM isolation methods at any clinical stage of GOC. In 93% of patients, where EpCAM selected CTCs were identified, a proportion also co-expressed surface uPAR (CK+/EpCAM+/DAPI+/CD45-/uPAR+ CTCs) [130]. In further analyses, we found that where more than 60% of these EpCAM selected uPAR+ CTCs also co-expressed uPAR, histological tumour uPAR IHC scoring was also increased (Figure 3). Metastasis formation and OS was not associated with proportional assessment of CTCs (more than 60% of EpCAM-selected showed uPAR-positivity) in this cohort of patients (Figure 4b). There was a trend to poorer OS in this highly selected group of patients where absolute number of EpCAM+/uPAR+ CTCs was greater than 10, but this would likely be attributed to absolute higher CTC numbers opposed to proportional cut offs (Figure 4a). Intriguingly, higher CTC numbers may be linked to uPAR-positivity; however, any such connection needs to be more closely investigated.

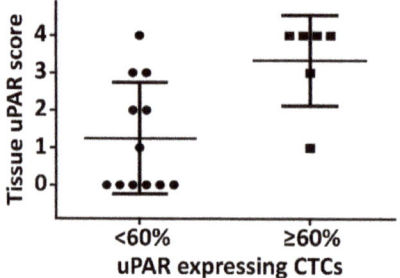

Figure 3. Tissue expression of uPAR is increased in patients where more than 60% of their epithelial cell adhesion molecule (EpCAM) selected circulating tumour cells (CTCs) co-expressed uPAR. Mean score in the lower group 1.3, higher group 3.3 (n = 18, p = 0.0008).

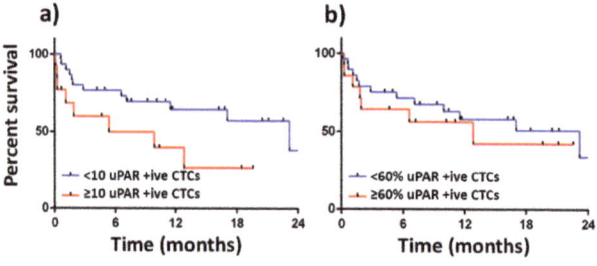

Figure 4. Kaplan Meier curves showing OS demonstrating (n = 43): (**a**) a trend of improved survival seen in patients with less than 10 EpCAM+/uPAR+ CTCs (p = 0.06); (**b**) no survival benefit seen where more than 60% of EpCAM+ CTCs also co-expressed uPAR (p = 0.5).

6. Therapeutics and Diagnostics Directed towards the uPAS Pathway

It is clear that in many carcinoma types, including GOC, the uPAS is a driver of tumour aggressiveness. Not surprisingly, several experimental anti-cancer and imaging approaches targeting various components of the uPAS have been pursued (reviewed in detail by Lin et al. [131], Mahmood and Rabbani [15] and Yuan et al. [132]). Briefly, anti-uPAS therapeutic approaches include antagonists of uPAR and various uPAR ligand (e.g., uPA, vitronectin, integrins, etc) interactions, small molecule and antibody inhibitors directed against uPA protease activity, PAI-1 inhibitors and uPA-therapeutic drug conjugates [15,131,132]. Our group has previously described the use of PAI-2 conjugated cytotoxins and therapeutic radioisotopes, which were effective in mouse models of human breast and colon cancer [133–137]. We have also recently described novel amiloride analogues with low nanomolar uPA inhibitory activity, high target selectivity and potent antimetastatic activity in mouse models of human lung and orthotopic pancreatic cancer metastasis [138,139]. To date, most of these experimental approaches have not progressed beyond pre-clinical models and very few have utilised models of GOC [68,140,141]. One orally active small molecule uPA inhibitor upamostat (the prodrug form of WX-UK1) was efficacious in a Phase 2 trial for locally advanced non-resectable pancreatic cancer in combination with gemcitabine showing a 17% increase in 1-year survival over gemcitabine or upamostat alone and an acceptable safety profile [142]. However, upamostat shows broad activity across many serine proteases and is currently being tested in other indications including a Phase 2/3 study for patients with symptomatic COVID-19 (NCT04723537). Nevertheless, this highlights the promise of perhaps more selective uPAS drugs for the treatment of advanced disease. Small molecule uPAR binding peptides and antibodies targeting uPAR and uPA conjugated to imaging radioisotopes are also being developed that have been shown to successfully detect primary tumours and metastases (which overexpress uPA/uPAR) with ongoing clinical trials aiming to determine the utility of these approaches for prognostication and/or response to therapy (reviewed in Mahmood and Rabbani [15]). To the best of our knowledge, none of these trials yet includes patients with GOC.

7. Conclusions

The uPAS is an important pathway whose upregulation contributes to uncontrolled ECM remodelling and cell signalling resulting in increased tumour, invasion and metastasis. uPA, uPAR and PAI-1 all have clear prognostic associations with GOCs, with evidence supported by a multitude of individual studies and a meta-analysis. Further, the expression of uPAS is associated with adverse clinicopathological features of GOCs. Therefore, GOC tumour levels of uPA, uPAR and PAI-1 can be considered a significant prognostic biomarker, with increased expression resulting in worse outcomes for patients.

Tumour-associated stroma is infiltrated with immune cells; the role of this stroma is the focus of ongoing research uncovering a deeper understanding of its role in tumour progression. uPAS expression is elevated in macrophages and myofibroblasts in GOC. GOC (except distal gastric) stromal macrophage uPAR expression is associated with a poorer prognosis. The role of the uPAS in the stroma is under-investigated in GOCs; larger cohorts and prognostic assessment are required to understand the role of the uPAS protein expression in the stroma.

An optimal biomarker for GOCs would offer real time prognostic and/or predictive qualities, as such liquid biopsy is of keen interest. suPAR shows promise as a diagnostic biomarker with increased expression reported in patients with GOCs. Unfortunately, to date, suPAR has failed to yield a prognostic association in GOCs in the same way as it has for colon cancer. For this reason, it is not currently considered a useful predictive biomarker. uPAR mRNA isolated from circulating immune cells from the peripheral blood monocyte layer has been shown to have prognostic potential, when assessing reduction in OS. These findings offer potential of a uPAS-related prognostic biomarker being identified in the circulating blood.

In summary, uPAS has a highly active role in the progression of GOC, and compelling evidence of its relationship with prognosis and clinicopathological features regardless of its assessment in the primary tissue or as a circulating biomarker. GOC uPAS expression in tumour-associated stroma requires further investigation to further specify the stromal role in tumour progression. We have demonstrated primary tissue assessment of the uPAS as a useful prognostic biomarker in GOCs and highlighted the exciting potential of liquid biopsies to be added to the list of prognostic biomarkers. Through ongoing investigation and drug development to target this pathway, there is significant potential for the uPAS as a predictive biomarker of uPAS directed therapies.

Author Contributions: G.T. performed literature review, discussion and manuscript draft. D.B. and M.R. conceived the idea, assisted in drafting and editing the manuscript. A.-K.P., K.L.V., T.B. and M.A. reviewed and edited the manuscript. All authors have read and agreed to the published version of the manuscript.

Funding: G.T. is a recipient of University of Wollongong matching scholarship.

Institutional Review Board Statement: The study was conducted according to the guidelines of the Declaration of Helsinki, and approved by the South Western Sydney Local Health District Human Research and Ethics Committee (HREC/15/LPOOL/121, 12 May 2015).

Informed Consent statement: Informed consent was obtained from all subjects involved in the study.

Data Availability Statement: The data presented in this study are available on request from the corresponding author.

Conflicts of Interest: The authors declare no conflict of interest.

References

1. Bray, F.; Ferlay, J.; Soerjomataram, I.; Siegel, R.L.; Torre, L.A.; Jemal, A. Global cancer statistics 2018: GLOBOCAN estimates of incidence and mortality worldwide for 36 cancers in 185 countries. *CA Cancer J. Clin.* **2018**, *68*, 394–424. [CrossRef]
2. Enzinger, P.C.; Mayer, R.J. Esophageal cancer. *N. Engl. J. Med.* **2003**, *349*, 2241–2252. [CrossRef] [PubMed]
3. Riihimaki, M.; Hemminki, A.; Sundquist, K.; Sundquist, J.; Hemminki, K. Metastatic spread in patients with gastric cancer. *Oncotarget* **2016**, *7*, 52307–52316. [CrossRef] [PubMed]
4. Wilkinson, N.; Howe, J.; Gay, G.; Patel-Parekh, L.; Scott-Conner, C.; Donohue, J. Differences in the pattern of presentation and treatment of proximal and distal gastric cancer: Results of the 2001 gastric patient care evaluation. *Ann. Surg. Oncol.* **2008**, *15*, 1644–1650. [CrossRef]
5. Andreasen, P.A.; Kjøller, L.; Christensen, L.; Duffy, M.J. The urokinase-type plasminogen activator system in cancer metastasis: A review. *Int. J. Cancer* **1997**, *72*, 1–22. [CrossRef]
6. Ranson, M.; Andronicos, N.M. Plasminogen binding and cancer: Promises and pitfalls. *Front. Biosci.* **2003**, *8*, s294–s304. [CrossRef]
7. Laufs, S.; Schumacher, J.; Allgayer, H. Urokinase-receptor (u-PAR): An essential player in multiple games of cancer: A review on its role in tumor progression, invasion, metastasis, proliferation/dormancy, clinical outcome and minimal residual disease. *Cell Cycle* **2006**, *5*, 1760–1771.
8. Duffy, M.J. The urokinase plasminogen activator system: Role in malignancy. *Curr. Pharm. Des.* **2004**, *10*, 39–49. [CrossRef]
9. Dano, K.; Behrendt, N.; Hoyer-Hansen, G.; Johnsen, M.; Lund, L.R.; Ploug, M.; Romer, J. Plasminogen activation and cancer. *Thromb. Haemost.* **2005**, *93*, 676–681.
10. McMahon, B.; Kwaan, H.C. The plasminogen activator system and cancer. *Pathophysiol. Haemost. Thromb.* **2008**, *36*, 184–194. [CrossRef]
11. Croucher, D.R.; Saunders, D.N.; Lobov, S.; Ranson, M. Revisiting the biological roles of PAI2 (SERPINB2) in cancer. *Nat. Rev. Cancer* **2008**, *8*, 535–545. [CrossRef] [PubMed]
12. Alpízar-Alpízar, W.; Christensen, I.J.; Santoni-Rugiu, E.; Skarstein, A.; Ovrebo, K.; Illemann, M.; Laerum, O.D. Urokinase plasminogen activator receptor on invasive cancer cells: A prognostic factor in distal gastric adenocarcinoma. *Int. J. Cancer* **2012**, *131*, E329–E336. [CrossRef] [PubMed]
13. Dass, K.; Ahmad, A.; Azmi, A.S.; Sarkar, S.H.; Sarkar, F.H. Evolving role of uPA/uPAR system in human cancers. *Cancer Treat. Rev.* **2008**, *34*, 122–136. [CrossRef] [PubMed]
14. Gårdsvoll, H.; Jacobsen, B.; Kriegbaum, M.C.; Behrendt, N.; Engelholm, L.; Østergaard, S.; Ploug, M. Conformational regulation of urokinase receptor function: Impact of receptor occupancy and epitope-mapped monoclonal antibodies on lamellipodia induction. *J. Biol. Chem.* **2011**, *286*, 33544–33556. [CrossRef] [PubMed]
15. Mahmood, N.; Rabbani, S.A. Fibrinolytic System and Cancer: Diagnostic and Therapeutic Applications. *Int. J. Mol. Sci.* **2021**, *22*, 4358. [CrossRef]

16. Scicolone, G.; Sanchez, V.; Vauthay, L.; Fuentes, F.; Scicolone, A.; Scicolone, L.; Rapacioli, M.; Flores, V. Tissue-type plasminogen activator activity in morphologically normal tissues adjacent to gastrointestinal carcinomas is associated with the degree of tumor progression. *J. Cancer Res. Clin. Oncol.* **2006**, *132*, 309–319. [CrossRef] [PubMed]
17. Brungs, D.; Chen, J.; Aghmesheh, M.; Vine, K.L.; Becker, T.M.; Carolan, M.G.; Ranson, M. The urokinase plasminogen activation system in gastroesophageal cancer: A systematic review and meta-analysis. *Oncotarget* **2017**, *8*, 23099–23109. [CrossRef]
18. Laerum, O.D.; Ovrebo, K.; Skarstein, A.; Christensen, I.J.; Alpizar-Alpizar, W.; Helgeland, L.; Dano, K.; Nielsen, B.S.; Illemann, M. Prognosis in adenocarcinomas of lower oesophagus, gastro-oesophageal junction and cardia evaluated by uPAR-immunohistochemistry. *Int. J. Cancer* **2012**, *131*, 558–569. [CrossRef]
19. Wang, S.N.; Miyauchi, M.; Koshikawa, N.; Maruyama, K.; Kubota, T.; Miura, K.; Kurosawa, Y.; Awaya, A.; Kanai, Y. Antigen expression associated with lymph node metastasis in gastric adenocarcinomas. *Pathol. Int.* **1994**, *44*, 844–849. [CrossRef]
20. Hong, S.I.; Park, I.C.; Son, Y.S.; Lee, S.H.; Kim, B.G.; Lee, J.I.; Lee, T.W.; Kook, Y.H.; Min, Y.I.; Hong, W.S. Expression of urokinase-type plasminogen activator, its receptor, and its inhibitor in gastric adenocarcinoma tissues. *J. Korean Med. Sci.* **1996**, *11*, 33–37. [CrossRef]
21. Kawasaki, K.; Hayashi, Y.; Wang, Y.; Suzuki, S.; Morita, Y.; Nakamura, T.; Narita, K.; Doe, W.; Itoh, H.; Kuroda, Y. Expression of urokinase-type plasminogen activator receptor and plasminogen activator inhibitor-1 in gastric cancer. *J. Gastroenterol. Hepatol.* **1998**, *13*, 936–944. [CrossRef] [PubMed]
22. Ito, H.; Yonemura, Y.; Fujita, H.; Tsuchihara, K.; Kawamura, T.; Nojima, N.; Fujimura, T.; Nose, H.; Endo, Y.; Sasaki, T. Prognostic relevance of urokinase-type plasminogen activator (uPA) and plasminogen activator inhibitors PAI-1 and PAI-2 in gastric cancer. *Virchows Arch.* **1996**, *427*, 487–496. [CrossRef]
23. Kaneko, T.; Konno, H.; Baba, M.; Tanaka, T.; Nakamura, S. Urokinase-type plasminogen activator expression correlates with tumor angiogenesis and poor outcome in gastric cancer. *Cancer Sci.* **2003**, *94*, 43–49. [CrossRef] [PubMed]
24. Nekarda, H.; Schlegel, P.; Schmitt, M.; Stark, M.; Mueller, J.D.; Fink, U.; Siewert, J.R. Strong prognostic impact of tumor-associated urokinase-type plasminogen activator in completely resected adenocarcinoma of the esophagus. *Clin. Cancer Res.* **1998**, *4*, 1755–1763.
25. Nekarda, H.; Schmitt, M.; Ulm, K.; Wenninger, A.; Vogelsang, H.; Becker, K.; Roder, J.D.; Fink, U.; Siewert, J.R. Prognostic impact of urokinase-type plasminogen activator and its inhibitor PAI-1 in completely resected gastric cancer. *Cancer Res.* **1994**, *54*, 2900–2907.
26. Beyer, B.C.; Heiss, M.M.; Simon, E.H.; Gruetzner, K.U.; Babic, R.; Jauch, K.W.; Schildberg, F.W.; Allgayer, H. Urokinase system expression in gastric carcinoma: Prognostic impact in an independent patient series and first evidence of predictive value in preoperative biopsy and intestinal metaplasia specimens. *Cancer* **2006**, *106*, 1026–1035. [CrossRef]
27. Boonstra, M.C.; Verbeek, F.P.R.; Mazar, A.P.; Prevoo, H.A.J.M.; Kuppen, P.J.K.; van de Velde, C.J.H.; Vahrmeijer, A.L.; Sier, C.F.M. Expression of uPAR in tumor-associated stromal cells is associated with colorectal cancer patient prognosis: A TMA study. *BMC Cancer* **2014**, *14*, 269. [CrossRef] [PubMed]
28. Ploug, M.; Gardsvoll, H.; Jorgensen, T.J.; Lonborg Hansen, L.; Dano, K. Structural analysis of the interaction between urokinase-type plasminogen activator and its receptor: A potential target for anti-invasive cancer therapy. *Biochem. Soc. Trans.* **2002**, *30*, 177–183. [CrossRef]
29. Deryugina, E.I.; Quigley, J. Cell surface remodeling by plasmin: A new function for an old enzyme. *J. Biomed. Biotechnol.* **2012**, *2012*, 564259. [CrossRef]
30. Stamenkovic, I. Extracellular matrix remodelling: The role of matrix metalloproteinases. *J. Pathol.* **2003**, *200*, 448–464. [CrossRef]
31. Smith, H.W.; Marshall, C.J. Regulation of cell signalling by uPAR. *Nat. Rev. Mol. Cell Biol.* **2010**, *11*, 23–36. [CrossRef] [PubMed]
32. Carriero, M.V.; Franco, P.; Votta, G.; Longanesi-Cattani, I.; Vento, M.T.; Masucci, M.T.; Mancini, A.; Caputi, M.; Iaccarino, I.; Stoppelli, M.P. Regulation of cell migration and invasion by specific modules of uPA: Mechanistic insights and specific inhibitors. *Curr. Drug Targets* **2011**, *12*, 1761–1771. [CrossRef]
33. Ferraris, G.M.S.; Schulte, C.; Buttiglione, V.; De Lorenzi, V.; Piontini, A.; Galluzzi, M.; Podestà, A.; Madsen, C.D.; Sidenius, N. The interaction between uPAR and vitronectin triggers ligand-independent adhesion signalling by integrins. *EMBO J.* **2014**, *33*, 2458–2472. [CrossRef]
34. Thuno, M.; Macho, B.; Eugen-Olsen, J. suPAR: The molecular crystal ball. *Dis. Markers* **2009**, *27*, 157–172. [CrossRef] [PubMed]
35. Fidan, E.; Mentese, A.; Ozdemir, F.; Deger, O.; Kavgaci, H.; Caner Karahan, S.; Aydin, F. Diagnostic and prognostic significance of CA IX and suPAR in gastric cancer. *Med. Oncol.* **2013**, *30*, 540. [CrossRef]
36. Rohrberg, K.S.; Skov, B.G.; Lassen, U.; Christensen, I.J.; Høyer-Hansen, G.; Buysschaert, I.; Pappot, H. Markers of angiogenesis and epidermal growth factor receptor signalling in patients with pancreatic and gastroesophageal junction cancer. *Cancer Biomark* **2010**, *7*, 141–151. [CrossRef] [PubMed]
37. Masucci, M.T.; Pedersen, N.; Blasi, F. A soluble, ligand binding mutant of the human urokinase plasminogen activator receptor. *J. Biol. Chem.* **1991**, *266*, 8655–8658. [CrossRef]
38. Høyer-Hansen, G.; Behrendt, N.; Ploug, M.; Danø, K.; Preissner, K.T. The intact urokinase receptor is required for efficient vitronectin binding: Receptor cleavage prevents ligand interaction. *FEBS Lett.* **1997**, *420*, 79–85. [CrossRef]
39. Ploug, M.; Rahbek-Nielsen, H.; Ellis, V.; Roepstorff, P.; Danø, K. Chemical modification of the urokinase-type plasminogen activator and its receptor using tetranitromethane. Evidence for the involvement of specific tyrosine residues in both molecules during receptor-ligand interaction. *Biochemistry* **1995**, *34*, 12524–12534. [CrossRef] [PubMed]

40. Fazioli, F.; Resnati, M.; Sidenius, N.; Higashimoto, Y.; Appella, E.; Blasi, F. A urokinase-sensitive region of the human urokinase receptor is responsible for its chemotactic activity. *EMBO J.* **1997**, *16*, 7279–7286. [CrossRef]
41. Selleri, C.; Montuori, N.; Ricci, P.; Visconte, V.; Carriero, M.V.; Sidenius, N.; Serio, B.; Blasi, F.; Rotoli, B.; Rossi, G.; et al. Involvement of the urokinase-type plasminogen activator receptor in hematopoietic stem cell mobilization. *Blood* **2005**, *105*, 2198–2205. [CrossRef]
42. Resnati, M.; Pallavicini, I.; Wang, J.M.; Oppenheim, J.; Serhan, C.N.; Romano, M.; Blasi, F. The fibrinolytic receptor for urokinase activates the G protein-coupled chemotactic receptor FPRL1/LXA4R. *Proc. Natl. Acad. Sci. USA* **2002**, *99*, 1359–1364. [CrossRef]
43. Placencio, V.R.; De Clerck, Y.A. Plasminogen Activator Inhibitor-1 in Cancer: Rationale and Insight for Future Therapeutic Testing. *Cancer Res.* **2015**, *75*, 2969–2974. [CrossRef]
44. Herz, J.; Strickland, D.K. LRP: A multifunctional scavenger and signaling receptor. *J. Clin. Invest.* **2001**, *108*, 779–784. [CrossRef]
45. Nykjær, A.; Conese, M.; Christensen, E.I.; Olson, D.; Cremona, O.; Gliemann, J.; Blasi, F. Recycling of the urokinase receptor upon internalization of the uPA:serpin complexes. *EMBO J.* **1997**, *16*, 2610–2620. [CrossRef] [PubMed]
46. Cochran, B.J.; Croucher, D.R.; Lobov, S.; Saunders, D.N.; Ranson, M. Dependence on endocytic receptor binding via a minimal binding motif underlies the differential prognostic profiles of SerpinE1 and SerpinB2 in cancer. *J. Biol. Chem.* **2011**, *286*, 24467–24475. [CrossRef] [PubMed]
47. Kubala, M.H.; DeClerck, Y.A. The plasminogen activator inhibitor-1 paradox in cancer: A mechanistic understanding. *Cancer Metastasis Rev.* **2019**, *38*, 483–492. [CrossRef] [PubMed]
48. Croucher, D.R.; Saunders, D.N.; Stillfried, G.E.; Ranson, M. A structural basis for differential cell signalling by PAI-1 and PAI-2 in breast cancer cells. *Biochem. J.* **2007**, *408*, 203–210. [CrossRef]
49. Harbeck, N.; Schmitt, M.; Meisner, C.; Friedel, C.; Untch, M.; Schmidt, M.; Sweep, C.G.; Lisboa, B.W.; Lux, M.P.; Beck, T.; et al. Ten-year analysis of the prospective multicentre Chemo-N0 trial validates American Society of Clinical Oncology (ASCO)-recommended biomarkers uPA and PAI-1 for therapy decision making in node-negative breast cancer patients. *Eur. J. Cancer* **2013**, *49*, 1825–1835. [CrossRef]
50. Behrendt, N.; List, K.; Andreasen, P.A.; Danø, K. The pro-urokinase plasminogen-activation system in the presence of serpin-type inhibitors and the urokinase receptor: Rescue of activity through reciprocal pro-enzyme activation. *Biochem. J.* **2003**, *371 Pt 2*, 277–287. [CrossRef]
51. Petersen, L.C.; Lund, L.R.; Nielsen, L.S.; Danø, K.; Skriver, L. One-chain urokinase-type plasminogen activator from human sarcoma cells is a proenzyme with little or no intrinsic activity. *J. Biol. Chem.* **1988**, *263*, 11189–11195. [CrossRef]
52. Almholt, K.; Wang, J.; Pass, J.; Røder, G.; Padkjær, S.B.; Hebsgaard, J.B.; Xia, W.; Yang, L.; Forsell, J.; Breinholt, V.M.; et al. Identification and preclinical development of an anti-proteolytic uPA antibody for rheumatoid arthritis. *J. Mol. Med.* **2020**, *98*, 585–593. [CrossRef] [PubMed]
53. Dow, M.P.D. Gonadotrophin surge-induced upregulation of mRNA for plasminogen activator inhibitors 1 and 2 within bovine periovulatory follicular and luteal tissue. *Reproduction* **2002**, *123*, 711–719. [CrossRef]
54. Xing, R.H.; Rabbani, S.A. Regulation of urokinase production by androgens in human prostate cancer cells: Effect on tumor growth and metastases in vivo. *Endocrinology* **1999**, *140*, 4056–4064. [CrossRef]
55. Long, B.J.; Rose, D. Invasive capacity and regulation of urokinase-type plasminogen activator in estrogen receptor (ER)-negative MDA-MB-231 human breast cancer cells, and a transfectant (S30) stably expressing ER. *Cancer Lett.* **1996**, *99*, 209–215. [CrossRef]
56. Casslén, B.; Nordengren, J.; Gustavsson, B.; Nilbert, M.; Lund, L.R. Progesterone stimulates degradation of urokinase plasminogen activator (u-PA) in endometrial stromal cells by increasing its inhibitor and surface expression of the u-PA receptor. *J. Clin. Endocrinol. Metab.* **1995**, *80*, 2776–2784. [PubMed]
57. Korczak, B.; Kerbel, R.S.; Dennis, J.W. Autocrine and paracrine regulation of tissue inhibitor of metalloproteinases, transin, and urokinase gene expression in metastatic and nonmetastatic mammary carcinoma cells. *Cell Growth Differ.* **1991**, *2*, 335–341.
58. Moriyama, T.; Kataoka, H.; Hamasuna, R.; Yoshida, E.; Sameshima, T.; Iseda, T.; Yokogami, K.; Nakano, S.; Koono, M.; Wakisaka, S. Simultaneous up-regulation of urokinase-type plasminogen activator (uPA) and uPA receptor by hepatocyte growth factor/scatter factor in human glioma cells. *Clin. Exp. Metastasis* **1999**, *17*, 873–879. [CrossRef] [PubMed]
59. Santibáñez, J.F.; Iglesias, M.; Frontelo, P.; Martínez, J.; Quintanilla, M. Involvement of the Ras/MAPK signaling pathway in the modulation of urokinase production and cellular invasiveness by transforming growth factor-beta(1) in transformed keratinocytes. *Biochem. Biophys. Res. Commun.* **2000**, *273*, 521–527. [CrossRef]
60. Kirchheimer, J.C.; Nong, Y.H.; Remold, H.G. IFN-gamma, tumor necrosis factor-alpha; urokinase regulate the expression of urokinase receptors on human monocytes. *J. Immunol.* **1988**, *141*, 4229–4234. [PubMed]
61. Kroon, M.E.; Koolwijk, P.; van der Vecht, B.; van Hinsbergh, V.W. Urokinase receptor expression on human microvascular endothelial cells is increased by hypoxia: Implications for capillary-like tube formation in a fibrin matrix. *Blood* **2000**, *96*, 2775–2783. [CrossRef]
62. Bell, S.M.; Brackenbury, R.W.; Leslie, N.D.; Degen, J.L. Plasminogen activator gene expression is induced by the src oncogene product and tumor promoters. *J. Biol. Chem.* **1990**, *265*, 1333–1338. [CrossRef]
63. Johnson, M.D.; Torri, J.A.; Lippman, M.E.; Dickson, R.B. Regulation of motility and protease expression in PKC-mediated induction of MCF-7 breast cancer cell invasiveness. *Exp. Cell Res.* **1999**, *247*, 105–113. [CrossRef]

64. Niiya, K.; Ozawa, T.; Tsuzawa, T.; Ueshima, S.; Matsuo, O.; Sakuragawa, N. Transcriptional regulation of urokinase-type plasminogen activator receptor by cyclic AMP in PL-21 human myeloid leukemia cells: Comparison with the regulation by phorbol myristate acetate. *Thromb. Haemost.* **1998**, *79*, 574–578.
65. Myohanen, H.; Vaheri, A. Regulation and interactions in the activation of cell-associated plasminogen. *Cell Mol. Life Sci.* **2004**, *61*, 2840–2858. [CrossRef] [PubMed]
66. Lee, K.; Choi, E.; Kim, M.; Kim, K.; Jang, B.; Kim, S.; Kim, S.; Song, S.; Kim, J.-R. Inhibition of histone deacetylase activity down-regulates urokinase plasminogen activator and matrix metalloproteinase-9 expression in gastric cancer. *Mol. Cell Biochem.* **2010**, *343*, 163–171. [CrossRef] [PubMed]
67. Kuga, H.; Morisaki, T.; Nakamura, K.; Onishi, H.; Noshiro, H.; Uchiyama, A.; Tanaka, M.; Katano, M. Interferon-gamma suppresses transforming growth factor-beta-induced invasion of gastric carcinoma cells through cross-talk of Smad pathway in a three-dimensional culture model. *Oncogene* **2003**, *22*, 7838–7847. [CrossRef] [PubMed]
68. Wang, J.; Chen, X.; Su, L.; Zhu, Z.; Wu, W.; Zhou, Y. Suppressive effects on cell proliferation and motility in gastric cancer SGC-7901 cells by introducing ulinastatin in vitro. *Anticancer Drugs* **2016**, *27*, 651–659. [CrossRef]
69. Gong, M.; Lu, Z.; Fang, G.; Bi, J.; Xue, X. A small interfering RNA targeting osteopontin as gastric cancer therapeutics. *Cancer Lett.* **2008**, *272*, 148–159. [CrossRef]
70. Lee, K.H.; Choi, E.Y.; Koh, S.A.E.; Kim, M.K.; Jang, B.I.; Kim, S.W.; Kim, J.-R. IL-1beta-stimulated urokinase plasminogen activator expression through NF-kappaB in gastric cancer after HGF treatment. *Oncol Rep.* **2014**, *31*, 2123–2130. [CrossRef]
71. Onwuegbusi, B.; Rees, J.; Lao-Sirieix, P.; Fitzgerald, R. Selective loss of TGFbeta Smad-dependent signalling prevents cell cycle arrest and promotes invasion in oesophageal adenocarcinoma cell lines. *PLoS ONE* **2007**, *2*, e177. [CrossRef] [PubMed]
72. Wang, P.; Ma, M.; Zhang, S. EGF-induced urokinase plasminogen activator receptor promotes epithelial to mesenchymal transition in human gastric cancer cells. *Oncol. Rep.* **2017**, *38*, 2325–2334. [CrossRef] [PubMed]
73. Kyung Hee, L.; Eun Young, C.; Min Kyoung, K.; Myung Soo, H.; Byung Ik, J.; Tae Nyeun, K.; Sang Woon, K.; Sun Kyo, S.; Jung Hye, K.; Jae-Ryong, K. Regulation of hepatocyte growth factor-mediated urokinase plasminogen activator secretion by MEK/ERK activation in human stomach cancer cell lines. *Exp. Mol. Med.* **2006**, *38*, 27–35.
74. Lian, S.; Xia, Y.; Ung, T.T.; Khoi, P.N.; Yoon, H.J.; Lee, S.G.; Kim, K.K.; Jung, Y.D. Prostaglandin E2 stimulates urokinase-type plasminogen activator receptor via EP2 receptor-dependent signaling pathways in human AGS gastric cancer cells. *Mol. Carcinog.* **2017**, *56*, 664–680. [CrossRef] [PubMed]
75. Shin, V.Y.; Wu, W.K.K.; Chu, K.-M.; Wong, H.P.S.; Lam, E.K.Y.; Tai, E.K.K.; Koo, M.W.L.; Cho, C.-H. Nicotine induces cyclooxygenase-2 and vascular endothelial growth factor receptor-2 in association with tumor-associated invasion and angiogenesis in gastric cancer. *Mol. Cancer Res.* **2005**, *3*, 607–615. [CrossRef]
76. Lee, D.H.; Yang, Y.; Lee, S.J.; Kim, K.-Y.; Koo, T.H.; Shin, S.M.; Song, K.S.; Lee, Y.H.; Kim, Y.-J.; Lee, J.J.; et al. Macrophage inhibitory cytokine-1 induces the invasiveness of gastric cancer cells by up-regulating the urokinase-type plasminogen activator system. *Cancer Res.* **2003**, *63*, 4648–4655. [PubMed]
77. Li, P.-Y.; Lv, J.; Qi, W.-W.; Zhao, S.-F.; Sun, L.-B.; Liu, N.; Sheng, J.; Qiu, W.-S. Tspan9 inhibits the proliferation, migration and invasion of human gastric cancer SGC7901 cells via the ERK1/2 pathway. *Oncol. Rep.* **2016**, *36*, 448–454. [CrossRef]
78. Kyung Hee, L.; Eun Young, C.; Sung Ae, K.; Min Kyoung, K.; Kyeong Ok, K.; Si Hyung, L.; Byung Ik, J.; Se Won, K.; Sang Woon, K.; Sun Kyo, S.; et al. Down-regulation of survivin suppresses uro-plasminogen activator through transcription factor JunB. *Exp. Mol. Med.* **2011**, *43*, 501–509.
79. Liu, L.; Sun, L.; Zhao, P.; Yao, L.; Jin, H.; Liang, S.; Wang, Y.; Zhang, D.; Pang, Y.; Shi, Y.; et al. Hypoxia promotes metastasis in human gastric cancer by up-regulating the 67-kDa laminin receptor. *Cancer Sci.* **2010**, *101*, 1653–1660. [CrossRef]
80. Jin, H.; Pan, Y.; He, L.; Zhai, H.; Li, X.; Zhao, L.; Sun, L.; Liu, J.; Hong, L.; Song, J.; et al. p75 neurotrophin receptor inhibits invasion and metastasis of gastric cancer. *Mol. Cancer Res.* **2007**, *5*, 423–433. [CrossRef]
81. Hewin, D.F.; Savage, P.B.; Alderson, D.; Vipond, M.N. Plasminogen activators in oesophageal carcinoma. *Br. J. Surg.* **1996**, *83*, 1152–1155. [CrossRef]
82. Hourihan, R.N.; O'Sullivan, G.C.; Morgan, J.G. Transcriptional gene expression profiles of oesophageal adenocarcinoma and normal oesophageal tissues. *Anticancer Res.* **2003**, *23*, 161–165.
83. Gouri, A.; Dekaken, A.; El Bairi, K.; Aissaoui, A.; Laabed, N.; Chefrour, M.; Ciccolini, J.; Milano, G.; Benharkat, S. Plasminogen Activator System and Breast Cancer: Potential Role in Therapy Decision Making and Precision Medicine. *Biomark Insights* **2016**, *11*, 105–111. [CrossRef]
84. Umehara, Y.; Kimura, T.; Yoshida, M.; Oba, N.; Harada, Y. Relationship between plasminogen activators and stomach carcinoma stage. *Acta Oncol* **1991**, *30*, 815–818. [CrossRef] [PubMed]
85. Suh, Y.-S.; Yu, J.; Kim, B.C.; Choi, B.; Han, T.-S.; Ahn, H.S.; Kong, S.-H.; Lee, H.-J.; Kim, W.H.; Yang, H.-K. Overexpression of Plasminogen Activator Inhibitor-1 in Advanced Gastric Cancer with Aggressive Lymph Node Metastasis. *Cancer Res. Treat.* **2015**, *47*, 718–726. [CrossRef] [PubMed]
86. Maeda, K.; Chung, Y.; Sawada, T.; Ogawa, Y.; Onoda, N.; Nakata, B.; Kato, Y.; Sowa, M. Combined evaluation of urokinase-type plasminogen activator and plasminogen activator inhibitor-2 expression in gastric carcinoma. *Int. J. Oncol.* **1996**, *8*, 499–503. [CrossRef] [PubMed]

87. Nakamura, M.; Konno, H.; Tanaka, T.; Maruo, Y.; Nishino, N.; Aoki, K.; Baba, S.; Sakaguchi, S.; Takada, Y.; Takada, A. Possible role of plasminogen activator inhibitor 2 in the prevention of the metastasis of gastric cancer tissues. *Thromb. Res.* **1992**, *65*, 709–719. [CrossRef]
88. Ding, Y.; Zhang, H.; Zhong, M.; Zhou, Z.; Zhuang, Z.; Yin, H.; Wang, X.; Zhu, Z. Clinical significance of the uPA system in gastric cancer with peritoneal metastasis. *Eur. J. Med. Res.* **2013**, *18*, 28. [CrossRef] [PubMed]
89. Ding, Y.; Zhang, H.; Lu, A.; Zhou, Z.; Zhong, M.; Shen, D.; Wang, X.; Zhu, Z. Effect of urokinase-type plasminogen activator system in gastric cancer with peritoneal metastasis. *Oncol. Lett.* **2016**, *11*, 4208–4216. [CrossRef]
90. Nishioka, N.; Matsuoka, T.; Yashiro, M.; Hirakawa, K.; Olden, K.; Roberts, J.D. Plasminogen activator inhibitor 1 RNAi suppresses gastric cancer metastasis in vivo. *Cancer Sci.* **2012**, *103*, 228–232. [CrossRef]
91. Heiss, M.M.; Babic, R.; Allgayer, H.; Gruetzner, K.U.; Jauch, K.W.; Loehrs, U.; Schildberg, F.W. Tumor-associated proteolysis and prognosis: New functional risk factors in gastric cancer defined by the urokinase-type plasminogen activator system. *J. Clin. Oncol.* **1995**, *13*, 2084–2093. [CrossRef]
92. Brungs, D.; Lochhead, A.; Iyer, A.; Illemann, M.; Colligan, P.; Hirst, N.G.; Splitt, A.; Liauw, W.; Vine, K.L.; Pathmanandavel, S.; et al. Expression of cancer stem cell markers is prognostic in metastatic gastroesophageal adenocarcinoma. *Pathology* **2019**, *51*, 474–480. [CrossRef]
93. Plava, J.; Cihova, M.; Burikova, M.; Matuskova, M.; Kucerova, L.; Miklikova, S. Recent advances in understanding tumor stroma-mediated chemoresistance in breast cancer. *Mol. Cancer* **2019**, *18*, 67. [CrossRef] [PubMed]
94. Valkenburg, K.C.; de Groot, A.E.; Pienta, K.J. Targeting the tumour stroma to improve cancer therapy. *Nat. Rev. Clin. Oncol.* **2018**, *15*, 366–381. [CrossRef]
95. Bussard, K.M.; Mutkus, L.; Stumpf, K.; Gomez-Manzano, C.; Marini, F.C. Tumor-associated stromal cells as key contributors to the tumor microenvironment. *Breast Cancer Res.* **2016**, *18*, 84. [CrossRef] [PubMed]
96. Sounni, N.E.; Noel, A. Targeting the tumor microenvironment for cancer therapy. *Clin. Chem.* **2013**, *59*, 85–93. [CrossRef] [PubMed]
97. Gambardella, V.; Castillo, J.; Tarazona, N.; Gimeno-Valiente, F.; Martínez-Ciarpaglini, C.; Cabeza-Segura, M.; Roselló, S.; Roda, D.; Huerta, M.; Cervantes, A.; et al. The role of tumor-associated macrophages in gastric cancer development and their potential as a therapeutic target. *Cancer Treat. Rev.* **2020**, *86*, 102015. [CrossRef] [PubMed]
98. Nielsen, B.S.; Sehested, M.; Duun, S.; Rank, F.; Timshel, S.; Rygaard, J.; Johnsen, M.; Danø, K. Urokinase plasminogen activator is localized in stromal cells in ductal breast cancer. *Lab. Invest.* **2001**, *81*, 1485–1501. [CrossRef] [PubMed]
99. Pyke, C.; Graem, N.; Ralfkiaer, E.; Ronne, E.; Hoyerhansen, G.; Brunner, N.; Dano, K. Receptor for Urokinase Is Present in Tumor-Associated Macrophages in Ductal Breast-Carcinoma. *Cancer Res.* **1993**, *53*, 1911–1915.
100. Bianchi, E.; Cohen, R.L.; Thor, A.T.; Todd, R.F.; Mizukami, I.F.; Lawrence, D.A.; Ljung, B.M.; Shuman, M.A.; Smith, H.S. The urokinase receptor is expressed in invasive breast cancer but not in normal breast tissue. *Cancer Res.* **1994**, *54*, 861–866.
101. Bianchi, E.; Cohen, R.L.; Dai, A.; Thor, A.T.; Shuman, M.A.; Smith, H.S. Immunohistochemical localization of the plasminogen activator inhibitor-1 in breast cancer. *Int. J. Cancer* **1995**, *60*, 597–603. [CrossRef]
102. Costantini, V.; Sidoni, A.; Deveglia, R.; Cazzato, O.A.; Bellezza, G.; Ferri, I.; Bucciarelli, E.; Nenci, G.G. Combined overexpression of urokinase, urokinase receptor; plasminogen activator inhibitor-1 is associated with breast cancer progression-An immunohistochemical comparison of normal, benign; malignant breast tissues. *Cancer* **1996**, *77*, 1079–1088. [CrossRef]
103. Ohtani, H.; Pyke, C.; Dan Ø, K.; Nagura, H. Expression of urokinase receptor in various stromal-cell populations in human colon cancer: Immunoelectron microscopical analysis. *Int. J. Cancer* **1995**, *62*, 691–696. [CrossRef] [PubMed]
104. Pyke, C.; Kristensen, P.; Ralfkiaer, E.; Grondahlhansen, J.; Eriksen, J.; Blasi, F.; Dano, K. Urokinase-Type Plasminogen-Activator Is Expressed in Stromal Cells and Its Receptor in Cancer-Cells at Invasive Foci in Human Colon Adenocarcinomas. *Am. J. Pathol.* **1991**, *138*, 1059–1067.
105. Nakstad, B.; Lyberg, T. Immunohistochemical localization of coagulation, fibrinolytic and antifibrinolytic markers in adenocarcinoma of the lung. *APMIS* **1991**, *99*, 981–988. [CrossRef]
106. Noruzi, S.; Azizian, M.; Mohammadi, R.; Hosseini, S.A.; Rashidi, B.; Mohamadi, Y.; Nesaei, A.; Seiri, P.; Sahebkar, A.; Salarinia, R.; et al. Micro-RNAs as critical regulators of matrix metalloproteinases in cancer. *J. Cell Biochem.* **2018**, *119*, 8694–8712. [CrossRef] [PubMed]
107. Zhao, Z.S.; Wang, Y.Y.; Ye, Z.Y.; Tao, H.Q. Prognostic value of tumor-related molecular expression in gastric carcinoma. *Pathol. Oncol. Res.* **2009**, *15*, 589–596. [CrossRef]
108. Allgayer, H.; Babic, R.; Beyer, B.C.; Grützner, K.U.; Tarabichi, A.; Schildberg, F.W.; Heiss, M.M. Prognostic relevance of MMP-2 (72-kD collagenase IV) in gastric cancer. *Oncology* **1998**, *55*, 152–160. [CrossRef]
109. Ji, F.; Chen, Y.L.; Jin, E.Y.; Wang, W.L.; Yang, Z.L.; Li, Y.M. Relationship between matrix metalloproteinase-2 mRNA expression and clinicopathological and urokinase-type plasminogen activator system parameters and prognosis in human gastric cancer. *World J. Gastroenterol.* **2005**, *11*, 3222–3226. [CrossRef]
110. Mijanović, O.; Branković, A.; Panin, A.N.; Savchuk, S.; Timashev, P.; Ulasov, I.; Lesniak, M.S. Cathepsin B: A sellsword of cancer progression. *Cancer Lett.* **2019**, *449*, 207–214. [CrossRef]
111. Gondi, C.S.; Rao, J.S. Cathepsin B as a cancer target. *Expert Opin Ther Targets* **2013**, *17*, 281–291. [CrossRef]
112. Kobayashi, H.; Moniwa, N.; Sugimura, M.; Shinohara, H.; Ohi, H.; Terao, T. Effects of membrane-associated cathepsin B on the activation of receptor-bound prourokinase and subsequent invasion of reconstituted basement membranes. *Biochim. Biophys. Acta* **1993**, *1178*, 55–62. [CrossRef]

113. Herszényi, L.; István, G.; Cardin, R.; De Paoli, M.; Plebani, M.; Tulassay, Z.; Farinati, F. Serum cathepsin B and plasma urokinase-type plasminogen activator levels in gastrointestinal tract cancers. *Eur. J. Cancer Prev.* **2008**, *17*, 438–445. [CrossRef] [PubMed]
114. Kita, Y.; Fukagawa, T.; Mimori, K.; Kosaka, Y.; Ishikawa, K.; Aikou, T.; Natsugoe, S.; Sasako, M.; Mori, M. Expression of uPAR mRNA in peripheral blood is a favourite marker for metastasis in gastric cancer cases. *Br. J. Cancer* **2009**, *100*, 153–159. [CrossRef] [PubMed]
115. Vidal, Ó.; Metges, J.P.; Elizalde, I.; Valentíni, M.; Volant, A.; Molina, R.; Castells, A.; Pera, M. High preoperative serum vascular endothelial growth factor levels predict poor clinical outcome after curative resection of gastric cancer. *Br. J. Surg.* **2009**, *96*, 1443–1451. [CrossRef]
116. Rao, J.S.; Gujrati, M.; Chetty, C. Tumor-associated soluble uPAR-directed endothelial cell motility and tumor angiogenesis. *Oncogenesis* **2013**, *2*, e53. [CrossRef] [PubMed]
117. Rolff, H.C.; Christensen, I.J.; Svendsen, L.B.; Wilhelmsen, M.; Lund, I.K.; Thurison, T.; Høyer-Hansen, G.; Illemann, M.; Nielsen, H.J. The concentration of the cleaved suPAR forms in pre- and postoperative plasma samples improves the prediction of survival in colorectal cancer: A nationwide multicenter validation and discovery study. *J. Surg. Oncol.* **2019**, *120*, 1404–1411. [CrossRef]
118. Olingy, C.E.; Dinh, H.Q.; Hedrick, C.C. Monocyte heterogeneity and functions in cancer. *J. Leukoc. Biol.* **2019**, *106*, 309–322. [CrossRef] [PubMed]
119. Hodges, G.; Lyngbaek, S.; Selmer, C.; Ahlehoff, O.; Theilade, S.; Sehestedt, T.B.; Abildgaard, U.; Eugen-Olsen, J.; Galloe, A.M.; Hansen, P.R.; et al. SuPAR is associated with death and adverse cardiovascular outcomes in patients with suspected coronary artery disease. *Scand. Cardiovasc. J.* **2020**, *54*, 339–345. [CrossRef] [PubMed]
120. Hamie, L.; Daoud, G.; Nemer, G.; Nammour, T.; El Chediak, A.; Uthman, I.W.; Kibbi, A.G.; Eid, A.; Kurban, M. SuPAR, an emerging biomarker in kidney and inflammatory diseases. *Postgrad. Med. J.* **2018**, *94*, 517–524. [CrossRef]
121. Ho, C.H.; Chao, Y.; Lee, S.D.; Chau, W.K.; Wu, C.W.; Liu, S.M. Diagnostic and prognostic values of plasma levels of fibrinolytic markers in gastric cancer. *Thromb. Res.* **1998**, *91*, 23–27. [CrossRef]
122. Banys-Paluchowski, M.; Witzel, I.; Aktas, B.; Fasching, P.A.; Hartkopf, A.; Janni, W.; Kasimir-Bauer, S.; Pantel, K.; Schon, G.; Rack, B.; et al. The prognostic relevance of urokinase-type plasminogen activator (uPA) in the blood of patients with metastatic breast cancer. *Sci. Rep.* **2019**, *9*, 2318. [CrossRef]
123. Piironen, T.; Laursen, B.; Pass, J.; List, K.; Gårdsvoll, H.; Ploug, M.; Danø, K.; Høyer-Hansen, G. Specific Immunoassays for Detection of Intact and Cleaved Forms of the Urokinase Receptor. *Clin. Chem.* **2004**, *50*, 2059–2068. [CrossRef]
124. Loosen, S.H.; Tacke, F.; Binnebosel, M.; Leyh, C.; Vucur, M.; Heitkamp, F.; Schoening, W.; Ulmer, T.F.; Alizai, P.H.; Trautwein, C.; et al. Serum levels of soluble urokinase plasminogen activator receptor (suPAR) predict outcome after resection of colorectal liver metastases. *Oncotarget* **2018**, *9*, 27027–27038. [CrossRef]
125. Tang, Z.Z.; Sheng, H.Y.; Zheng, X.; Ying, L.S.; Wu, L.; Liu, D.; Liu, G. Upregulation of circulating cytokeratin 20, urokinase plasminogen activator and C-reactive protein is associated with poor prognosis in gastric cancer. *Mol. Clin. Oncol.* **2015**, *3*, 1213–1220. [CrossRef] [PubMed]
126. Zou, K.; Yang, S.; Zheng, L.; Wang, S.; Xiong, B. Prognostic Role of the Circulating Tumor Cells Detected by Cytological Methods in Gastric Cancer: A Meta-Analysis. *Biomed. Res. Int.* **2016**, *2016*, 2765464. [CrossRef] [PubMed]
127. Lee, M.W.; Kim, G.H.; Jeon, H.K.; Park, S.J. Clinical Application of Circulating Tumor Cells in Gastric Cancer. *Gut Liver* **2019**, *13*, 394–401. [CrossRef]
128. Po, J.W. *Importance and Detection of Epithelial-to-Mesenchymal Transition (EMT) Phenotype in CTCs, in Tumour Metastasis*; Xu, K., Ed.; IntechOpen: London, UK, 2016.
129. Jo, M.; Lester, R.D.; Montel, V.; Eastman, B.; Takimoto, S.; Gonias, S.L. Reversibility of epithelial-mesenchymal transition (EMT) induced in breast cancer cells by activation of urokinase receptor-dependent cell signaling. *J. Biol. Chem.* **2009**, *284*, 22825–22833. [CrossRef]
130. Brungs, D.; Lynch, D.; Luk, A.W.; Minaei, E.; Ranson, M.; Aghmesheh, M.; Vine, K.L.; Carolan, M.; Jaber, M.; de Souza, P.; et al. Cryopreservation for delayed circulating tumor cell isolation is a valid strategy for prognostic association of circulating tumor cells in gastroesophageal cancer. *World J. Gastroenterol.* **2018**, *24*, 810–818. [CrossRef] [PubMed]
131. Lin, H.; Xu, L.; Yu, S.; Hong, W.; Huang, M.; Xu, P. Therapeutics targeting the fibrinolytic system. *Exp. Mol. Med.* **2020**, *52*, 367–379. [CrossRef]
132. Yuan, C.; Guo, Z.; Yu, S.; Jiang, L.; Huang, M. Development of inhibitors for uPAR: Blocking the interaction of uPAR with its partners. *Drug Discov. Today* **2021**, *26*, 1076–1085. [CrossRef]
133. Belfiore, L.; Saunders, D.N.; Ranson, M.; Vine, K.L. N-Alkylisatin-Loaded Liposomes Target the Urokinase Plasminogen Activator System in Breast Cancer. *Pharmaceutics* **2020**, *12*, 641. [CrossRef]
134. Vine, K.L.; Lobov, S.; Indira Chandran, V.; Harris, N.L.; Ranson, M. Improved pharmacokinetic and biodistribution properties of the selective urokinase inhibitor PAI-2 (SerpinB2) by site-specific PEGylation: Implications for drug delivery. *Pharm. Res.* **2015**, *32*, 1045–1054. [CrossRef]
135. Vine, K.L.; Indira Chandran, V.; Locke, J.M.; Matesic, L.; Lee, J.; Skropeta, D.; Bremner, J.B.; Ranson, M. Targeting urokinase and the transferrin receptor with novel, anti-mitotic N-alkylisatin cytotoxin conjugates causes selective cancer cell death and reduces tumor growth. *Curr. Cancer Drug Targets* **2012**, *12*, 64–73. [CrossRef]

136. Stutchbury, T.K.; Al-Ejeh, F.; Stillfried, G.E.; Croucher, D.R.; Andrews, J.; Irving, D.; Links, M.; Ranson, M. Preclinical evaluation of 213Bi-labeled plasminogen activator inhibitor type 2 in an orthotopic murine xenogenic model of human breast carcinoma. *Mol. Cancer Ther.* **2007**, *6*, 203–212. [CrossRef]
137. Hang, M.T.N.; Ranson, M.; Saunders, D.N.; Liang, X.M.; Bunn, C.L.; Baker, M.S. Pharmacokinetics and biodistribution of recombinant human plasminogen activator inhibitor type 2 (PAI-2) in control and tumour xenograft-bearing mice. *Fibrinolysis Proteolysis* **1998**, *12*, 145–154. [CrossRef]
138. Buckley, B.J.; Aboelela, A.; Minaei, E.; Jiang, L.X.; Xu, Z.; Ali, U.; Fildes, K.; Cheung, C.Y.; Cook, S.M.; Johnson, D.C.; et al. 6-Substituted Hexamethylene Amiloride (HMA) Derivatives as Potent and Selective Inhibitors of the Human Urokinase Plasminogen Activator for Use in Cancer. *J. Med. Chem.* **2018**, *61*, 8299–8320. [CrossRef]
139. Buckley, B.J.; Majed, H.; Aboelela, A.; Minaei, E.; Jiang, L.; Fildes, K.; Cheung, C.Y.; Johnson, D.; Bachovchin, D.; Cook, G.M.; et al. 6-Substituted amiloride derivatives as inhibitors of the urokinase-type plasminogen activator for use in metastatic disease. *Bioorg. Med. Chem. Lett.* **2019**, *29*, 126753. [CrossRef] [PubMed]
140. Li, H.; Chen, C. Quercetin Has Antimetastatic Effects on Gastric Cancer Cells via the Interruption of uPA/uPAR Function by Modulating NF-κb, PKC-δ, ERK1/2; AMPKα. *Integr. Cancer Ther.* **2017**, *17*, 511–523. [CrossRef]
141. Ding, Y.; Zhang, H.; Zhou, Z.; Zhong, M.; Chen, Q.; Wang, X.; Zhu, Z. u-PA inhibitor amiloride suppresses peritoneal metastasis in gastric cancer. *World J. Surg. Oncol.* **2012**, *10*, 270. [CrossRef] [PubMed]
142. Heinemann, V.; Ebert, M.P.; Laubender, R.P.; Bevan, P.; Mala, C.; Boeck, S. Phase II randomised proof-of-concept study of the urokinase inhibitor upamostat (WX-671) in combination with gemcitabine compared with gemcitabine alone in patients with non-resectable, locally advanced pancreatic cancer. *Br. J. Cancer* **2013**, *108*, 766–770. [CrossRef] [PubMed]

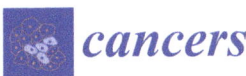

Systematic Review

Risk-Predictive and Diagnostic Biomarkers for Colorectal Cancer; a Systematic Review of Studies Using Pre-Diagnostic Blood Samples Collected in Prospective Cohorts and Screening Settings

Sophia Harlid [1], Marc J. Gunter [2] and Bethany Van Guelpen [1,3,*]

1. Department of Radiation Sciences, Oncology, Umeå University, 90187 Umeå, Sweden; sophia.harlid@umu.se
2. Nutrition and Metabolism Branch, International Agency for Research on Cancer, 69372 Lyon, France; gunterm@iarc.fr
3. Wallenberg Centre for Molecular Medicine, Umeå University, 90187 Umeå, Sweden
* Correspondence: bethany.vanguelpen@umu.se

Citation: Harlid, S.; Gunter, M.J.; Van Guelpen, B. Risk-Predictive and Diagnostic Biomarkers for Colorectal Cancer; a Systematic Review of Studies Using Pre-Diagnostic Blood Samples Collected in Prospective Cohorts and Screening Settings. *Cancers* 2021, *13*, 4406. https://doi.org/10.3390/cancers13174406

Academic Editor: Takaya Shimura

Received: 30 June 2021
Accepted: 25 August 2021
Published: 31 August 2021

Publisher's Note: MDPI stays neutral with regard to jurisdictional claims in published maps and institutional affiliations.

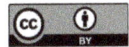

Copyright: © 2021 by the authors. Licensee MDPI, Basel, Switzerland. This article is an open access article distributed under the terms and conditions of the Creative Commons Attribution (CC BY) license (https://creativecommons.org/licenses/by/4.0/).

Simple Summary: Currently, colorectal cancer screening typically involves stool tests, but a blood test might be more acceptable for screening participants. Most research on blood biomarkers for colorectal cancer has been conducted using samples from patients and may not be as predictive for early-stage cancer or pre-cancerous tumors. This systematic review summarizes the evidence from studies that used samples collected before the onset of symptoms. The quality of the studies was generally high, but very few potential biomarkers showed consistent, clinically relevant results across more than one study. Of these, the anti-p53 antibody was the most promising marker. Panels of biomarkers performed better than single markers. The results of this review underscore the need for validation of promising colorectal cancer biomarkers in independent pre-diagnostic settings.

Abstract: This systematic review summarizes the evidence for blood-based colorectal cancer biomarkers from studies conducted in pre-diagnostic, asymptomatic settings. Of 1372 studies initially identified, the final selection included 30 studies from prospective cohorts and 23 studies from general screening settings. Overall, the investigations had high quality but considerable variability in data analysis and presentation of results, and few biomarkers demonstrated a clinically relevant discriminatory ability. One of the most promising biomarkers was the anti-p53 antibody, with consistent findings in one screening cohort and in the 3–4 years prior to diagnosis in two prospective cohort studies. Proteins were the most common type of biomarker assessed, particularly carcinoembryonic antigen (CEA) and C-reactive protein (CRP), with modest results. Other potentially promising biomarkers included proteins, such as AREG, MIC-1/GDF15, LRG1 and FGF-21, metabolites and/or metabolite profiles, non-coding RNAs and DNA methylation, as well as re-purposed routine lab tests, such as ferritin and the triglyceride–glucose index. Biomarker panels generally achieved higher discriminatory performance than single markers. In conclusion, this systematic review highlighted anti-p53 antibodies as a promising blood-based biomarker for use in colorectal cancer screening panels, together with other specific proteins. It also underscores the need for validation of promising biomarkers in independent pre-diagnostic settings.

Keywords: colorectal neoplasms; cancer screening tests; biomarkers; liquid biopsy; early detection of cancer; precision medicine

1. Introduction

Colorectal cancer is the second most common cancer in men and women globally [1], affecting roughly one in twenty people over the course of their lifetime. Largely a disease of older age, colorectal cancer incidence rates can be expected to rise as life expectancy increases in a population, but trends have been reversed in some countries, including the United States [2], largely due to the implementation of age-based general screening programs [3].

The gold standard for colorectal cancer screening is full colonoscopy. In addition to providing the best chance of detecting colorectal cancer through, ideally, inspection of the entire colorectal epithelium, colonoscopy has important advantages as a screening technique. In particular, diagnostic biopsies can be taken directly from tumors found, and many precancerous lesions can be removed. Screening colonoscopy is, therefore, a tool not only for early detection of asymptomatic colorectal cancer, but also for primary prevention. However, the implementation of colonoscopy for general screening is limited by several factors. The procedure is resource demanding, dependent on qualified personnel, uncomfortable for the patient and entails a small, but non-negligible, risk of complications such as bleeding or intestinal perforation. Achieving adequate uptake is a challenge, which is further hampered by inabilities to adequately capture all socioeconomic and ethnic groups [4].

Many countries have implemented fecal blood testing into colorectal cancer screening programs, using guaiac-based fecal occult blood tests (gFOBT) or, increasingly, quantitative fecal immunochemical tests (FIT). FIT can also be supplemented with a multitargeted tumor DNA test (FIT-DNA) that is approved for use in the United States [5]. Fecal blood testing is generally followed by sigmoidoscopy in patients with a positive result and sometime extended to full colonoscopy upon detection of polyps. Whereas full colonoscopy is effective at 10-year intervals, fecal testing is generally performed every one to three years. Moreover, limiting to sigmoidoscopy misses the roughly one third or more of colorectal cancer occurring in the proximal colon, which is more common at higher ages and in women [6,7].

In order to optimize colorectal cancer screening, there is a need for continued improvement of testing methods with respect to acceptability (i.e., less invasive tests), accessibility (i.e., lower costs and staffing demands) and performance. Blood-based biomarkers represent an enticing avenue toward achieving these goals. To date, one blood test, entailing measurement of methylated *Septin 9* gene (*mSEPT9*) in plasma, has been approved for colorectal cancer screening in some regions including the United States (in people who decline other screening methods). Although the discriminatory performance of *mSEPT9* is lower than for other screening methods currently in use [8,9], this may be compensated by an increased willingness of potential screening participants to undergo phlebotomy compared to stool testing or colonoscopy. The discriminatory ability of biomarkers is typically evaluated using measures such as sensitivity, specificity and receiver-operating characteristics (ROC) probability curves, in which the false positive rate is plotted on the x-axis against the true positive rate on the y-axis. The area under the ROC curve (AUC, or AUROC) ranges from 0.5, indicative of no power to separate cases from non-cases, to 1, indicative of perfect discrimination. To be clinically meaningful, biomarkers should have an AUC value as close to 1 as possible. There are no pre-defined performance thresholds for screening tests; the accuracy of novel biomarkers is generally evaluated in comparison with existing, approved tests. For FIT, the most recent systematic review from the US Preventive Services Task Force reported a pooled sensitivity of 0.74 for colorectal cancer and 0.23 for advanced adenoma, both with a specificity of approximately 0.95 [10], though the discriminatory performance varies depending on setting, test and cut-off.

Blood-based testing has several potential uses, not only as diagnostic biomarkers to help select people most likely to benefit from endoscopy and avoid unnecessary endoscopy in general screening programs, but also for risk stratification to help refine and individualize screening recommendations [11]. Risk-predictive biomarkers, in contrast to diagnostic biomarkers, would not necessarily indicate the presence of a tumor, but rather the risk of colorectal cancer over a longer time period. Such a test could be used, for example, at younger ages (e.g., 30–45 years, prior to the typical screening start at 50–60 years), to help decide when a person should enter a general screening program and perhaps what modality and frequency of screening would be most appropriate. Although colorectal cancer at ages under 50 years is rare, rates are increasing, especially for rectal cancer, and younger age groups are therefore an emerging target population for risk stratification and precision screening [12]. Risk-prediction algorithms using age, family history of cancer, genetic risk variants and lifestyle-related factors show some promise for colorectal cancer risk stratification [13–16], but have not achieved sufficient performance to guide precision screening. Novel blood-based biomarkers could, therefore, have clinical value for both risk prediction and diagnosis of colorectal cancer.

Research into blood-based biomarkers for colorectal cancer has expanded rapidly in recent years, as summarized in recent reviews [17,18]. The types of biomarkers assessed vary widely, and some of the most promising findings have been based on tumor DNA [19,20], either genetic or epigenetic. Other types of biomarkers, such as proteins, microRNA, antibodies and metabolites have also been reported to distinguish between colorectal cancer patients and controls. However, the bulk of research to date has used samples collected from patients diagnosed in clinical settings. Although such biomarkers could be very valuable for disease monitoring, their ability to detect colorectal cancer may not apply in the asymptomatic, pre-diagnostic period targeted by general screening. Studies conducted to identify and/or validate biomarkers in settings directly relevant for colorectal cancer screening, i.e., true screening settings or prospective cohorts, may be particularly valuable for the translation of findings from observational research to randomized trials and, ultimately, to clinical implementation.

The aim of this systematic review was to summarize the evidence for blood-based risk-predictive and diagnostic biomarkers of colorectal cancer identified in studies using pre-diagnostic samples from asymptomatic individuals, i.e., samples collected in prospective cohorts or general screening settings. Overall, few biomarkers demonstrated a clinically relevant discriminatory ability, especially with consistent results in more than one study. Proteins were the most common type of marker investigated, whereas markers including anti-p53 antibodies and DNA methylation at specific sites showed more consistent and stronger results, respectively. Multi-marker panels generally achieved higher discriminatory performance than single markers.

2. Materials and Methods
2.1. Eligibility Criteria

We included original, peer-reviewed, human studies presented in English and published in the past 10 years, i.e., between 1 January 2011 and 4 February 2021. Under these conditions, short reports, null results in brief and letters could be considered eligible, whereas pre-prints and conference abstracts were ineligible. The time period was chosen to balance a broad search intent with a manageable return of papers to assess for inclusion. In line with the intent of the review, only studies of blood-based biomarkers, analyzed in pre-diagnostic samples, i.e., collected in prospective cohorts or general screening settings, for the purpose of risk prediction or early diagnosis of colorectal cancer were considered eligible. Given the importance of precancerous lesions in colorectal cancer, studies including colorectal adenoma were included. Survival and therapeutic response outcomes were ineligible. We set a generous, arbitrary lower limit for sample size of 25 study subjects in at least one relevant endpoint group and in the comparison (control) group. Hereditary colorectal cancer, such as hereditary non-polyposis colorectal cancer or familial adenomatous polyposis, was an exclusion criterion, as were non-general screening settings including high-risk groups, such as familial cancer, inflammatory bowel disease and surveillance due to previous adenoma.

2.2. Information Sources

Searches were carried out in PubMed on 4 February 2021 and, with a modified search string, on 9 February 2021. Review articles, the reference lists of papers found in the searches, the article collections of the authors as well as post hoc searches of PubMed were used to identify additional studies not captured by the original search strings.

2.3. Search Strategy

The initial search string run was:

"(Marker OR Biomarker) AND (Serum OR Plasma OR Blood OR Circulating) AND (Diagnosis OR Screening OR "Early Detection of Cancer" [Mesh]) AND (Prospective OR "Prediagnostic" OR "prediagnostic" OR "Pre-diagnostic" OR "pre-diagnostic") AND (Colorectal OR Colon OR Rectal) AND (Cancer OR Adenocarcinoma OR Carcinoma OR Adenoma)".

In an informal quality check using the authors' collections, we found that the search string missed relevant papers lacking the prospective/pre-diagnostic term. Adding the word "screening" to the term resolved the issue, but returned a dramatically higher number of hits. Therefore, we used both search strings, but for the second string including the word "screening", we filtered the search to title and abstract only:

"(Marker [Title/Abstract] OR Biomarker [Title/Abstract]) AND (Serum [Title/Abstract] OR Plasma [Title/Abstract] OR Blood OR Circulating [Title/Abstract]) AND (Diagnosis [Title/Abstract] OR Screening [Title/Abstract] OR "Early Detection of Cancer" [Mesh]) AND (Screening [Title/Abstract] OR Prospective [Title/Abstract] OR "Prediagnostic" [Title/Abstract] OR "prediagnostic" [Title/Abstract] OR "Pre-diagnostic" [Title/Abstract] OR "pre-diagnostic" [Title/Abstract]) AND (Colorectal [Title/Abstract] OR Colon [Title/Abstract] OR Rectal [Title/Abstract]) AND (Cancer [Title/Abstract] OR Adenocarcinoma [Title/Abstract] OR Carcinoma [Title/Abstract] OR Adenoma [Title/Abstract])."

2.4. Selection Process

The study selection process is summarized in Figure 1. Two of the authors (S.H. and B.V.G.) perused all study titles independently of each other and marked clearly ineligible studies for exclusion, due to obviously wrong endpoint (e.g., wrong disease, response to therapy), obviously post-diagnostic samples, samples that were not blood or studies that were completely off topic. Articles with congruent exclusion decisions were excluded. Articles with incongruent assessments or congruent short-list assessments underwent abstract examination. The same two authors then read the abstracts of all remaining studies and provided comments on why a study should be excluded. Studies with incongruent abstract assessments were discussed, and in some cases, the methods section of the full paper was checked, and if agreement was not immediately reached, we erred on the side of shortlisting for examination of the full paper. All remaining papers were read in full by either S.H. or B.V.G., and papers with uncertainties were read by all authors to reach a consensus decision. Additional studies fulfilling the inclusion criteria were identified from reference lists, reviews, article collections of the authors and post hoc searches of PubMed.

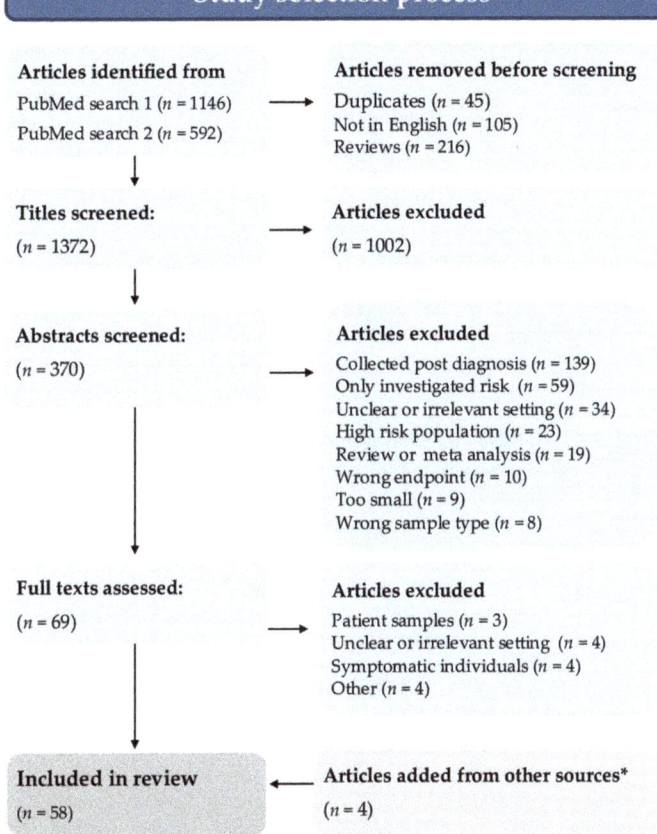

Figure 1. Flow diagram illustrating the selection of studies assessing blood-based risk-predictive and diagnostic biomarkers of colorectal cancer using pre-diagnostic samples from asymptomatic individuals, i.e., samples collected in prospective cohorts or general screening settings. During data extraction, an additional five studies were excluded due to lack of key information ($n = 1$), too small sample size ($n = 2$) or non-general screening population ($n = 2$). * Other sources included reference lists, review articles, the article collections of the authors and post hoc searches of PubMed.

2.5. Data Collection Process

For data extraction and presentation, studies were classified according to setting, either prospective cohort (hereafter sometimes referred to simply as prospective) or general screening, from which data were extracted by S.H. and B.V.G, respectively. Additionally, the extracted data for a random selection of approximately 10% of the studies from both settings were checked by M.G., with no corrections.

2.6. Data Items

Data on study design, numbers of study participants, sample medium, biomarker analyses and main findings were tabulated, separately for prospective cohort and screening studies. Effect measures extracted were limited to area under the receiver operating curve (AUC), sensitivity and specificity (highest specificity presented in the study) and estimates of risk (odds ratio (OR), hazard ratio (HR), relative risk (RR)). Results for colorectal cancer and advanced adenoma endpoints were prioritized in the summary of main findings. For studies including multiple data sets, e.g., discovery, internal validation and/or external validation, results were extracted only for data sets meeting the criteria for inclusion in the systematic review.

2.7. Quality Assessment

In order to provide an overview of study quality, we used the Newcastle–Ottawa Scale (NOS) for assessing the quality of non-randomized studies in meta-analyses [21], which we adapted for biomarker studies in prospective cohorts (including nested case-control studies) and screening settings. Categories and rating scales, i.e., maximum numbers of stars per category, were retained. In the case-control scale, high-quality record linkage or registry data for case definition were considered adequate. For ascertainment of exposure in both the case-control and cohort scales, we made an overall assessment of sample handling and analytical method quality. For the comparability of cases and controls, age was considered the most important factor, whereas other factors could include sex, follow-up time from sampling to diagnosis, lifestyle factors, etc. The systematic review was registered in PROSPERO (registration number CRD42021236073), including a brief presentation of the review process.

3. Results and Interpretation

3.1. Study Selection

Searches yielded 1146 and 592 hits for search string 1 and 2, respectively. After exclusions for duplicates, articles not in English and review articles, 1372 articles remained. Based on a generous assessment of their titles (excluding only articles that were deemed clearly irrelevant by both S.H. and B.V.G.), 370 were selected for abstract screening. Among the screened abstracts, 69 were selected for full article assessment. The most common reason for excluding an abstract was the use of post-diagnostic blood samples (n = 139). In addition, several studies used an approach focused on risk and etiology, with no clear intent to identify or validate biomarkers from the perspective of risk prediction or early detection (n = 59) or had an unclear or irrelevant study setting (n = 34), which was confirmed by a specific check of the methods section of the full paper when the independent author assessments were incongruent. Interrater congruence was 84% at the title stage and 88% at the abstract stage. Four additional articles were identified from other sources, including reference lists, reviews, the article collections of the authors and post hoc searches of PubMed, for a total of 58 studies selected for data extraction (Figure 1).

3.2. Study Characteristics

We identified 31 studies conducted in a prospective cohort setting, of which one was excluded due to lack of key information (number of cases and outcome measure) [22]. Of the remaining 30 studies fulfilling the inclusion criteria, one [23] investigated adenoma and the remainder colorectal cancer. The majority of the prospective studies (n = 23) utilized a nested case-control design, and a few used a cohort or case-cohort design. The number of cases ranged from 32 to 4210 cases, rarely more than 500.

A total of 27 studies included data potentially stemming from a general screening setting, of which four were excluded due to small sample size or non-general screening [24–27]. Of the remaining 23 studies, 17 presented results for colorectal cancer, and 15 presented results for advanced adenoma. Case-control design was most common, of which six studies used matched controls and the remainder unmatched. Two studies used a cohort design. The number of colorectal cancer cases ranged from 25 to 59, and the number of advanced adenoma cases ranged from 37 to 420, generally fewer than 150. Half of the screening studies were based on the BliTz (Begleitende Evaluierung innovativer Testverfahren zur Darmkrebsfrüherkennung) study, a well-characterized cohort in southern Germany.

For both the prospective and screening studies, plasma or serum were the most common sample media. A few studies used other media such as extracted nucleic acids or circulating white blood cells. Most prospective studies reported either OR, AUC or both, whereas in the screening studies AUC, sensitivity and specificity were most common.

The quality of the studies included in the review was evaluated using an adaptation of the NOS score. All studies scored high, in part because studies with a weak design, or performed in an unclear setting, were excluded at an earlier stage of the article selection process. Some studies received a lower score on selection due to lack of information on how the cases were ascertained, what the matching factors were and, for the prospective cohort studies, whether the controls were free from cancer at the start of the study.

3.3. Biomarkers

3.3.1. Proteins

Protein markers represented the most common target in both the prospective cohort-based studies (11 of 30 selected studies) and in the screening studies (11 of 23 selected studies) (Table 1). The most frequently evaluated protein was carcinoembryonic antigen (CEA), which was included in six studies [28–33]. CEA is a known marker of colorectal cancer progression, used for surveillance of colorectal cancer patients [34]. As a single marker, CEA performed modestly well when colorectal cancer was the outcome, with AUCs ranging from 0.59 in samples collected prospectively between 3–4 years before diagnosis [31] to 0.63 for samples collected in a screening setting [30]. It performed best when included in multi-marker panels; for example, CEA combined with p53 auto antibodies yielded an AUC of 0.85 for colorectal cancer from samples collected in a screening setting [33]. However, for detecting adenomas, the highest reported AUC for panels including CEA was 0.56, which indicates that it does not have sufficient discriminatory ability to be useful for early detection or risk stratification.

Other proteins identified as potentially promising colorectal cancer biomarkers were proteins known to be either directly involved in or strongly associated with inflammation. They included C-reactive protein (CRP) (five studies [23,30,35–37]), macrophage chemoattractant protein-1 (MCP-1) (two studies [36,38]), interleukin-6 (IL-6) (two studies [23,28]), macrophage inhibitory cytokine 1, also known as growth differentiation factor 15, (MIC-1/GDF15) (three studies, [23,28,39]), amphiregulin (AREG) (three studies [28,39,40]) and Leucine-rich alpha-2-glycoprotein-1 (LRG1) (two studies [29,41]). The inflammatory protein included in most studies was CRP, a common marker of acute inflammation [42]. However, CRP failed to reach the top markers in two of the five studies that included it [23,36]; did not detect advanced adenoma in Tao et al., with an AUC of 0.5 [37]; and performed only modestly as an early detection biomarker in the remaining two studies, with an AUC of 0.64 for advanced adenoma in Lim et al. [30], and a combined AUC (CRP+SAA) of 0.62 for colorectal cancer in Toriola et al. [35].

Of the remaining inflammatory proteins, those that showed the strongest potential as future colorectal cancer biomarkers were AREG, LRG1 and potentially MIC-1/GDF15. AREG performed well on its own, with an AUC consistently above 0.6 [28,39,40]. When included in a multi-marker panel (that also included MIC-1/GDF15), the AUC was above 0.8 for colorectal cancer and reached 0.6 for advanced adenomas in two of the three studies [39,40]. However, AREG was evaluated as part of three screening studies that all stemmed from the BliTz screening trial. Therefore, before any general conclusions can be drawn about its performance, it would need to be evaluated in samples collected in an independent setting.

LRG1, on the other hand, was included as a marker in one prospective study based on samples from the Women's Health Initiative (WHI) cohort [29], and in a screening study from 2020 [41]. In the case-control setting, using samples collected at least 3 months before colorectal cancer diagnosis, a panel containing LRG1 reached an AUC of 0.72. In the screening setting, a multi-marker panel containing HP, LRG1 and PON3 had an AUC of 0.65 for detection of advanced adenomas and another panel, optimized for detecting colorectal cancer, reached an AUC of 0.79.

MIC-1/GDF15 was evaluated as part of several larger panels without reaching the top-ranked markers. It was included as a separate marker for adenomas in Song et al. [23], where it performed reasonably well with an OR of 1.55 (95% CI: 1.03–2.32), AUC not shown. It is noteworthy that MIC-1/GDF15 had also been favorably evaluated in a study of recurrent adenoma, not included in the systematic review selection [43].

Some studies assessed candidate protein biomarkers that have shown promise in clinical colonoscopy settings. One such example is CYFRA 21-1 (cytokeratin 19 fragment) [44–46], which showed an AUC of 0.73 for detecting advanced adenomas in a general cancer screening setting [30]. CYFRA 21-1 was also selected for inclusion in at least one multi-marker panel tested in a screening setting [32], whereas in a prospective cohort setting, it was deemed unsuitable as a screening marker [31].

Several studies used a proteomics approach, measuring large panels of proteins in their first phases (sometimes a clinical or patient setting) and typically proceeding with validation of top hits. For example, one prospective study [47] nested within the North Sweden Health and Disease Study and five studies from the BliTz screening cohort [28,38–40,48] used Proseek Multiplex immunoassays (Olink Proteomics, Uppsala, Sweden), though most top hits differed. Many of the highest ranked proteins were only included in one study, making it difficult to assess reproducibility. One notable exception was fibroblast growth factor 21 (FGF-21), elevated levels of which were associated with a higher risk of colorectal cancer in the Swedish study, in which both the discovery and validation phases used prediagnostic samples [47], and in the BliTz validation set [48]. However, the discriminatory ability of FGF 21-1 in both studies was insufficient for clinical implementation.

Table 1. Studies of inflammatory markers and other proteins, sometimes supplemented by antibodies, analyzed in pre-diagnostic blood samples (collected in prospective cohort or general screening settings) for the purpose of risk prediction or early diagnosis of colorectal cancer.

Reference	Cohort (Design)	Time from Sampling to Diagnosis (Cohort Setting Only)	CRC	Adenoma	Contr./Cohort	Biomarker/Platform	Main Findings	Adapted NOS Scale ** Max: Selection = ★★★★ Comp. = ★★ Exp./Outc. = ★★★
				Cohort setting				
Ladd et al. Cancer Prev. Res, 2012 [29]	WHI (Nested case control)	245 days (mean) 109 days (mean)	90 32	– –	90 * 32 *	Proteomics (MS): (1) 5022 unique protein IDs (2) 1779 quantified (3) 6 significant ($p < 0.05$)	Top markers: MAPRE1, LRG1, IGFBP2, Enolase 1, ARMET, PDIA3 Panel: MAPRE1, LRG1, IGFBP2 + CEA Validation set (4 marker panel): AUC: 0.72 Sensitivity: 41% Specificity: 95%	★★★ ★★★ ★★★
Touvier et al. World J Gastroentero, 2012 [36]	SUVIMAX (Nested case control)	6.5 years (median)	50	–	100 *	Proteins: hs-CRP, Adiponectin, Leptin, sVCAM-1, sICAM-1, sE-selectin, MCP-1	Top markers: Adiponectin Panel: Adiponectin, sVCAM Adiponectin: OR: 0.45 (95% CI: 0.22–0.91. $p = 0.03$) Panel (Adiponectin, sVCAM): AUC: 0.98	★★★ ★★★ ★★★
Toriola et al. Int J Cancer, 2013 [35]	WHI (Nested case control)	3 years (cutoff, follow up)	988	–	988 *	CRP, SAA	CRP (5th vs. 1st quintile, colon) OR: 1.37 (95% CI: 0.95–1.97) SAA (5th vs. 1st quintile, colon) OR: 1.26 (95% CI: 0.88–1.80) AUC (Both): 0.62 (95% CI: 0.55–0.68)	★★★ ★★ ★★★
Thomas et al. Brit J Cancer, 2015 [31]	UKCTOCS (Nested case control)	4 years (cutoff, serial samples)	40	–	40 *	CEA, CYFRA21-1, CA12	Top marker: CEA All stages AUC (CEA): 0–1 year before diagnosis: 0.74 1–2 years before diagnosis: 0.64 2–3 years before diagnosis: 0.61 3–4 years before diagnosis: 0.59	★★★★ ★★ ★★★

Table 1. *Cont.*

Reference	Cohort (Design)	Time from Sampling to Diagnosis (Cohort Setting Only)	CRC	Adenoma	Contr./Cohort	Biomarker/Platform	Main Findings	Adapted NOS Scale ** Max: Selection = ★★★★ Comp. = ★★ Exp./Outc. = ★★★
Bertuzzi et al. BMC Cancer, 2015 [49]	EPIC-FLORENCE (Nested case control)	3 years (mean)	48	-	48 *	Global proteome analysis (phase 1 + 2) Targeted proteome analysis (phase 3): APOC2, CLU, CO4-B, CO9, FETUA, MASP2, MBL2, GRP2	CLU (men only) AUC: 0.72 Sensitivity: 95% Specificity: 75%	★★★ ★★ ★★★
Song et al. Cancer Prev Res, 2016 [23]	NHS (Nested case control)	10 years (median)	757	-	757 *	MIC-1, CRP, IL-6, sTNFR-2	MIC-1: (5th vs. 1st quintile) OR: 1.55 (95% CI: 1.03–2.32)	★★★★ ★★ ★★★
Shao et al. Cancer Epidemiol Biomarkers Prev, 2017 [50]	AFHSC/DoDSR (Nested case control)	8 years (cutoff, serial samples)	397	-	397 *	Proteomics (MALDI-TOF MS)	Proteomic peaks: 2886.67, 2939.24, 3119.32, and 5078.81 The 4 peaks associated with CRC 1 year before diagnosis. Sensitivity: 69% Specificity: 67%	★★★★ ★★ ★★★
Song et al. Int. J Cancer, 2018 [51]	JPHC (Case-cohort)	9.5 years (median)	457	-	751	67 inflammatory and immunity markers	Top markers: CCL2/MCP1, CCL3/MIP1A, CCL15/MIP1D, CCL27/CTACK, CXCL6/GCP2, sTNFR2 HR (4th vs. 1st quartile) CCL2/MCP1: 1.69 sTNFR2: 1.61 CCL15/MIP1D: 1.39 CCL27/CTACK: 1.35 CXCL6/GCP2: 0.70 CCL3/MIP1A: 0.61 Significance lost after adjustments	★★★★ ★★ ★★★

Table 1. Cont.

Reference	Cohort (Design)	Time from Sampling to Diagnosis (Cohort Setting Only)	CRC/Adenoma	Contr. Cohort	Biomarker/Platform	Main Findings	Adapted NOS Scale ** Max: Selection = ★★★★ Comp. = ★★ Exp./Outc. = ★★★
Rho et al. Gut 2018 [52]	CHS (Nested case control)	0–1 years (31 cases) 1–3 years (35 cases)	79	–	79 *	Discovery: 1100 markers Pre validation: 78 markers	Final panel: BAG4, IL6ST, VWF, EGFR, CD44 Panel, all cancers versus all controls: AUC: 0.86 Sensitivity: 73% Specificity: 90%	★★★ ★★★
Harlid et al. Sci Rep, 2021 [47]	NSHDS (Nested case control)	0.7 years (median) 6.7 years (median)	58 450	–	58 * 450 *	Olink proteomic panels (Inflammation and Oncology II)	Top markers: FGF-21, PPY FGF-21, colon OR: 1.23 95% CI 1.03–1.47 6 marker panel, colon AUC: 0.63 PPY, rectum OR: 1.47 95% CI 1.12–1.9 AUC: 0.61	★★★★ ★★ ★★★

Screening setting

Reference	Cohort (Design)	Time from Sampling to Diagnosis (Cohort Setting Only)	CRC/Adenoma	Contr. Cohort	Biomarker/Platform	Main Findings	Adapted NOS Scale **
Chen H et al. Clin Cancer Res, 2015 [28]	BliTz (discovery set)	–	35	–	54	PEA (Olink Oncology I), 92 proteins	Top markers: (AUC > 6): AREG, CEA, GDF-15, IL-6 Multi-marker (8 proteins): AUC 0.76 (0.65–0.85), sensitivity 44% at 90% specificity	★★★★ – ★★★
Wen Y-H et al. Clin Chim Acta, 2015 [32]	General health screening at patient's expense, Taoyuan, Taiwan	–	26	–	See footnote ***	AFP, CA 15-3, CA 125, PSA, SCC, CEA, CA 19-9, CYFRA 21-1	Top markers: CEA, sensitivity 53.8%, CYFRA 21-1 sensitivity 38.9 Multi-marker panel (all 8 markers): sensitivity 76.9%	★★★★ – ★★★
Tao S, et al. Br J. Cancer, 2015 [37]	BliTz	–	AA: 193	–	225	CRP, sCD26, complement C3a anaphylatoxin, TIMP-1	CRP: AUC 0.50 (0.45–0.55) C3a: AUC 0.52 (0.47–0.57) sCD26: AUC 0.54 (0.49–0.59) TIMP-1: AUC 0.58 (0.53–0.63)	★★★★ ★ ★★★

Table 1. Cont.

Reference	Cohort (Design)	Time from Sampling to Diagnosis (Cohort Setting Only)	CRC	Adenoma	Contr/Cohort	Biomarker/Platform	Main Findings	Adapted NOS Scale ** Max: Selection = ★★★★ Comp. = ★★ Exp./Outc. = ★★★
Werner S, et al. Clin Cancer Res, 2016 [33]	BliTz (validation study)	-	36	AA: 420	1200	CEA, ferritin, seprase, osteopontin, anti-p53 antibody ****	5-marker panel, CRC: AUC 0.78 (0.68–0.87), sensitivity 42% (26–59) at 95% specificity 5-marker panel, AA: AUC 0.56 (0.53–0.59), sensitivity 9% (6–12) at 95% specificity CEA+anti-p53, CRC: AUC 0.85 (0.78–0.91), sensitivity 45% at 95% specificity CEA+anti-p53, AA: AUC 0.56 (0.53–0.59), sensitivity 6% at 95% specificity	★★★★ - ★★★
Butt J et al. Int J Cancer, 2017 [53]	BliTz	-	50	AA: 100 NAA: 30	228	Multiplex serology (11 proteins) for *Streptococcus gallolyticus* subsp. *gallolyticus* Tested: individual proteins, any protein, ≥2 of 6-protein panel, Gallo2178-Gallo217 double-positivity	CRC: Gallo2178: OR 3.19 (1.11–9.21) AA: Gallo0933: OR 2.02 (CI: 1.01–4.04)	★★★★ ★★ ★★★

Table 1. Cont.

Reference	Cohort (Design)	Time from Sampling to Diagnosis (Cohort Setting Only)	CRC	Adenoma	Contr./Cohort	Biomarker/Platform	Main Findings	Adapted NOS Scale ** Max: Selection = ★★★★ Comp. = ★★ Exp./Outc. = ★★★
Chen H et al. Clin Epidemiol, 2017 [39]	BliTz (validation set)	-	41	AA: 106	107	PEA (Olink Oncology I v.2, 92 proteins) and serum p53 antibodies	Top markers, CRC: 12 proteins in both discovery and validation sets using Wilcoxon (10 with AUC > 6) Multi-marker (GDF-15, AREG, FasL, Flt3L), CRC: AUC 0.81 (0.73–0.88), sensitivity 53.6% at 90% specificity, AA: AUC 0.58 (0.51–0.65), sensitivity 18.9 at 90% specificity Multi-marker + p53, CRC: AUC 0.82 (0.74–0.90), sensitivity 56.4 at 90% specificity, AA: 0.60 (0.52–0.69), sens. 22.0 at 90% specificity	★★★★ ★★ ★★★
Qian J et al. Br J Cancer 2018 [48]	BliTz (validation set)	-	45	AA: 80 NAA: 72	250 *	PEA (Olink Inflammation I, 92 proteins)	FGF-21, CRC: AUC 0.71 (0.61–0.81), sensitivity 37.1% at 90% specificity, OR highest vs. lowest tertile 3.92 (1.51–12.18) FGF-21, AA: 0.57 (0.50–0.63), sensitivity 11.1% at 90% specificity, OR highest vs. lowest tertile 2.24 (1.18–4.44)	★★★★ ★★ ★★★

Table 1. Cont.

Reference	Cohort (Design)	Time from Sampling to Diagnosis (Cohort Setting Only)	CRC	Adenoma	Contr./Cohort	Biomarker/ Platform	Main Findings	Adapted NOS Scale ** Max: Selection = ★★★★ Comp. = ★★ Exp./Outc. = ★★★
Qian et al. J Clin Epidemiol, 2018 [38]	BliTz (validation set)	-	42	-	84 *	PEA (Olink Inflammation I, 92 proteins)	Individual proteins: AUC > 6 for 13 proteins, of which 5 overlapped with discovery set results. Sensitivity >25% at 90% specificity for 5 proteins, of which one overlapped with discovery results. 5-protein panel (FGF-23, CSF-1, Flt3L, DNER, MCP-1): AUC 0.59 (0.47–0.70), sensitivity 28.6% and 11.9% at 90% and 95% specificity, respectively	★★★★ ★★ ★★★
Lim DH, et al. J Clin Lab Anal, 2018 [30]	Screening patients, Cheonan, South Korea	-	-	AA: 59 NAA: 232	223	CYFRA 21-1, CEA, CA19-9, AFP, hsCRP	Top markers, AA: CYFRA 21-1: AUC 0.732 (0.656–0.809), sensitivity 30.5%, CEA: AUC 0.628 (0.542–0.714) sensitivity 11.8%, hsCRP: AUC 0.637 (0.559–0.715), sensitivity not presented	★★★ - ★★
Bhardwaj M et al. Cancers, 2019 [40]	BliTz (validation set)	-	56	AA: 101	102 *	PEA. Tested 12 overlapping proteins from LC/MRM-MS and PEA (Olink Oncology II, Immune response and Cardiovascular III): CDH5, Gal, IGFBP2, MASP1, MMP9, MPO, OPN, PON3, PRTN3, SPARC, TFRC (TR), AREG	Top markers, CRC (AUC > 6): CDH5, OPN, TR, AREG Multi-marker, CRC (MASP1, OPN, PON3, TR, AREG): AUC 0.82 (0.74–0.89), sensitivity 50% at 90% specificity Multi-marker, AA (MASP1, OPN, PON3, TR, AREG): AUC 0.60 (0.51–0.69)	★★★★ ★★ ★★★

Table 1. Cont.

Reference	Cohort (Design)	Time from Sampling to Diagnosis (Cohort Setting Only)	CRC	Adenoma	Contr./Cohort	Biomarker/ Platform	Main Findings	Adapted NOS Scale ** Max: Selection = ★★★★ Comp. = ★★ Exp./Outc. = ★★★
Bhardwaj M et al. Eur J Cancer, 2020 [41]	BliTz (validation set)	-	56	AA: 99	99 *	LC/MRM-MS, 270 proteins	Individual markers, CRC (44 proteins): AUC range 0.53 (0.44–0.63) to 0.77 (0.69–0.84) Multi-marker, CRC (A1AT, APOA1, HP, LRG1, PON3): AUC 0.79 (0.70–0.86), sensitivity 46% at 90% specificity Multi-marker, AA (early-stage CRC panel: HP, LRG1, PON3): AUC 0.65 (0.56–0.73), sensitivity 25% at 90% specificity	★★★★ ★★ ★★★
Li B, et al. Cancer Biomarkers, 2020 [54]	Health exam project, not otherwise specified, Jiangsu, China	-	50	AA: 50	150 *	Netrin-1	CRC: OR highest vs. lowest (optimal cut-off) = 7.731 (3.618–16.519), AUC 0.759 (0.680–0.837), sensitivity 46% at 90% specificity AA: null	★★ ★★ ★★★

Abbreviations (not including biomarker names, for which the reader is referred to the original study article): **AA**, Advanced Adenoma; **AFHSC**, Armed Forces Health Surveillance Center; **AUC**, Area Under the Curve: **BliTz**, Begleitende Evaluierung innovativer Testverfahren zur Darmkrebs-Früherkennun, Germany; **CHS**, Cardiovascular Health Study; **CRC**, Colorectal Cancer; **DoDSR**, Department of Defense Serum Repository; **EPIC**, European Prospective Investigation into Cancer and Nutrition; **HR**, Hazard Ratio: **JPHC**, Japan Public Health Center-based Prospective Study; **LC/MRM-MS**, liquid chromatography/multiple reaction monitoring-mass spectrometry; **MS**, Mass Spectrometry; **NAA**, non-advanced adenoma; **NHS**, Nurses' Health Study; **NSHDS**, North Sweden Health and Disease Study; **OR**, odds ratio; **PEA**, proximity extension assay; **SUVIMAX**, Supplémentation en Vitamines et Minéraux AntioXydants; **SWHS**, Shanghai Women's Health Study; **UKCTOCS**, UK Collaborative Trial of Ovarian Cancer Screening; **WHI**, Women's Health Initiative. * Matched controls. ** Newcastle-Ottawa Quality Assessment Scale for case-control studies, adapted for use for assessment of biomarker studies conducted in a screening setting. For case-control studies: selection (max 4 stars), comparability (max 2 stars), exposure (max 3 stars). For cohort studies: selection (max 4 stars), comparability (max 2 stars), outcome (max 3 stars). *** Cohort design, total $n = 41,516$, NOS assessment using the cohort scale. **** CYFRA 21-1 from the original panel was described in the statistics section as having been found to be "dispensable" in an extra colorectal cancer enriched re-optimization study and it was therefore not included in further analyses.

3.3.2. Metabolites

The metabolome was evaluated in four of the cohort-based studies [55–58] and one of the screening studies [59] included in this review (Table 2). Methods and materials differed between studies and included both liquid and gas chromatography, as well as both plasma and serum samples. One of the earlier prospective studies used a combination of methods to measure 676 metabolites in serum samples from 254 case-control pairs collected at a median of approximately 8 years prior to diagnosis [55]. Of 447 metabolites successfully identified, none were significantly associated with colorectal cancer risk. In contrast, an AUC of 0.81 was reported for a panel of 14 metabolites identified in serum by gas chromatography in a study of 31 advanced adenoma patients and 254 healthy controls from a screening program, using an approach with a training and test set [59].

A prospective study based on samples from two Shanghai cohorts, the Shanghai Women's Health Study (SWHS) and the Shanghai Men's Health Study (SMHS), identified metabolites using both Gas Chromatography-Time of Flight Mass Spectrometry (GC-TOFMS) and Ultra-performance Liquid Chromatography and Quadrupole Time-of-flight Tandem Mass Spectrometry (UPLC-QTOFMS) for global metabolic profiling of plasma samples from 250 case-control pairs [58]. In that study, 35 metabolites were significantly associated with colorectal cancer, nine of which retained significance after multivariable adjustments. A panel containing the top nine produced an AUC of 0.76.

The two remaining metabolomics studies both used samples collected as part of the EPIC cohort. One was a case-cohort study from EPIC-Heidelberg [56], and the other was a nested case-control study with samples from EPIC-Turin [57]. The EPIC-Heidelberg study, which included 163 colorectal cancer cases and a subcohort of 774 participants [56], analyzed levels of 120 metabolites in plasma, of which one (lysophosphatidylcholine 18:0) was inversely associated, and another (phosphatidylcholine PC ae C30:0) was positively associated, with colorectal cancer risk. Both metabolic markers may be more likely to function as risk factors rather than early disease biomarkers. The study from EPIC-Turin analyzed serum from 66 case-control pairs [57], using an untargeted metabolomics approach focused on lipophilic molecules, and identified nine features that they deemed to be of further future interest.

Important to note is that although some metabolomics studies yielded high enough AUCs to be clinically useful, there is a lack of replication of individual metabolites. Until more studies evaluating the same targets are produced, metabolomic markers are more likely to contribute to the understanding of colorectal cancer etiology, rather than be used as biomarkers for risk prediction and early diagnosis.

Table 2. Studies of metabolites analyzed in pre-diagnostic blood samples (collected in prospective cohort or general screening settings) for the purpose of risk prediction or early diagnosis of colorectal cancer.

Reference	Cohort (Design)	Time from Sampling to Diagnosis (Cohort Setting Only)	CRC	Adenoma	Contr./Cohort	Biomarker/Platform	Main Findings	Adapted NOS Scale ** Max: Selection = ★★★★ Comp. = ★★ Exp./Outc. = ★★★
Cohort setting								
Kühn et al. BMC Med, 2016 [56]	EPIC-HEIDELBERG (Case-cohort)	6.6 years (median)	163	-	774	120 metabolites: (acylcarnitines, amino acids, biogenic amines, phosphatidyl-cholines, sphingolipids, and hexoses)	Top markers: LysoPC a C18:0, PC ae C30:0 LysoPC a C18:0 (4th vs. 1st quartile) OR: 1.84 (95% CI: 1.02–3.34) PC ae C30:0 (4th vs. 1st quartile) OR: 0.50 (95% CI: 0.28–0.90)	★★★ ★★ ★★★
Shu et al. Int J Cancer, 2018 [58]	SWHS/SMHS (Nested case control)	Time stratification: <4 years and >4 years	250	-	250 *	Metabolites in plasma: 35 metabolites associated with CRC at FDR-p < 0.05	Top 9 panel: AUC: 0.76 Top 2 single metabolites: Picolinic acid: OR: 5.11 (95% CI: 2.33–11.20) PE(20:0/18:2): OR: 0.45 (95% CI: 0.29–0.70)	★★★★ ★★ ★★★
Cross et al. Cancer, 2014 [55]	PLCO (Nested case control)	7.8 years (median)	254	-	254 *	676 serum metabolites (metabolon)	Leucyl-leucine (90th vs. 10th percentile) OR: 0.50 (95% CI: 0.32–0.80) Glycochenodeoxycholate (90th vs. 10th percentile, sex stratified) OR: 5.34 (95% CI: 2.09–13.68) Significance lost after adjustments	★★★★ ★★ ★★★
Perttula et al. BMC Cancer, 2018 [57]	EPIC-TURIN (Nested case control)	7.5 years (median)	66	-	66 *	Lipophilic metabolites incl. (ULCFAs): 8690 features, 9 selected	Top markers: IDs: 5080, 3207, 6054 and 839 Classification rate: 72%	★★ ★★ ★★★

Table 2. *Cont.*

Reference	Cohort (Design)	Time from Sampling to Diagnosis (Cohort Setting Only)	CRC	Adenoma	Contr./Cohort	Biomarker/Platform	Main Findings	Adapted NOS Scale ** Max: Selection = ★★★★ Comp. = ★★ Exp./Outc. = ★★★
Screening setting								
Farshidfar F et al. Br J Cancer, 2016 [59]	Screening patients, Calgary, Canada (discovery)	-	-	A: 31	254	GC-MS untargeted metabolomics	Multi-marker profile: (14 metabolites): AUC 0.81 (0.70–0.92)	★★★ ★★ ★★★

Abbreviations (not including biomarker names, for which the reader is referred to the original study article): **CI**, confidence interval; **CRC**, colorectal cancer; **EPIC**, European Prospective Investigation into Cancer and Nutrition; **GC-MS**, gas chromatography–mass spectrometry; **OR**, odds ratio; **PLCO**, Prostate, Lung, Colorectal, and Ovarian cancer screening trial; **SMHS**, Shanghai Men's Health Study; **SWHS**, Shanghai Women's Health Study. * Matched controls. ** Newcastle–Ottawa Quality Assessment Scale for case-control studies, adapted for use for assessment of biomarker studies conducted in a screening setting. For case-control studies: selection (max 4 stars), comparability (max 2 stars), exposure (max 3 stars). For cohort studies: selection (max 4 stars), comparability (max 2 stars), outcome (max 3 stars).

3.3.3. Antibodies

Among the studies selected for this review, seven included evaluations of antibodies [33,39,60–64], five evaluated antibodies only (listed in Table 3) and two evaluated combinations of protein panels and antibodies (listed in Table 1). A majority of the studies analyzed auto-antibodies to p53. Antibodies towards this tumor suppressor have lately attained increasing interest as a promising early detection biomarker for colorectal cancer. In the studies included in this review, two evaluated the independent association between levels of p53 autoantibodies and colorectal cancer risk [61,64], whereas an additional three included it in a multi-marker panel [33,39,62]. Teras et al. used a nested case control design with 392 cases and 774 controls drawn from the Cancer Prevention Study-II Nutrition Cohort. They found significant associations for the full case set, which were strengthened when limiting the analysis to participants diagnosed within 3 years of blood draw (RR = 2.26, 95% CI = 1.06–4.83). This time dependency was corroborated by Butt et al. in 2020 [61], using a much larger dataset including 3702 colorectal cancer cases and an equal number of controls. When stratified by follow-up time, the association in this study was significant only among cases diagnosed within 4 years of blood draw, with similar risk estimates to those presented in Teras et al. (OR = 2.27, 95% CI = 1.62–3.19).

Table 3. Studies of antibodies analyzed in pre-diagnostic blood samples (collected in prospective cohort or general screening settings) for the purpose of risk prediction or early diagnosis of colorectal cancer.

Reference	Cohort (Design)	Time from Sampling to Diagnosis (Cohort Setting Only)	CRC	Adenoma	Contr/Cohort	Biomarker/Platform	Main Findings	Adapted NOS Scale ** Max: Selection = ★★★★ Comp. = ★★ Exp./Outc. = ★★★
				Cohort setting				
Pedersen et al. Int J Cancer, 2014 [63]	UKCTOCS (Nested case control)	6.8 years (median)	97	-	94 *	Autoantibodies: MUC1, MUC2 and MUC4	Top markers: MUC1-STn, MUC1-Core3 MUC1-STn Sensitivity: 8.2% Specificity: 95% MUC1-Core3 Sensitivity: 13.4% Specificity: 95%	★★★★ ★ ★★★
Butt et al. Cancer Epidemiol Biomarkers Prev, 2018 [60]	CLUE, CPSII, HPFS, MEC, NHS, NYUWHS, PHS, PLCO, SCCS and WHI (Nested case control)	4–18 years (median, different studies)	4210	-	4210 *	Antibody responses to 9 Streptococcus gallolyticus (SGG) proteins	Top marker: Gallo2178 Gallo2178 All cases: OR: 1.23 (95% CI: 0.99–1.52) Diagnosed <10 years after blood draw: OR: 1.40 (95% CI: 1.09–1.79)	★★★ ★★ ★★★
Teras et al. Cancer Epidemiol Biomarkers Prev, 2018 [64]	CPSII (Nested case control)	11 years (follow up)	392	-	774 *	p53 autoantibodies	All cases: RR: 1.77 (95% CI: 1.12–2.78) Diagnosed <3 years after blood draw: RR: 2.26 (95% CI: 1.06–4.83)	★★★★ ★★ ★★★
Butt et al. Cancer Epidemiol Biomarkers Prev, 2020 [61]	CLUE, CPSII, HPFS, MEC, NHS, NYUWHS, PHS, PLCO, SCCS and WHI (Nested case control)	7 years (median)	3702	-	3702 *	p53 autoantibodies	All cases: OR: 1.33 (95% CI: 1.09–1.61) Diagnosed <4 years after blood draw: OR: 2.27 (95% CI: 1.62–3.19)	★★★ ★★ ★★★

Table 3. Cont.

Reference	Cohort (Design)	Time from Sampling to Diagnosis (Cohort Setting Only)	CRC	Adenoma	Contr./Cohort	Biomarker/Platform	Main Findings	Adapted NOS Scale ** Max: Selection = ★★★★ Comp. = ★★ Exp./Outc. = ★★★
Screening setting								
Chen H et al. Oncotarget, 2016 [62]	BliTz (validation study)	-	49	AA: 99 NAA: 29	100	Autoantibodies to 64 tumor associated antigens Tested: individual proteins and 2- to 6-marker panels	Top hits: TP53, anti-IMPDH2, anti-MDM2, anti-MAGEA4 Best 2-marker panel (TP53, anti-IMPDH2): sensitivity CRC 10% (4–22), sensitivity AA 7 (3–14), specificity 95 (89–98) Best 6-marker panel (TP53+IMPDH2+MDM2 +MAGEA4+CTAG1 +MTDH), Sensitivity CRC 24% (15–38), sensitivity AA 25% (18–35), specificity 85% (77–91)	★★★★ - ★★★

Abbreviations (not including biomarker names, for which the reader is referred to the original study article): **AA**, advanced adenoma; **BliTz**, Begleitende Evaluierung innovativer Testverfahren zur Darmkrebs-Früherkennun, Germany; **CLUE**, Campaign Against Cancer and Stroke; **CPSII**, Cancer Prevention Study-II; **CRC**, colorectal cancer; **EPIC**, European Prospective Investigation into Cancer and Nutrition; **HPFS**, Health Professionals Follow-up study; **MEC**, Multiethnic Cohort Study; **NAA**, non-advanced adenoma; **NHS**, Nurses' Health Study; **NYUWHS**, NYU Women's Health Study; **OR**, odds ratio; **PHS**, Physicians' Health Study; **PLCO**, Prostate, Lung, Colorectal, and Ovarian Screening Study; **SCCS**, Southern Community Cohort Study; **UKCTOCS**, UK Collaborative Trial of Ovarian Cancer Screening; **WHI**, Women's Health Initiative. * Matched controls. ** Newcastle-Ottawa Quality Assessment Scale for case-control studies, adapted for use for assessment of biomarker studies conducted in a screening setting. For case-control studies: selection (max 4 stars), comparability (max 2 stars), exposure (max 3 stars). For cohort studies: selection (max 4 stars), comparability (max 2 stars), outcome (max 3 stars).

3.3.4. Nucleic Acids

In the category nucleic acids, we included all studies evaluating non-coding RNAs (five in total, [65–69]), as well as studies evaluating DNA markers, such as DNA methylation [8,70–74], mitochondrial DNA [75] and circulating tumor DNA [19] (Table 4).

Among the non-coding RNA studies, microRNAs have been most extensively investigated, but few have produced significant results. The earliest study identified in our search used a TaqMan microRNA array, as well as an in-depth literature search, to identify 12 potential microRNA targets [65], none of which reached significance in validation tests including samples from adenoma patients. Of the four studies of microRNAs, three used samples collected in screening settings [65,67,69] and one [68] used prospective samples from the Northern Sweden Health and Disease Study. In the prospective study, 12 candidate microRNAs were measured in plasma samples collected at both pre- and post-diagnostic time points from the same patients, with the top four giving an AUC for colorectal cancer detection of 0.93. However, only one (miR-21) showed a time trajectory consistent with potential use as an early detection marker for colorectal cancer, elevated approximately three years prior to diagnosis. The other two microRNA studies [67,69] both used an approach including FIT-positive and unselected patients from general screening. Using a multi-marker microRNA panel containing six markers Marcuello et al. reached an AUC of 0.80, while Zanuttoa et al., using a similarly sized panel with different microRNAs, observed an AUC of 0.61, in both studies for the detection of advanced adenomas.

One recent cohort-based study [66] analyzed a PIWI interacting RNA (piR-54265) in serum samples from 307 colorectal cancer cases and 614 matched controls from the prospective cohort study of Dongfeng-Tongji (DFTJ) in China. They found it to be significantly associated with colorectal cancer risk, primarily in individuals diagnosed within 2–3 years after blood draw. For other non-coding RNA studies included in this review, independent validation of results is lacking.

Among DNA-based markers, the most well studied is DNA methylation of *Septin 9*, with somewhat mixed results [76]. Our search identified two studies that included *SEPT9* methylation, both based on samples collected at screening [8,74] and both published before 2015. More recent studies on DNA methylation included one that evaluated genome-wide DNA methylation in leukocytes and identified three CpG sites (cg04036920, cg14472551 and cg12459502) that together produced a c-statistic of 0.74 [72]. Another DNA methylation study specifically evaluated methylation in four genes (*SFRP1*, *SFRP2*, *SDC2* and *PRIMA1*) [70], with an AUC of 0.93 for the multi-marker panel for detecting adenoma. DNA methylation in circulating tumor DNA was also the focus of a recent study using a newly constructed panel (PanSeer) with the ability to detect multiple different cancer types [19]. For colorectal cancer, a pre-diagnostic sensitivity of 94.9% was reported for samples collected up to four years before diagnosis.

Table 4. Studies of nucleic acids analyzed in pre-diagnostic blood samples (collected in prospective cohort or general screening settings) for the purpose of risk prediction or early diagnosis of colorectal cancer.

Reference	Cohort (Design)	Time from Sampling to Diagnosis (Cohort Setting Only)	CRC	Adenoma	Contr./Cohort	Biomarker/Platform	Main Findings	Adapted NOS Scale ** Max: Selection = ★★★★ Comp. = ★★ Exp./Outc. = ★★★
			Cohort setting					
Wikberg et al. Cancer Med, 2018 [68]	NSHDS/VIP (Nested case control)	20 years (maximum follow up)	58	-	147 *	12 miRNAs	Top panel: miRNA-21, miR-18a, miR-22, miR-25 4 marker panel: AUC: 0.93 Sensitivity: 67% Specificity: 90%	★★★★ ★★ ★★★
Mai et al. Theranostics, 2020 [66]	DFTJ (Nested case control)	9 years (follow up)	307	-	614 *	Serum piR-54265	All cases: OR: 2.10 (95% CI: 1.66–2.65) Diagnosed <1 years after blood draw: OR: 2.80 (95% CI: 1.60–4.89) Diagnosed <2 years after blood draw: OR: 2.45 (95% CI: 1.49–4.03) Diagnosed <3 years after blood draw: OR: 1.24 (95% CI: 0.90–1.72)	★★ ★★★
Huang et al. Cancer Epidemiol Biomarkers Prev, 2014 [75]	SWHS (Nested case control)	Time stratification: <5 years and >5 years	444	-	1423	mtDNA copy number	OR (2nd vs. 3rd tertile): 1.26 (95% CI: 0.93–1.70) OR (1st vs. 3rd tertile): 1.44 (95% CI: 1.06–1.94)	★★★★ ★ ★★★
Dietmar Barth et al. J Natl Cancer Inst, 2015 [71]	EPIC-HEIDELBERG (Nested case control)	6.4 years (mean)	185	-	807	"ImmunoCRIT" Cell type specific DNA methylation in Foxp3, CD3 and GAPDH loci	ImmunoCRIT HR (3rd vs. 1st tertile): 1.59 (95% CI: 0.99–2.54)	★★★★ ★★ ★★★

Table 4. Cont.

Reference	Cohort (Design)	Time from Sampling to Diagnosis (Cohort Setting Only)	CRC Cohort	Adenoma Cohort	Contr. Cohort	Biomarker/Platform	Main Findings	Adapted NOS Scale ** Max: Selection = ★★★★ Comp. = ★★★ Exp./Outc. = ★★★
Onwuka et al. BMC Cancer, 2020 [73]	EPIC-TURIN (Nested case control)	6.2 years (mean)	166	-	424 *	Blood DNA methylation CpG-sites	Methylation risk score (MRS), based on 16 CpGs. OR (original dataset): 2.68 (95% CI: 2.13–3.38) OR (testing dataset): 2.02 (95% CI: 1.48–2.74) AUC: 0.82	★★★ ★ ★★
Chen et al. Nat Commun, 2020 [19]	TZL (Nested case control)	4 years (cutoff, follow up)	35	-	414	PanSeer panel: Circulating tumor DNA from pre-diagnostic stomach, esophageal, colorectal, lung or liver cancer patients	Pre-diagnosis sensitivity (all cancers): 94.9 (95% CI: 88.5–98.3)	★★★★ ★★ ★★★
Screening setting								
Warren JD, et al. BMC Med, 2011 [74]	Screening patients, single community clinic, USA (validation)	-	-	A: 78	See footnote ***ttPCR in triplicate	$SEPT9$ methylation, ttPCR in triplicate	Sensitivity 10%	★★★★ - ★★★
Luo X, et al., PLoS ONE, 2013 [65]	BliTz (validation set)	-	-	AA: 50	50	Five miRNAs from discovery phase (miR-29a, -106b, -133a, -342-3p, -532-3p), seven candidate miRNAs (miR-18a, -20a, -21, -92a, -143, -145, -181b)	Null	★★★ - ★★★

Table 4. Cont.

Reference	Cohort (Design)	Time from Sampling to Diagnosis (Cohort Setting Only)	CRC	Adenoma	Contr. Cohort	Biomarker/ Platform	Main Findings	Adapted NOS Scale ** Max: Selection = ★★★★ Comp. = ★★ Exp./Outc. = ★★★
Church T, et al., Gut, 2014 [8]	PRESEPT **** (validation study)	-	53	AA: 314 NAA: 209	934	SEPT9 methylation (Epi proColon Assay)	≥1/2 runs positive, CRC: Sensitivity 48.2% (32.4–63.6), specificity 91.5% (89.7–93.1) ≥1/3 runs positive, CRC (post hoc): Sensitivity 63.9% (47.5–79.2), specificity 88.4% (86.2–90.4) ≥1/2 runs positive, AA: Sensitivity 11.2% (7.2–15.7) compared to 9.2% positive rate in controls	★★★★ ★★ ★★★
Maffei et al. Mutagenesis, 2014 [77]	FOB+ screening patients, Bologna, Italy	-	25	26 "polyps"	31	Micronucleus frequency in peripheral blood lymphocytes	Mean micronucleus frequency in CRC > polyps > controls (all 3 t-tests $p < 0.001$)	★★ ★★★ ★★★
Heiss JA, Brenner H Clin Epigenetics, 2017 [72]	BliTz (clinical+screening for discovery, divided for modelling)	-	46	-	46 *	Leucocyte DNA methylation array	Top markers: cg04036920, cg14472551, cg12459502 Multi-marker (3 markers): C-statistic 0.74 (0.57–0.87)	★★★★ ★★ ★★★
Myint NNM, et al. Cell Death Dis, 2018 [78]	FOBT+ patients, BCSP	-	-	Pre-neoplastic lesions: 76	37	Total cfDNA, and tumor-related mutations (BRAF, KRAS by ddPCR) and patient-specific assays for trunk mutations identified by multiregional targeted NGS of adenoma tissues	Null	★★ - ★★★

225

Table 4. Cont.

Reference	Cohort (Design)	Time from Sampling to Diagnosis (Cohort Setting Only)	CRC	Adenoma	Contr./Cohort	Biomarker/Platform	Main Findings	Adapted NOS Scale ** Max: Selection = ★★★★ Comp. = ★★ Exp./Outc. = ★★★
Barták BK, et al. Epigenetics, 2018 [70]	Screening patients, not otherwise specified (validation study)	-	47	AA: 37	37	DNA methylation of SFRP1, SFRP2, SDC2 and PRIMA1	Individual markers, CRC: all AUC >8, adenoma: all AUC > 6 Multi-marker (4 genes), CRC: AUC 0.978 (0.954–1.000), sensitivity 91.5%, specificity 97.3% Multi-marker (4 genes), adenoma: AUC 0.937 (0.885–0.989), sensitivity 89.2%, specificity 86.5%	★★–★★★★
Marcuello M et al. Cancers, 2019 [67]	FIT+ screening patients, Barcelona, Spain (validation study)	-	59	AA: 74	80	miR-29a-3p, miR-15b-5p, miR-18a-5p, miR-19a-3p, miR-19b-3p, miR-335-5p	Multi-marker (6 miRNAs), CRC: AUC 0.74 (0.65–0.82), sensitivity 81%, specificity 56% Multi-marker (6 miRNAs), AA: AUC 0.80 (0.72–0.87), sensitivity 81%, specificity 63%	★★ - ★★
Zanutto S, et al. Int J Cancer, 2020 [69]	FIT+ screening patients, Milan, Italy (discovery and validation sets)	-	Ext. valid. 33	Ext. valid. AA:18 NAA: 313	Ext. valid. 568	miRNA Taqman array 13 miRNAS selected for validation (of which 4 excluded after hemolysis experiments) plus one candidate from a previous study	Individual markers, CRC: AUC ~0.6 for 5 best miRNAs, AA: AUC range for all miRNAs 0.589–0.608 Multi-marker, CRC (hsa-miR-378, hsa-miR-342-3p): AUC 0.604 (0.504–0.704) Multi-marker, AA (hsa-miR-106b-5p, hsa-miR-483-5p, hsa-miR-323a-3p, hsa-miR-335-5p, hsa-miR-186-5p, hsa-miR-342-3p): AUC 0.608 (0.560–0.656)	★★ ★★ ★★★

Abbreviations (not including biomarker names, for which the reader is referred to the original study article): **A**, adenoma; **AA**, advanced adenoma; **AUC**, Area Under the Curve; **BCST**, Bowel Cancer Screening Programme; **BliTz**, Begleitende Evaluierung innovativer Testverfahren zur Darmkrebs-Früherkennun, Germany; **DFTJ**, Dongfeng–Tongji cohort; **EPIC**, European Prospective Investigation into Cancer and Nutrition; **FIT**, fecal immunochemical test; **FOB**, fecal occult blood; **FOBT**, fecal occult blood test; **miRNA**, micro-RNA; **NAA**, non-advanced adenoma; **NSHDS**, North Sweden Health and Disease Study; **PRESEPT**, PRospective Evaluation of SEPTin 9, United States and Germany; **rtPCR**, real-time PCR; **SWHS**: Shanghai Women's Health Study; **TZL**, Taizhou Longitudinal Study; **USA**, United States of America. * Matched controls. ** Newcastle–Ottawa Quality Assessment Scale for case-control studies, adapted for use for assessment of biomarker studies conducted in a screening setting. For case-control studies: selection (max 4 stars), comparability (max 2 stars), exposure (max 3 stars). For cohort studies: selection (max 4 stars), comparability (max 2 stars), outcome (max 3 stars). *** Cohort design. Total screening colonoscopy cohort: 195 of which 34 completely normal NOS assessment using the cohort scale. **** Commercially sponsored.

3.3.5. Other Markers

Aside from the types of markers already described, which were included in multiple studies, some types of biomarkers were only included in single studies (Table 5). One example is a recent investigation of the triglyceride–glucose index (TyG index) published in 2020 [79]. This easily accessible marker gave an AUC of 0.69, which is not as high as some biomarkers but would be much easier to implement. Another example of re-purposing of routine lab tests is the iron-storage protein and inflammatory marker ferritin, which was included in a promising multi-marker panel [33].

Table 5. Studies of other biomarkers analyzed in pre-diagnostic blood samples (collected in prospective cohort or general screening settings) for the purpose of risk prediction or early diagnosis of colorectal cancer.

Reference	Cohort (Design)	Time from Sampling to Diagnosis (Cohort Setting Only)	CRC	Adenoma	Contr/Cohort	Biomarker/Platform	Main Findings	Adapted NOS Scale ** Max: Selection = ★★★★ Comp. = ★★ Exp./Outc. = ★★★
				Cohort setting				
Perttula et al. Cancer Epidemiol Biomarkers Prev, 2016 [80]	EPIC-TURIN (Nested case control)	7.1 years (baseline)	95	-	95 *	Ultra-long Chain Fatty Acids (ULCFA)	Top markers: ULCFAs: 446, 466, 468, 492 and 494. Differences diminished with increasing time to diagnosis	★★ ★★ ★★★
Prizment et al. Cancer Epidemiol Biomarkers Prev, 2016 [81]	ARIC (Cohort)	14.8 years (median follow up)	255	-	12,300	Beta-2-microglobulin (B2M)	HR (4th vs. 1st quartile): 2.21 (95% CI: 1.32–3.70)	★★★ ★★ ★★★
Doherty et al. Sci Rep, 2018 [82]	FINRISK (Nested case control)	10 years (follow up)	40	-	80 *	Plasma N-glycans	Top markers: F(6)A2G2, F(6)A2G25(6)1 All peaks + age: AUC: 0.65 Sensitivity: 12.5% Specificity: 95%	★★★ ★★ ★★★
Pilling et al. Plos One, 2018 [83]	UK BIOBANK (Cohort)	9 years (follow up)	1327	-	240,477	Red Blood Cell Distribution Width (RDW)	Higher RDW: sHR: 1.92 (95% CI: 1.36 to 2.72)	★★★ ★★ ★★★
Okamura et al. Bmc Endocr Disord, 2020 [79]	NAGALA (Cohort)	4.4 years (median)	116	-	27,921	Triglyceride–glucose index (TyG index)	HR (TyG index): 1.38 (95% CI: 1.0–1.9) AUC: 0.69 Sensitivity: 62% Specificity: 67%	★★ ★★ ★★★

Table 5. *Cont.*

Reference	Cohort (Design)	Time from Sampling to Diagnosis (Cohort Setting Only)	CRC	Adenoma	Contr./Cohort	Biomarker/Platform	Main Findings	Adapted NOS Scale ** Max: Selection = ★★★★ Comp. = ★★ Exp./Outc. = ★★★
Le Cornet et al. Cancer Res, 2020 [84]	EPIC-HEIDELBERG (Case cohort)	6.7 years (mean)	111	-	465	Immune cell counts (neutrophils, monocytes, and lymphocytes)	Top finding: FOXP3+ T-cell counts HR: 1.59 (95% CI: 1.04–2.42)	★★★★ ★★ ★★★

Abbreviations (not including biomarker names, for which the reader is referred to the original study article): **A**, adenoma; **AA**, advanced adenoma; **ARIC**, Atherosclerosis Risk in Communities; **AUC**, Area Under the Curve; **CRC**, Colorectal Cancer; **EPIC**, European Prospective Investigation into Cancer and Nutrition; **FINRISK**, The National FINRISK Study; **HR**, Hazard Ratio; **NAGALA**, NAfld in the Gifu Area, Longitudinal Analysis; **RDW**, Red Blood Cell Distribution Width; **UK BIOBANK**, United Kingdom Biobank. * Matched controls. ** Newcastle–Ottawa Quality Assessment Scale for case-control studies, adapted for use for assessment of biomarker studies conducted in a screening setting. For case-control studies: selection (max 4 stars), comparability (max 2 stars), exposure (max 3 stars). For cohort studies: selection (max 4 stars), comparability (max 2 stars), outcome (max 3 stars).

All markers, including top findings, are presented in Tables 1–5.

4. Discussion

4.1. Limitations of the Evidence

The investigations identified in this review were generally of high quality but varied considerably with respect to data analysis and presentation of results, and few biomarkers demonstrated a consistent, clinically relevant discriminatory ability across more than one study. As expected, the performance of the biomarkers summarized in this review was generally not sufficient for clinical implementation. The ideal circulating biomarker for screening would be released from the tumor into the bloodstream in sufficient quantities to achieve high discriminatory ability. Colorectal tumors present in asymptomatic people, particularly if they are early-stage carcinoma or advanced adenoma, may not release adequate amounts for detection, even as technological advances achieve increasingly high sensitivity. Perhaps even more importantly, not all tumors are likely to possess a given biomarker, such as a specific genetic or epigenetic alteration, or produce a specific marker protein. Testing a panel including different types of biomarkers could help overcome this limitation, as exemplified by studies including panels with both proteins and p53 autoantibodies [33,39].

Some studies presented results stratified for early- and late-stage colorectal cancer. Since detection of early-stage colorectal cancer is a premise of effective colorectal cancer screening, such analyses are highly relevant, particularly for studies conducted in a screening setting. Stage-specific results were not presented in the results tables in this review, mainly because of the generally small subgroup sizes. Colorectal cancer screening also targets the detection and removal of advanced adenoma. Of the studies included in this review, a majority of those with samples collected in general screening settings presented results for advanced adenoma as an endpoint. In contrast, only one of the studies conducted in a prospective cohort setting investigated advanced adenoma [23]. In general, findings for precancerous lesions were weak to null, with some exceptions, such as in Marcuello et al. [67], in which a panel of six microRNAs reached an AUC of 0.80 for detecting advanced adenomas in FIT+ participants in a screening setting.

A major challenge in biomarker discovery is the risk of over-fitting and chance findings. At the very least, bootstrapping, cross-validation, consideration of multiple testing and/or other statistical methods to reduce the risk of false positive findings should be applied, which was not always conducted rigorously in the studies identified for this review. Validation of discovery-stage findings is also a critical step in biomarker development, though not always possible within the same study setting as the discovery analyses. For example, the rarity of colorectal cancer events in general screening programs typically prevents division into separate discovery and validation sets. This issue can be addressed through collaborative efforts, as in most of the BliTz studies included in this review, for example, by joining forces with clinical cohorts. However, few to no biomarkers have a demonstrated clinically relevant discriminatory ability in more than one pre-diagnostic data set.

An advantage of studies set in prospective cohorts is the opportunity to address the temporality of biomarker performance. A biomarker that becomes detectable or demonstrates altered levels close to diagnosis would be a strong candidate for a screening test to supplement or replace fecal testing, whereas a biomarker that differentiates future cases from controls but without a clear time trajectory would more likely be a biomarker of risk. The latter could still have relevance for screening, primarily to improve risk-prediction algorithms to inform precision screening protocols with respect to starting age and screening frequency.

In order to distinguish between potential risk-predictive and diagnostic biomarkers, repeated pre-diagnostic samples represent a particularly valuable resource. We previously used such a design in a validation study inspired by promising findings from the Alpha-Tocopherol, Beta-Carotene (ATBC) cohort for the gut hormone ghrelin [85]. Murphy et al.

observed dramatically higher colorectal cancer risk in ATBC participants with low circulating total ghrelin concentrations in samples collected within 10 years prior to case diagnosis (OR: 10.86, 95% CI 5.01 to 23.55), whereas an inverse association was observed at longer follow-up times. This relationship was not replicated in our analysis of a unique set of 60 matched case-control pairs with repeated, pre-diagnostic plasma samples (one sample collected within 5 years prior to case diagnosis and one sample collected 10 years earlier), despite adequate statistical power [86]. There was no obvious explanation for the diverging findings, which demonstrates the value of validation studies in observational settings prior to clinical testing.

A major disadvantage of prospective cohorts for cancer biomarker research is the inherently limited sample volumes available for analysis. Whereas plasma/serum volumes of several milliliters are typically required for analyses of circulating tumor DNA, especially for asymptomatic patients with low tumor burden, analyses in biobank samples must usually be limited to sample volumes of 500 µL or less.

4.2. Limitations of Review Processes

A major limitation of the review process was the use of general search strings for a broad topic, which included many different types of exposures. Studies using the specific name of the biochemical analyte or platform, without referring to them as biomarkers or markers, would be missed in our searches. Furthermore, search string 2 could potentially miss relevant research published in a form with no abstract, such as a short report or letter. The aforementioned ghrelin publication by the authors was missed for this reason [86].

We also found it difficult to establish defined criteria to distinguish between studies focusing on etiology versus studies aimed towards identifying suitable biomarkers for screening. This problem was especially prominent for the prospective cohort studies. Although biomarkers investigated to help elucidate etiological mechanisms could certainly have relevance as biomarkers for screening, we recognize that the studies identified in our searches represent a minute fraction of all such publications. Therefore, we only included studies for which risk prediction or early diagnosis was clearly in focus, for example, as a specified aim or with calculation of discriminatory ability. Although this is in line with the stated purpose of this review, it was not noted specifically as a restriction in the PROSPERO registration.

Limiting the review to papers published from 2011 and onward may have led to relevant studies being missed. We accepted this risk based on the consideration that important novel biomarkers identified more than 10 years ago would likely have been validated in studies during the past 10 years. Our eligibility criteria will also have missed any promising biomarkers published only in non-English papers.

In order to assess the quality of the studies included in this review, we applied the Newcastle–Ottawa Scale (NOS) for assessing the quality of non-randomized studies in meta-analyses. We adapted the scale for use in assessing biomarker studies, making an effort to minimize the modifications. This may have introduced a bias toward higher scores, particularly with respect to the scoring category for exposure in the case-control scale. For example, using the same method of exposure ascertainment for cases and controls is standard procedure in this type of biomarker study design. However, the generally high scores noted also reflect the inclusion criteria for the review, which were set to ensure selection of studies with sampling prior to diagnosis, i.e., high-quality study designs. Most studies also accounted for factors such as age, typically by matching of cases and controls or by multivariable adjustment, and were thus awarded two NOS stars for the category on comparability of cases and controls. However, for cancer screening, the practice of matching controls has been called into question [87], and some studies, therefore, made an active decision not to use matched controls [28,39,53].

4.3. Implications for Practice and Policy

Taken together, this systematic review did not identify any single biomarker or biomarker panel that consistently demonstrated a discriminatory ability on par with FIT, suggesting that stool testing in general colorectal cancer screening is unlikely to be replaced by a blood test in the foreseeable future. Though not accurate enough to be used alone, autoantibodies to p53 showed consistently promising results as a marker for early diagnosis of colorectal cancer and might serve as a supplement to methylated *Septin 9* testing or in a future multi-marker panel. In general, panels of biomarkers performed better than single markers. The results of this review underscore the need for validation of promising colorectal cancer biomarkers in independent pre-diagnostic settings prior to clinical testing and implementation.

Translation of biomarkers to clinical implementation requires consideration of factors beyond discriminatory ability. The optimal biomarker would be insensitive to variable pre-analytical conditions, such as time of day for sample collection, fasting status and sample handling. It would be collected in standard phlebotomy tubes and be analyzed on equipment available at larger hospital laboratories. Many of the more promising biomarkers in this review, including anti-p53 antibodies, could be developed to fulfill these considerations. However, these are not absolute requirements for a clinical blood test. For example, interleukins degrade rapidly at room temperature, but IL-6 is routinely analyzed in clinical practice. Metabolites are often sensitive to fasting status [88], which could be a disadvantage if samples are to be used in biomarker panels for risk stratification, but a metabolomics-based diagnostic biomarker reflecting the tumor itself might be less likely to be affected by food intake. The results of a biomarker test should also be easy to interpret, which does not exclude the possibility of multi-marker or omics-based tests requiring advanced data analyses to generate results. The explosion of genomic and transcriptomic tumor testing in recent years, such as FoundationOne and PAM50, and the rapid implementation in clinical oncology practice, illustrate the willingness of clinicians to adopt and familiarize themselves with modern, data-heavy analyses.

A health-economical evaluation is central to the implementation of any medical testing, including cancer screening. Demonstrating cost effectiveness for a colorectal cancer screening test with a discriminatory performance on par with current fecal testing alternatives should not be difficult given the high and increasing costs of therapy, as the drug arsenal expands and survival during therapy continues to improve. However, for a test with a high positivity rate, cost effectiveness approaching that of colonoscopy screening might be achieved simply by chance, i.e., by the high proportion of screening participants selected for colonoscopy. This issue has been raised for annual *SEPT9* testing, which would send 70% of screenees to colonoscopy within 5 years [89]. Conversely, the potential of a highly discriminatory biomarker test to reduce unnecessary colonoscopy, beneficial from both a patient and health-economy perspective, should not be overlooked. Risk stratification, using prediction algorithms, potentially supplemented with biomarkers, might not only be helpful to select and encourage high-risk individuals to attend earlier or more frequent screening, but also to identify very low-risk individuals who might safely postpone their screening start.

Risk-prediction and diagnostic biomarkers could also have value in the clinical setting, to help shorten the time to diagnosis in patients with symptoms potentially consistent with a colorectal tumor but otherwise low suspicion of malignancy. Such an aid to clinical decision could be implemented in referral guidelines [90], similar to the recent addition of FIT to the NICE guidelines for example [91]. From a secondary prevention perspective, effective and personalized risk stratification could help guide surveillance strategies after adenoma removal.

In addition, there are other potential preventative benefits of blood-based biomarkers (Figure 2). The minimally invasive nature of blood testing should be conducive not only to improving overall screening uptake, but ideally also to reducing socioeconomic disparities in participation rates. A biomarker panel indicative of risk over a longer time period could be used for precision lifestyle counselling and/or pharmacoprevention, especially if it could detect specific negative physiological effects of poor lifestyle behaviors or metabolic health. Candidate pharmacopreventive drugs exist, for example the antidiabetic drug Metformin and aspirin and other non-steroidal anti-inflammatory drugs [92–94] and a targeted approach might improve both compliance and numbers needed to treat/harm.

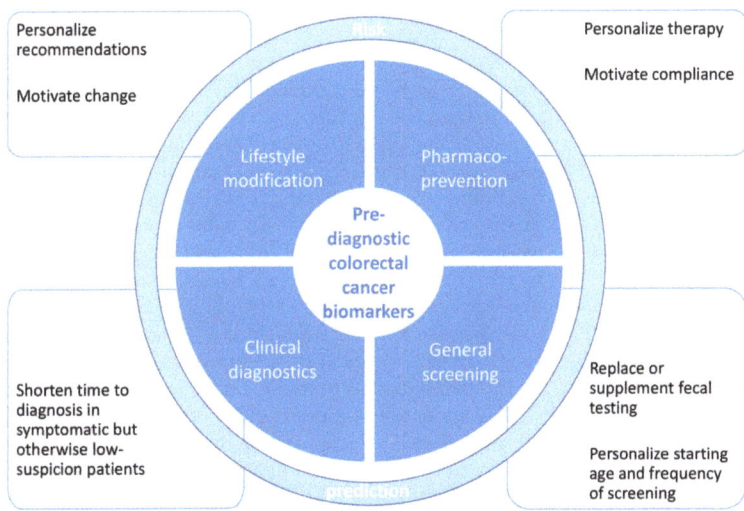

Figure 2. Potential applications of pre-diagnostic biomarkers for prevention and early detection of colorectal cancer.

4.4. Future Research Perspectives

The numbers of studies using pre-diagnostic blood samples to investigate colorectal cancer biomarker is limited compared to the overwhelming volume of publications based on patient samples. In part, this is likely due to the relatively large volumes of blood required for some types of biomarkers, such as tumor DNA-based markers and extra-cellular vesicles (especially in asymptomatic tumor bearers), rendering such analyses generally unfeasible in prospective cohort biobanks. Prospective cohorts have also traditionally focused primarily on etiological biomarker studies, with the aim of elucidating how colorectal cancer arises and grows, including mechanistic links between lifestyle-based exposures and carcinogenesis. However, with the rapid expansion of large-scale proteomics and other technologies using smaller sample volumes, prospective cohorts seem poised to become a key asset for translating biomarkers to the clinic. Furthermore, novel collaborative efforts such as the international Colorectal Cancer Pooling Project (C2P2, originally planned with a risk factor and etiology focus) may prove invaluable as a resource for research of blood-based risk-predictive and diagnostic biomarkers, with large sample sizes allowing for analyses of various time points prior to diagnosis and of clinical and molecular tumor subgroups. Such resources could also provide opportunities for validation in various geographical, ethnic and socioeconomic settings. The extensive etiological biomarker data previously collected in many prospective cohorts might also be revisited to identify multi-marker panels for risk stratification, using, for example, machine learning methods.

For future studies, we would stress the importance of a clear and complete description of the samples used, in particular distinguishing between screening, clinical and mixed colonoscopy settings. In new etiological studies in prospective cohorts, scientists might consider the possible additional value of evaluating the biomarkers also from the perspective of risk prediction, with appropriate statistical analyses and lag-time stratification as pre-specified analyses. We also support standardized reporting of results according to published guidelines and checklists, such as the Standards for Reporting Diagnostic Accuracy (STARD) statement [95], and the Transparent Reporting of a multivariable prediction model for Individual Prognosis Or Diagnosis (TRIPOD) Statement [96], to aid interpretation of findings.

5. Conclusions

In this systematic review, we evaluated 53 articles that investigated risk-predictive or diagnostic biomarkers of colorectal cancer using blood samples collected in a pre-diagnostic, asymptomatic setting. All studies used samples collected either in prospective cohorts (months to years before diagnosis) or in general screening settings. The quality of the studies was generally high, but very few potential biomarkers showed consistent results in more than one study. The vast majority focused on protein biomarkers in plasma or serum, but even when combined into multi-marker panels, proteins alone did not achieve sufficient discriminatory ability to be clinically useful as an alternative to FIT in general colorectal cancer screening. However, one of the most promising biomarkers, p53 autoantibodies, consistently performed well, especially in combination with protein markers, which may warrant development as a supplement to current screening tests. In general, panels of biomarkers performed better than single markers.

The search for colorectal cancer biomarkers that can detect early carcinomas or advanced adenomas, or aid in the identification of high-risk individuals, has relied too heavily on samples collected from patients after diagnosis, whose tumor burden and systemic response may not be representative of the general screening setting. The findings of this review underscore the need for discovery and validation of biomarkers in independent, pre-diagnostic, asymptomatic settings, in order to improve the chances of successful translation to clinical implementation.

Author Contributions: Conceptualization, S.H. and B.V.G.; methodology, S.H., M.J.G. and B.V.G.; investigation, S.H. and B.V.G.; data curation, S.H. and B.V.G.; writing—original draft preparation, S.H. and B.V.G.; writing—review and editing, S.H., M.J.G. and B.V.G.; visualization, S.H.; project administration, S.H. and B.V.G.; funding acquisition, B.V.G. All authors have read and agreed to the published version of the manuscript.

Funding: This work was funded by the Swedish Cancer Society (20 1154 PjF), the Knut and Alice Wallenberg Foundation, the Cancer Research Foundation in Northern Sweden, the Faculty of Medicine at Umeå University and a regional agreement between Umeå University and Region Västerbotten.

Acknowledgments: The authors thank Janaki Brolin for valuable feedback.

Conflicts of Interest: The authors declare no conflict of interest. The funders had no role in the design of the study; in the collection, analyses or interpretation of data; in the writing of the manuscript, or in the decision to publish the results.**Disclaimer:** Where authors are identified as personnel of the International Agency for Research on Cancer/World Health Organization, the authors alone are responsible for the views expressed in this article and they do not necessarily represent the decisions, policy or views of the International Agency for Research on Cancer/World Health Organization.

References

1. Sung, H.; Ferlay, J.; Siegel, R.L.; Laversanne, M.; Soerjomataram, I.; Jemal, A.; Bray, F. Global Cancer Statistics 2020: GLOBOCAN Estimates of Incidence and Mortality Worldwide for 36 Cancers in 185 Countries. *CA Cancer J. Clin.* **2021**, *71*, 209–249. [CrossRef]
2. Siegel, R.L.; Miller, K.D.; Goding Sauer, A.; Fedewa, S.A.; Butterly, L.F.; Anderson, J.C.; Cercek, A.; Smith, R.A.; Jemal, A. Colorectal cancer statistics, 2020. *CA Cancer J. Clin.* **2020**, *70*, 145–164. [CrossRef] [PubMed]
3. Brenner, H.; Stock, C.; Hoffmeister, M. Effect of screening sigmoidoscopy and screening colonoscopy on colorectal cancer incidence and mortality: Systematic review and meta-analysis of randomised controlled trials and observational studies. *BMJ* **2014**, *348*, g2467. [CrossRef] [PubMed]
4. De Klerk, C.M.; Gupta, S.; Dekker, E.; Essink-Bot, M.L. Socioeconomic and ethnic inequities within organised colorectal cancer screening programmes worldwide. *Gut* **2018**, *67*, 679–687. [CrossRef]
5. Imperiale, T.F.; Ransohoff, D.F.; Itzkowitz, S.H.; Levin, T.R.; Lavin, P.; Lidgard, G.P.; Ahlquist, D.A.; Berger, B.M. Multitarget stool DNA testing for colorectal-cancer screening. *N. Engl. J. Med.* **2014**, *370*, 1287–1297. [CrossRef] [PubMed]

6. Kim, S.E.; Paik, H.Y.; Yoon, H.; Lee, J.E.; Kim, N.; Sung, M.K. Sex- and gender-specific disparities in colorectal cancer risk. *World J. Gastroenterol.* **2015**, *21*, 5167–5175. [CrossRef]
7. Yang, L.; Xiong, Z.; He, W.; Xie, K.; Liu, S.; Kong, P.; Jiang, C.; Guo, G.; Xia, L. Proximal shift of colorectal cancer with increasing age in different ethnicities. *Cancer Manag. Res.* **2018**, *10*, 2663–2673. [CrossRef]
8. Church, T.R.; Wandell, M.; Lofton-Day, C.; Mongin, S.J.; Burger, M.; Payne, S.R.; Castanos-Velez, E.; Blumenstein, B.A.; Rosch, T.; Osborn, N.; et al. Prospective evaluation of methylated SEPT9 in plasma for detection of asymptomatic colorectal cancer. *Gut* **2014**, *63*, 317–325. [CrossRef]
9. Potter, N.T.; Hurban, P.; White, M.N.; Whitlock, K.D.; Lofton-Day, C.E.; Tetzner, R.; Koenig, T.; Quigley, N.B.; Weiss, G. Validation of a real-time PCR-based qualitative assay for the detection of methylated SEPT9 DNA in human plasma. *Clin. Chem.* **2014**, *60*, 1183–1191. [CrossRef]
10. Lin, J.S.; Perdue, L.A.; Henrikson, N.B.; Bean, S.I.; Blasi, P.R. Screening for Colorectal Cancer: Updated Evidence Report and Systematic Review for the US Preventive Services Task Force. *JAMA* **2021**, *325*, 1978–1998. [CrossRef]
11. Hull, M.A.; Rees, C.J.; Sharp, L.; Koo, S. A risk-stratified approach to colorectal cancer prevention and diagnosis. *Nat. Rev. Gastroenterol. Hepatol.* **2020**, *17*, 773–780. [CrossRef] [PubMed]
12. Akimoto, N.; Ugai, T.; Zhong, R.; Hamada, T.; Fujiyoshi, K.; Giannakis, M.; Wu, K.; Cao, Y.; Ng, K.; Ogino, S. Rising incidence of early-onset colorectal cancer—A call to action. *Nat. Rev. Clin. Oncol.* **2021**, *18*, 230–243. [CrossRef]
13. Aleksandrova, K.; Reichmann, R.; Kaaks, R.; Jenab, M.; Bueno-de-Mesquita, H.B.; Dahm, C.C.; Eriksen, A.K.; Tjonneland, A.; Artaud, F.; Boutron-Ruault, M.C.; et al. Development and validation of a lifestyle-based model for colorectal cancer risk prediction: The LiFeCRC score. *BMC Med.* **2021**, *19*, 1. [CrossRef] [PubMed]
14. Jeon, J.; Du, M.; Schoen, R.E.; Hoffmeister, M.; Newcomb, P.A.; Berndt, S.I.; Caan, B.; Campbell, P.T.; Chan, A.T.; Chang-Claude, J.; et al. Determining Risk of Colorectal Cancer and Starting Age of Screening Based on Lifestyle, Environmental, and Genetic Factors. *Gastroenterology* **2018**, *154*, 2152–2164.e2119. [CrossRef] [PubMed]
15. Schmit, S.L.; Edlund, C.K.; Schumacher, F.R.; Gong, J.; Harrison, T.A.; Huyghe, J.R.; Qu, C.; Melas, M.; Van Den Berg, D.J.; Wang, H.; et al. Novel Common Genetic Susceptibility Loci for Colorectal Cancer. *J. Natl. Cancer Inst.* **2019**, *111*, 146–157. [CrossRef] [PubMed]
16. Smith, T.; Muller, D.C.; Moons, K.G.M.; Cross, A.J.; Johansson, M.; Ferrari, P.; Fagherazzi, G.; Peeters, P.H.M.; Severi, G.; Husing, A.; et al. Comparison of prognostic models to predict the occurrence of colorectal cancer in asymptomatic individuals: A systematic literature review and external validation in the EPIC and UK Biobank prospective cohort studies. *Gut* **2019**, *68*, 672–683. [CrossRef]
17. Bhardwaj, M.; Gies, A.; Werner, S.; Schrotz-King, P.; Brenner, H. Blood-Based Protein Signatures for Early Detection of Colorectal Cancer: A Systematic Review. *Clin. Transl. Gastroenterol.* **2017**, *8*, e128. [CrossRef]
18. Nikolaou, S.; Qiu, S.; Fiorentino, F.; Rasheed, S.; Tekkis, P.; Kontovounisios, C. Systematic review of blood diagnostic markers in colorectal cancer. *Tech. Coloproctol.* **2018**, *22*, 481–498. [CrossRef]
19. Chen, X.; Gole, J.; Gore, A.; He, Q.; Lu, M.; Min, J.; Yuan, Z.; Yang, X.; Jiang, Y.; Zhang, T.; et al. Non-invasive early detection of cancer four years before conventional diagnosis using a blood test. *Nat. Commun.* **2020**, *11*, 3475. [CrossRef]
20. Cohen, J.D.; Li, L.; Wang, Y.; Thoburn, C.; Afsari, B.; Danilova, L.; Douville, C.; Javed, A.A.; Wong, F.; Mattox, A.; et al. Detection and localization of surgically resectable cancers with a multi-analyte blood test. *Science* **2018**, *359*, 926–930. [CrossRef] [PubMed]
21. Wells, G.A.; Shea, B.; O'Connell, D.; Peterson, J.; Welch, V.; Losos, M.; Tugwell, P. The Newcastle-Ottawa Scale (NOS) for assessing the quality of nonrandomised studies in meta-analyses. Available online: http://www.ohri.ca/programs/clinical_epidemiology/oxford.asp (accessed on 26 June 2021).
22. Bailey, S.E.; Ukoumunne, O.C.; Shephard, E.A.; Hamilton, W. Clinical relevance of thrombocytosis in primary care: A prospective cohort study of cancer incidence using English electronic medical records and cancer registry data. *Br. J. Gen. Pract.* **2017**, *67*, e405–e413. [CrossRef]
23. Song, M.; Mehta, R.S.; Wu, K.; Fuchs, C.S.; Ogino, S.; Giovannucci, E.L.; Chan, A.T. Plasma Inflammatory Markers and Risk of Advanced Colorectal Adenoma in Women. *Cancer Prev. Res.* **2016**, *9*, 27–34. [CrossRef] [PubMed]
24. Cock, C.; Anwar, S.; Byrne, S.E.; Meng, R.; Pedersen, S.; Fraser, R.J.L.; Young, G.P.; Symonds, E.L. Low Sensitivity of Fecal Immunochemical Tests and Blood-Based Markers of DNA Hypermethylation for Detection of Sessile Serrated Adenomas/Polyps. *Dig. Dis. Sci.* **2019**, *64*, 2555–2562. [CrossRef]
25. De Chiara, L.; Paez de la Cadena, M.; Rodriguez-Berrocal, J.; Alvarez-Pardinas, M.C.; Pardinas-Anon, M.C.; Varela-Calvino, R.; Cordero, O.J. CD26-Related Serum Biomarkers: sCD26 Protein, DPP4 Activity, and Anti-CD26 Isotype Levels in a Colorectal Cancer-Screening Context. *Dis. Markers* **2020**, *2020*, 4347936. [CrossRef] [PubMed]
26. Ivancic, M.M.; Anson, L.W.; Pickhardt, P.J.; Megna, B.; Pooler, B.D.; Clipson, L.; Reichelderfer, M.; Sussman, M.R.; Dove, W.F. Conserved serum protein biomarkers associated with growing early colorectal adenomas. *Proc. Natl. Acad. Sci. USA* **2019**, *116*, 8471–8480. [CrossRef] [PubMed]
27. King, W.D.; Ashbury, J.E.; Taylor, S.A.; Tse, M.Y.; Pang, S.C.; Louw, J.A.; Vanner, S.J. A cross-sectional study of global DNA methylation and risk of colorectal adenoma. *BMC Cancer* **2014**, *14*, 488. [CrossRef]
28. Chen, H.; Zucknick, M.; Werner, S.; Knebel, P.; Brenner, H. Head-to-Head Comparison and Evaluation of 92 Plasma Protein Biomarkers for Early Detection of Colorectal Cancer in a True Screening Setting. *Clin. Cancer Res.* **2015**, *21*, 3318–3326. [CrossRef] [PubMed]

29. Ladd, J.J.; Busald, T.; Johnson, M.M.; Zhang, Q.; Pitteri, S.J.; Wang, H.; Brenner, D.E.; Lampe, P.D.; Kucherlapati, R.; Feng, Z.; et al. Increased plasma levels of the APC-interacting protein MAPRE1, LRG1, and IGFBP2 preceding a diagnosis of colorectal cancer in women. *Cancer Prev Res.* **2012**, *5*, 655–664. [CrossRef]
30. Lim, D.H.; Lee, J.H.; Kim, J.W. Feasibility of CYFRA 21-1 as a serum biomarker for the detection of colorectal adenoma and advanced colorectal adenoma in people over the age of 45. *J. Clin. Lab. Anal.* **2018**, *32*. [CrossRef]
31. Thomas, D.S.; Fourkala, E.O.; Apostolidou, S.; Gunu, R.; Ryan, A.; Jacobs, I.; Menon, U.; Alderton, W.; Gentry-Maharaj, A.; Timms, J.F. Evaluation of serum CEA, CYFRA21-1 and CA125 for the early detection of colorectal cancer using longitudinal preclinical samples. *Br. J. Cancer* **2015**, *113*, 268–274. [CrossRef]
32. Wen, Y.H.; Chang, P.Y.; Hsu, C.M.; Wang, H.Y.; Chiu, C.T.; Lu, J.J. Cancer screening through a multi-analyte serum biomarker panel during health check-up examinations: Results from a 12-year experience. *Clin. Chim. Acta* **2015**, *450*, 273–276. [CrossRef]
33. Werner, S.; Krause, F.; Rolny, V.; Strobl, M.; Morgenstern, D.; Datz, C.; Chen, H.; Brenner, H. Evaluation of a 5-Marker Blood Test for Colorectal Cancer Early Detection in a Colorectal Cancer Screening Setting. *Clin. Cancer Res.* **2016**, *22*, 1725–1733. [CrossRef] [PubMed]
34. Hall, C.; Clarke, L.; Pal, A.; Buchwald, P.; Eglinton, T.; Wakeman, C.; Frizelle, F. A Review of the Role of Carcinoembryonic Antigen in Clinical Practice. *Ann. Coloproctol.* **2019**, *35*, 294–305. [CrossRef]
35. Toriola, A.T.; Cheng, T.Y.; Neuhouser, M.L.; Wener, M.H.; Zheng, Y.; Brown, E.; Miller, J.W.; Song, X.; Beresford, S.A.; Gunter, M.J.; et al. Biomarkers of inflammation are associated with colorectal cancer risk in women but are not suitable as early detection markers. *Int. J. Cancer* **2013**, *132*, 2648–2658. [CrossRef] [PubMed]
36. Touvier, M.; Fezeu, L.; Ahluwalia, N.; Julia, C.; Charnaux, N.; Sutton, A.; Mejean, C.; Latino-Martel, P.; Hercberg, S.; Galan, P.; et al. Pre-diagnostic levels of adiponectin and soluble vascular cell adhesion molecule-1 are associated with colorectal cancer risk. *World J. Gastroenterol.* **2012**, *18*, 2805–2812. [CrossRef]
37. Tao, S.; Haug, U.; Kuhn, K.; Brenner, H. Comparison and combination of blood-based inflammatory markers with faecal occult blood tests for non-invasive colorectal cancer screening. *Br. J. Cancer* **2012**, *106*, 1424–1430. [CrossRef]
38. Qian, J.; Tikk, K.; Werner, S.; Balavarca, Y.; Saadati, M.; Hechtner, M.; Brenner, H. Biomarker discovery study of inflammatory proteins for colorectal cancer early detection demonstrated importance of screening setting validation. *J. Clin. Epidemiol.* **2018**, *104*, 24–34. [CrossRef]
39. Chen, H.; Qian, J.; Werner, S.; Cuk, K.; Knebel, P.; Brenner, H. Development and validation of a panel of five proteins as blood biomarkers for early detection of colorectal cancer. *Clin. Epidemiol.* **2017**, *9*, 517–526. [CrossRef]
40. Bhardwaj, M.; Gies, A.; Weigl, K.; Tikk, K.; Benner, A.; Schrotz-King, P.; Borchers, C.H.; Brenner, H. Evaluation and Validation of Plasma Proteins Using Two Different Protein Detection Methods for Early Detection of Colorectal Cancer. *Cancers* **2019**, *11*, 1426. [CrossRef]
41. Bhardwaj, M.; Weigl, K.; Tikk, K.; Holland-Letz, T.; Schrotz-King, P.; Borchers, C.H.; Brenner, H. Multiplex quantitation of 270 plasma protein markers to identify a signature for early detection of colorectal cancer. *Eur. J. Cancer* **2020**, *127*, 30–40. [CrossRef] [PubMed]
42. Vermeire, S.; Van Assche, G.; Rutgeerts, P. The role of C-reactive protein as an inflammatory marker in gastrointestinal diseases. *Nat. Clin. Pract. Gastroenterol. Hepatol.* **2005**, *2*, 580–586. [CrossRef]
43. Brown, D.A.; Hance, K.W.; Rogers, C.J.; Sansbury, L.B.; Albert, P.S.; Murphy, G.; Laiyemo, A.O.; Wang, Z.; Cross, A.J.; Schatzkin, A.; et al. Serum macrophage inhibitory cytokine-1 (MIC-1/GDF15): A potential screening tool for the prevention of colon cancer? *Cancer Epidemiol. Biomark. Prev.* **2012**, *21*, 337–346. [CrossRef]
44. Wilhelmsen, M.; Christensen, I.J.; Rasmussen, L.; Jorgensen, L.N.; Madsen, M.R.; Vilandt, J.; Hillig, T.; Klaerke, M.; Nielsen, K.T.; Laurberg, S.; et al. Detection of colorectal neoplasia: Combination of eight blood-based, cancer-associated protein biomarkers. *Int. J. Cancer* **2017**, *140*, 1436–1446. [CrossRef] [PubMed]
45. Rasmussen, L.; Nielsen, H.J.; Christensen, I.J. Early Detection and Recurrence of Colorectal Adenomas by Combination of Eight Cancer-Associated Biomarkers in Plasma. *Clin. Exp. Gastroenterol.* **2020**, *13*, 273–284. [CrossRef] [PubMed]
46. Wild, N.; Andres, H.; Rollinger, W.; Krause, F.; Dilba, P.; Tacke, M.; Karl, J. A combination of serum markers for the early detection of colorectal cancer. *Clin. Cancer Res.* **2010**, *16*, 6111–6121. [CrossRef]
47. Harlid, S.; Harbs, J.; Myte, R.; Brunius, C.; Gunter, M.J.; Palmqvist, R.; Liu, X.; Van Guelpen, B. A two-tiered targeted proteomics approach to identify pre-diagnostic biomarkers of colorectal cancer risk. *Sci. Rep.* **2021**, *11*, 5151. [CrossRef]
48. Qian, J.; Tikk, K.; Weigl, K.; Balavarca, Y.; Brenner, H. Fibroblast growth factor 21 as a circulating biomarker at various stages of colorectal carcinogenesis. *Br. J. Cancer* **2018**, *119*, 1374–1382. [CrossRef] [PubMed]
49. Bertuzzi, M.; Marelli, C.; Bagnati, R.; Colombi, A.; Fanelli, R.; Saieva, C.; Ceroti, M.; Bendinelli, B.; Caini, S.; Airoldi, L.; et al. Plasma clusterin as a candidate pre-diagnosis marker of colorectal cancer risk in the Florence cohort of the European Prospective Investigation into Cancer and Nutrition: A pilot study. *BMC Cancer* **2015**, *15*, 56. [CrossRef] [PubMed]
50. Shao, S.; Neely, B.A.; Kao, T.C.; Eckhaus, J.; Bourgeois, J.; Brooks, J.; Jones, E.E.; Drake, R.R.; Zhu, K. Proteomic Profiling of Serial Prediagnostic Serum Samples for Early Detection of Colon Cancer in the U.S. Military. *Cancer Epidemiol. Biomark. Prev.* **2017**, *26*, 711–718. [CrossRef]
51. Song, M.; Sasazuki, S.; Camargo, M.C.; Shimazu, T.; Charvat, H.; Yamaji, T.; Sawada, N.; Kemp, T.J.; Pfeiffer, R.M.; Hildesheim, A.; et al. Circulating inflammatory markers and colorectal cancer risk: A prospective case-cohort study in Japan. *Int. J. Cancer* **2018**, *143*, 2767–2776. [CrossRef]

52. Rho, J.H.; Ladd, J.J.; Li, C.I.; Potter, J.D.; Zhang, Y.; Shelley, D.; Shibata, D.; Coppola, D.; Yamada, H.; Toyoda, H.; et al. Protein and glycomic plasma markers for early detection of adenoma and colon cancer. *Gut* **2018**, *67*, 473–484. [CrossRef]
53. Butt, J.; Werner, S.; Willhauck-Fleckenstein, M.; Michel, A.; Waterboer, T.; Zornig, I.; Boleij, A.; Dramsi, S.; Brenner, H.; Pawlita, M. Serology of Streptococcus gallolyticus subspecies gallolyticus and its association with colorectal cancer and precursors. *Int. J. Cancer* **2017**, *141*, 897–904. [CrossRef]
54. Li, B.; Shen, K.; Zhang, J.; Jiang, Y.; Yang, T.; Sun, X.; Ma, X.; Zhu, J. Serum netrin-1 as a biomarker for colorectal cancer detection. *Cancer Biomark.* **2020**, *28*, 391–396. [CrossRef]
55. Cross, A.J.; Moore, S.C.; Boca, S.; Huang, W.Y.; Xiong, X.; Stolzenberg-Solomon, R.; Sinha, R.; Sampson, J.N. A prospective study of serum metabolites and colorectal cancer risk. *Cancer* **2014**, *120*, 3049–3057. [CrossRef] [PubMed]
56. Kuhn, T.; Floegel, A.; Sookthai, D.; Johnson, T.; Rolle-Kampczyk, U.; Otto, W.; von Bergen, M.; Boeing, H.; Kaaks, R. Higher plasma levels of lysophosphatidylcholine 18:0 are related to a lower risk of common cancers in a prospective metabolomics study. *BMC Med.* **2016**, *14*, 13. [CrossRef] [PubMed]
57. Perttula, K.; Schiffman, C.; Edmands, W.M.B.; Petrick, L.; Grigoryan, H.; Cai, X.; Gunter, M.J.; Naccarati, A.; Polidoro, S.; Dudoit, S.; et al. Untargeted lipidomic features associated with colorectal cancer in a prospective cohort. *BMC Cancer* **2018**, *18*, 996. [CrossRef]
58. Shu, X.; Xiang, Y.B.; Rothman, N.; Yu, D.; Li, H.L.; Yang, G.; Cai, H.; Ma, X.; Lan, Q.; Gao, Y.T.; et al. Prospective study of blood metabolites associated with colorectal cancer risk. *Int. J. Cancer* **2018**, *143*, 527–534. [CrossRef]
59. Farshidfar, F.; Weljie, A.M.; Kopciuk, K.A.; Hilsden, R.; McGregor, S.E.; Buie, W.D.; MacLean, A.; Vogel, H.J.; Bathe, O.F. A validated metabolomic signature for colorectal cancer: Exploration of the clinical value of metabolomics. *Br. J. Cancer* **2016**, *115*, 848–857. [CrossRef] [PubMed]
60. Butt, J.; Blot, W.J.; Teras, L.R.; Visvanathan, K.; Le Marchand, L.; Haiman, C.A.; Chen, Y.; Bao, Y.; Sesso, H.D.; Wassertheil-Smoller, S.; et al. Antibody Responses to Streptococcus gallolyticus Subspecies Gallolyticus Proteins in a Large Prospective Colorectal Cancer Cohort Consortium. *Cancer Epidemiol. Biomark. Prev.* **2018**, *27*, 1186–1194. [CrossRef]
61. Butt, J.; Blot, W.J.; Visvanathan, K.; Le Marchand, L.; Wilkens, L.R.; Chen, Y.; Sesso, H.D.; Teras, L.; Ryser, M.D.; Hyslop, T.; et al. Auto-antibodies to p53 and the Subsequent Development of Colorectal Cancer in a U.S. Prospective Cohort Consortium. *Cancer Epidemiol. Biomark. Prev.* **2020**, *29*, 2729–2734. [CrossRef] [PubMed]
62. Chen, H.; Werner, S.; Butt, J.; Zornig, I.; Knebel, P.; Michel, A.; Eichmuller, S.B.; Jager, D.; Waterboer, T.; Pawlita, M.; et al. Prospective evaluation of 64 serum autoantibodies as biomarkers for early detection of colorectal cancer in a true screening setting. *Oncotarget* **2016**, *7*, 16420–16432. [CrossRef] [PubMed]
63. Pedersen, J.W.; Gentry-Maharaj, A.; Nostdal, A.; Fourkala, E.O.; Dawnay, A.; Burnell, M.; Zaikin, A.; Burchell, J.; Papadimitriou, J.T.; Clausen, H.; et al. Cancer-associated autoantibodies to MUC1 and MUC4—A blinded case-control study of colorectal cancer in UK collaborative trial of ovarian cancer screening. *Int. J. Cancer* **2014**, *134*, 2180–2188. [CrossRef] [PubMed]
64. Teras, L.R.; Gapstur, S.M.; Maliniak, M.L.; Jacobs, E.J.; Gansler, T.; Michel, A.; Pawlita, M.; Waterboer, T.; Campbell, P.T. Prediagnostic Antibodies to Serum p53 and Subsequent Colorectal Cancer. *Cancer Epidemiol. Biomark. Prev.* **2018**, *27*, 219–223. [CrossRef]
65. Luo, X.; Stock, C.; Burwinkel, B.; Brenner, H. Identification and evaluation of plasma microRNAs for early detection of colorectal cancer. *PLoS ONE* **2013**, *8*, e62880. [CrossRef] [PubMed]
66. Mai, D.; Zheng, Y.; Guo, H.; Ding, P.; Bai, R.; Li, M.; Ye, Y.; Zhang, J.; Huang, X.; Liu, D.; et al. Serum piRNA-54265 is a New Biomarker for early detection and clinical surveillance of Human Colorectal Cancer. *Theranostics* **2020**, *10*, 8468–8478. [CrossRef]
67. Marcuello, M.; Duran-Sanchon, S.; Moreno, L.; Lozano, J.J.; Bujanda, L.; Castells, A.; Gironella, M. Analysis of A 6-Mirna Signature in Serum from Colorectal Cancer Screening Participants as Non-Invasive Biomarkers for Advanced Adenoma and Colorectal Cancer Detection. *Cancers* **2019**, *11*, 1542. [CrossRef]
68. Wikberg, M.L.; Myte, R.; Palmqvist, R.; van Guelpen, B.; Ljuslinder, I. Plasma miRNA can detect colorectal cancer, but how early? *Cancer Med.* **2018**, *7*, 1697–1705. [CrossRef]
69. Zanutto, S.; Ciniselli, C.M.; Belfiore, A.; Lecchi, M.; Masci, E.; Delconte, G.; Primignani, M.; Tosetti, G.; Dal Fante, M.; Fazzini, L.; et al. Plasma miRNA-based signatures in CRC screening programs. *Int. J. Cancer* **2020**, *146*, 1164–1173. [CrossRef] [PubMed]
70. Bartak, B.K.; Kalmar, A.; Peterfia, B.; Patai, A.V.; Galamb, O.; Valcz, G.; Spisak, S.; Wichmann, B.; Nagy, Z.B.; Toth, K.; et al. Colorectal adenoma and cancer detection based on altered methylation pattern of SFRP1, SFRP2, SDC2, and PRIMA1 in plasma samples. *Epigenetics* **2017**, *12*, 751–763. [CrossRef]
71. Barth, S.D.; Schulze, J.J.; Kuhn, T.; Raschke, E.; Husing, A.; Johnson, T.; Kaaks, R.; Olek, S. Treg-Mediated Immune Tolerance and the Risk of Solid Cancers: Findings From EPIC-Heidelberg. *J. Natl. Cancer Inst.* **2015**, *107*. [CrossRef]
72. Heiss, J.A.; Brenner, H. Epigenome-wide discovery and evaluation of leukocyte DNA methylation markers for the detection of colorectal cancer in a screening setting. *Clin. Epigenet.* **2017**, *9*, 24. [CrossRef] [PubMed]
73. Onwuka, J.U.; Li, D.; Liu, Y.; Huang, H.; Xu, J.; Liu, Y.; Zhang, Y.; Zhao, Y. A panel of DNA methylation signature from peripheral blood may predict colorectal cancer susceptibility. *BMC Cancer* **2020**, *20*, 692. [CrossRef]
74. Warren, J.D.; Xiong, W.; Bunker, A.M.; Vaughn, C.P.; Furtado, L.V.; Roberts, W.L.; Fang, J.C.; Samowitz, W.S.; Heichman, K.A. Septin 9 methylated DNA is a sensitive and specific blood test for colorectal cancer. *BMC Med.* **2011**, *9*, 133. [CrossRef] [PubMed]

75. Huang, B.; Gao, Y.T.; Shu, X.O.; Wen, W.; Yang, G.; Li, G.; Courtney, R.; Ji, B.T.; Li, H.L.; Purdue, M.P.; et al. Association of leukocyte mitochondrial DNA copy number with colorectal cancer risk: Results from the Shanghai Women's Health Study. *Cancer Epidemiol. Biomark. Prev.* **2014**, *23*, 2357–2365. [CrossRef]
76. Nian, J.; Sun, X.; Ming, S.; Yan, C.; Ma, Y.; Feng, Y.; Yang, L.; Yu, M.; Zhang, G.; Wang, X. Diagnostic Accuracy of Methylated SEPT9 for Blood-based Colorectal Cancer Detection: A Systematic Review and Meta-Analysis. *Clin. Transl. Gastroenterol.* **2017**, *8*, e216. [CrossRef] [PubMed]
77. Maffei, F.; Zolezzi Moraga, J.M.; Angelini, S.; Zenesini, C.; Musti, M.; Festi, D.; Cantelli-Forti, G.; Hrelia, P. Micronucleus frequency in human peripheral blood lymphocytes as a biomarker for the early detection of colorectal cancer risk. *Mutagenesis* **2014**, *29*, 221–225. [CrossRef]
78. Myint, N.N.M.; Verma, A.M.; Fernandez-Garcia, D.; Sarmah, P.; Tarpey, P.S.; Al-Aqbi, S.S.; Cai, H.; Trigg, R.; West, K.; Howells, L.M.; et al. Circulating tumor DNA in patients with colorectal adenomas: Assessment of detectability and genetic heterogeneity. *Cell Death Dis.* **2018**, *9*, 894. [CrossRef] [PubMed]
79. Okamura, T.; Hashimoto, Y.; Hamaguchi, M.; Obora, A.; Kojima, T.; Fukui, M. Triglyceride-glucose index (TyG index) is a predictor of incident colorectal cancer: A population-based longitudinal study. *BMC Endocr. Disord.* **2020**, *20*, 113. [CrossRef]
80. Perttula, K.; Edmands, W.M.; Grigoryan, H.; Cai, X.; Iavarone, A.T.; Gunter, M.J.; Naccarati, A.; Polidoro, S.; Hubbard, A.; Vineis, P.; et al. Evaluating Ultra-long-Chain Fatty Acids as Biomarkers of Colorectal Cancer Risk. *Cancer Epidemiol. Biomark. Prev.* **2016**, *25*, 1216–1223. [CrossRef]
81. Prizment, A.E.; Linabery, A.M.; Lutsey, P.L.; Selvin, E.; Nelson, H.H.; Folsom, A.R.; Church, T.R.; Drake, C.G.; Platz, E.A.; Joshu, C. Circulating Beta-2 Microglobulin and Risk of Cancer: The Atherosclerosis Risk in Communities Study (ARIC). *Cancer Epidemiol. Biomark. Prev.* **2016**, *25*, 657–664. [CrossRef] [PubMed]
82. Doherty, M.; Theodoratou, E.; Walsh, I.; Adamczyk, B.; Stockmann, H.; Agakov, F.; Timofeeva, M.; Trbojevic-Akmacic, I.; Vuckovic, F.; Duffy, F.; et al. Plasma N-glycans in colorectal cancer risk. *Sci. Rep.* **2018**, *8*, 8655. [CrossRef] [PubMed]
83. Pilling, L.C.; Atkins, J.L.; Kuchel, G.A.; Ferrucci, L.; Melzer, D. Red cell distribution width and common disease onsets in 240,477 healthy volunteers followed for up to 9 years. *PLoS ONE* **2018**, *13*, e0203504. [CrossRef]
84. Le Cornet, C.; Schildknecht, K.; Rossello Chornet, A.; Fortner, R.T.; Gonzalez Maldonado, S.; Katzke, V.A.; Kuhn, T.; Johnson, T.; Olek, S.; Kaaks, R. Circulating Immune Cell Composition and Cancer Risk: A Prospective Study Using Epigenetic Cell Count Measures. *Cancer Res.* **2020**, *80*, 1885–1892. [CrossRef]
85. Murphy, G.; Cross, A.J.; Dawsey, S.M.; Stanczyk, F.Z.; Kamangar, F.; Weinstein, S.J.; Taylor, P.R.; Mannisto, S.; Albanes, D.; Abnet, C.C.; et al. Serum ghrelin is associated with risk of colorectal adenocarcinomas in the ATBC study. *Gut* **2018**, *67*, 1646–1651. [CrossRef]
86. Sundkvist, A.; Myte, R.; Palmqvist, R.; Harlid, S.; Van Guelpen, B. Plasma ghrelin is probably not a useful biomarker for risk prediction or early detection of colorectal cancer. *Gut* **2018**. [CrossRef] [PubMed]
87. Brenner, H.; Altenhofen, L.; Tao, S. Matching of controls may lead to biased estimates of specificity in the evaluation of cancer screening tests. *J. Clin. Epidemiol.* **2013**, *66*, 202–208. [CrossRef]
88. Gertsman, I.; Barshop, B.A. Promises and pitfalls of untargeted metabolomics. *J. Inherit. Metab. Dis* **2018**, *41*, 355–366. [CrossRef] [PubMed]
89. Ransohoff, D.F. Evaluating a New Cancer Screening Blood Test: Unintended Consequences and the Need for Clarity in Policy Making. *J. Natl. Cancer Inst.* **2021**, *113*, 109–111. [CrossRef]
90. Williams, T.G.; Cubiella, J.; Griffin, S.J.; Walter, F.M.; Usher-Smith, J.A. Risk prediction models for colorectal cancer in people with symptoms: A systematic review. *BMC Gastroenterol.* **2016**, *16*, 63. [CrossRef]
91. National Institute for Health and Care Excellence. [NG12] Suspected Cancer: Recognition and Referral. Available online: https://www.nice.org.uk/guidance/ng12 (accessed on 29 January 2021).
92. Garcia-Albeniz, X.; Chan, A.T. Aspirin for the prevention of colorectal cancer. *Best Pract. Res. Clin. Gastroenterol.* **2011**, *25*, 461–472. [CrossRef]
93. Higurashi, T.; Hosono, K.; Takahashi, H.; Komiya, Y.; Umezawa, S.; Sakai, E.; Uchiyama, T.; Taniguchi, L.; Hata, Y.; Uchiyama, S.; et al. Metformin for chemoprevention of metachronous colorectal adenoma or polyps in post-polypectomy patients without diabetes: A multicentre double-blind, placebo-controlled, randomised phase 3 trial. *Lancet Oncol.* **2016**, *17*, 475–483. [CrossRef]
94. Rothwell, P.M.; Wilson, M.; Elwin, C.E.; Norrving, B.; Algra, A.; Warlow, C.P.; Meade, T.W. Long-term effect of aspirin on colorectal cancer incidence and mortality: 20-year follow-up of five randomised trials. *Lancet* **2010**, *376*, 1741–1750. [CrossRef]
95. Bossuyt, P.M.; Reitsma, J.B.; Bruns, D.E.; Gatsonis, C.A.; Glasziou, P.P.; Irwig, L.; Lijmer, J.G.; Moher, D.; Rennie, D.; de Vet, H.C.; et al. STARD 2015: An updated list of essential items for reporting diagnostic accuracy studies. *BMJ* **2015**, *351*, h5527. [CrossRef]
96. Collins, G.S.; Reitsma, J.B.; Altman, D.G.; Moons, K.G. Transparent Reporting of a multivariable prediction model for Individual Prognosis or Diagnosis (TRIPOD): The TRIPOD statement. *Ann. Intern. Med.* **2015**, *162*, 55–63. [CrossRef]

www.ingramcontent.com/pod-product-compliance
Lightning Source LLC
LaVergne TN
LVHW070439100526
838202LV00014B/1627

MDPI
St. Alban-Anlage 66
4052 Basel
Switzerland
Tel. +41 61 683 77 34
Fax +41 61 302 89 18
www.mdpi.com

Cancers Editorial Office
E-mail: cancers@mdpi.com
www.mdpi.com/journal/cancers

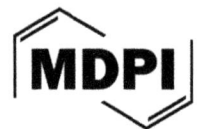